ELSEVIER

1600 John F. Ken

http://www.denta

DENTAL CLINIC
April, 2014 ISSN

Editor: John Vass
Developmental E

© **2014 Elsevier**

Dental Clinics of I
New York, NY 10
1600 John F. Ken,
NY and addition)
per year (domesti-
uals), $628.00 pe
tional institutions
delivery is include
Send address chr
Service, 3251 Riv
address): Elsevi
Heights, MO 63
service-usa@els

Reprints. For co
Department, Els
212-633-3820; E

The Dental Clinic
Medicine, ISI/BI

Printed in the Un

pp
uc
: P

CITO

C

A

ics.co

58 •

Contributors

EDITORS

THOMAS P. SOLLECITO, DMD, FDS RCSEd
Professor and Chair of Oral Medicine, University of Pennsylvania School of Dental Medicine, Philadelphia, Pennsylvania

ERIC T. STOOPLER, DMD, FDS RCSEd, FDS RCSEng
Associate Professor of Oral Medicine, Director, Postdoctoral Oral Medicine, Department of Oral Medicine, University of Pennsylvania School of Dental Medicine, Philadelphia, Pennsylvania

AUTHORS

SUNDAY O. AKINTOYE, BDS, DDS, MS
Associate Professor of Oral Medicine, Department of Oral Medicine, University of Pennsylvania School of Dental Medicine, Philadelphia, Pennsylvania

SUHER BAKER, BDS, DMD, MS
Section Chief and Program Director, Pediatric Dentistry Residency Program, Chair, Department of Dentistry, Assistant Clinical Professor (Surgery), Assistant Clinical Professor (Pediatrics), Yale School of Medicine, Yale-New Haven Hospital, New Haven, Connecticut

RAMESH BALASUBRAMANIAM, BDSc, MS
Clinical Associate Professor, Orofacial Pain Clinic, School of Dentistry, University of Western Australia, Perth; Perth Oral Medicine & Dental Sleep Centre, St John of God Hospital, Subiaco, Western Australia, Australia

COLONYA C. CALHOUN, DDS, PhD
Director of Dental Research, Division of Oral and Maxillofacial Surgery, Harbor UCLA, Torrance; Assistant Professor, Charles R. Drew University, Los Angeles, California

KATHARINE CIARROCCA, DMD, MSEd
Department of Oral Rehabilitation, College of Dental Medicine, Georgia Regents University, Augusta, Georgia

CARRIE ANN R. CUSACK, MD
Department of Dermatology, Drexel University College of Medicine, Philadelphia, Pennsylvania

SCOTT S. DE ROSSI, DMD
Department of Oral Health and Diagnostic Sciences, College of Dental Medicine, Georgia Regents University; Department of Otolaryngology/Head & Neck Surgery, Medical College of Georgia, Georgia Regents University; Department of Dermatology, Medical College of Georgia, Georgia Regents University, Augusta, Georgia

MARTIN S. GREENBERG, DDS, FDSRCS
Professor of Oral Medicine and Associate Dean for Hospital and Extramural Affairs, Department of Oral Medicine, University of Pennsylvania School of Dental Medicine, Philadelphia, Pennsylvania

CHRISTEL M. HABERLAND, DDS, MS
Attending Pediatric Dentist, Yale Hamden Dental Center, Clinical Instructor, Yale School of Medicine, Yale-New Haven Hospital, Hamden, Connecticut

A. ROSS KERR, DDS, MSD
Clinical Professor, Department of Oral & Maxillofacial Pathology, Radiology and Medicine, New York University, New York, New York

JOSEPH M. KIST, MD
Department of Dermatology, Perelman School of Medicine, University of Pennsylvania, Philadelphia, Pennsylvania

ARTHUR S. KUPERSTEIN, DDS
Assistant Professor of Oral Medicine, Director, Department of Oral Medicine, University of Pennsylvania School of Dental Medicine, Philadelphia, Pennsylvania

MICHAL KUTEN-SHORRER, DMD
Department of Oral Medicine, Infection, and Immunity, Harvard School of Dental Medicine, Boston, Massachusetts

RAJESH V. LALLA, DDS, PhD, CCRP
Section of Oral Medicine, University of Connecticut Health Center, Farmington, Connecticut

ANH D. LE, DDS, PhD
Adjunct Professor, Division of Oral and Maxillofacial Surgery, Herman Ostrow School of Dentistry of USC, Los Angeles, California; Chair and Norman Vine Endowed Professor of Oral Rehabilitation, Department of Oral and Maxillofacial Surgery and Pharmacology, University of Pennsylvania School of Dental Medicine, Penn Medicine Hospital of the University of Pennsylvania, Philadelphia, Pennsylvania

GEOFFREY F.S. LIM, BS
Department of Dermatology, Drexel University College of Medicine, Philadelphia, Pennsylvania

KETAN PATEL, DDS, PhD
Maxillofacial Oncology and Reconstructive Surgery Fellow, Division of Oral and Maxillofacial Surgery, University of Minnesota, Minneapolis, Minnesota

DOUGLAS E. PETERSON, DMD, PhD, FDS RCSEd
Section of Oral Medicine, University of Connecticut Health Center, Farmington, Connecticut

ANDRES PINTO, DMD, MPH, FDS RCSEd
Chairman, Department of Oral and Maxillofacial Medicine and Diagnostic Sciences, University Hospitals Case Medical Center, Case Western Reserve University School of Dental Medicine, Cleveland, Ohio

GORDON A. PRINGLE, DDS, PhD
Director, Oral Pathology Laboratory, Professor, Department of Pathology and Laboratory Medicine, Temple University Hospital, Temple University School of Medicine, Philadelphia, Pennsylvania

NELSON L. RHODUS, DMD, MPH, FICD
Morse Distinguished Professor and Director, Division of Oral Medicine, University of Minnesota, Minneapolis, Minnesota

DEBORAH P. SAUNDERS, BSc, DMD
Department of Dental Oncology, Northeast Cancer Centre, Health Sciences North, Northern Ontario School of Medicine, Sudbury, Ontario, Canada

ERIC T. STOOPLER, DMD, FDS RCSEd, FDS RCSEng
Associate Professor of Oral Medicine, Director, Postdoctoral Oral Medicine, Department of Oral Medicine, University of Pennsylvania School of Dental Medicine, Philadelphia, Pennsylvania

NATHANIEL S. TREISTER, DMD, DMSc
Division of Oral Medicine and Dentistry, Brigham and Women's Hospital, Boston, Massachusetts

JETTIE UYANNE, DDS
Assistant Professor, Division of Oral and Maxillofacial Surgery, Herman Ostrow School of Dentistry of USC, Los Angeles; Attending Staff, Division of Oral and Maxillofacial Surgery, Harbor UCLA, Torrance, California

SOOK-BIN WOO, DMD, MMSc
Division of Oral Medicine and Dentistry, Brigham and Women's Hospital, Boston, Massachusetts

Contents

Oral herpes virus infections (OHVIs) are among the most common mucosal disorders encountered by oral health care providers. These infections can affect individuals at any age, from infants to the elderly, and may cause significant pain and dysfunction. Immunosuppressed patients may be at increased risk for serious and potential life-threatening complications caused by OHVIs. Clinicians may have difficulty in diagnosing these infections because they can mimic other conditions of the oral mucosa. This article provides oral health care providers with clinically relevant information regarding etiopathogenesis, diagnosis, and management of OHVIs.

Recurrent aphthous stomatitis (RAS) is the most common ulcerative disease affecting the oral mucosa. RAS occurs mostly in healthy individuals and has an atypical clinical presentation in immunocompromised individuals. The etiology of RAS is still unknown, but several local, systemic, immunologic, genetic, allergic, nutritional, and microbial factors, as well as immunosuppressive drugs, have been proposed as causative agents. Clinical management of RAS using topical and systemic therapies is based on severity of symptoms and the frequency, size, and number of lesions. The goals of therapy are to decrease pain and ulcer size, promote healing, and decrease the frequency of recurrence.

Oral lichen planus (OLP) is commonly found in middle-aged women. Although the cause is unknown, research points to several complex immunologic events and cells that are responsible for the inflammatory destruction and chronicity of these lesions. Biopsy for histologic diagnosis is recommended. The mainstay of treatment remains topical corticosteroids; however, newer therapies such as immunomodulating agents are available for recalcitrant lesions. In cases of lichenoid mucositis or reactions, treatment should be directed at identifying and removing the presumed cause. Given the apparent risk of squamous cell carcinoma in these patients, frequent follow-up and repeat biopsy are vital.

In this article, the epidemiology, etiologic risk factors, clinical presentation, recognition, and diagnosis of oral precancer and cancer are reviewed.

Recommendations on clinical examination and early diagnostic techniques (including adjuncts) are presented. Treatment and complications from treatment of oral cancer are discussed.

Oral mucositis is a significant toxicity of systemic chemotherapy and of radiation therapy to the head and neck region. The morbidity of oral mucositis can include pain, nutritional compromise, impact on quality of life, alteration in cancer therapy, risk for infection, and economic costs. Management includes general symptomatic support and targeted therapeutic interventions for the prevention or treatment of oral mucositis. Evidence-based clinical practice guidelines are available to guide clinicians in the selection of effective management strategies.

Allogeneic hematopoietic cell transplantation (allo-HCT) is used for the treatment of a variety of disorders, primarily hematologic malignancies. Graft-versus-host disease (GVHD) is a significant complication following allo-HCT and a major cause of morbidity and mortality. The oral cavity is frequently involved in GVHD, leading to pain, functional impairment, and reduced quality of life. Early diagnosis, management, and long-term follow-up of oral GVHD are important components of overall patient care.

Nitrogen-containing and non–nitrogen-containing bisphosphonates have been implicated in the development of osteonecrosis of the jaw (ONJ), a condition termed bisphosphonate-related OHJ. Other antiresorptive drugs have been implicated in the development of OHJ, hence the new term antiresorptive drug–related ONJ. The underlying pathogenesis remains unclear, and no definite diagnosis or cure has been established for this debilitating condition. This article reviews some of the most common antiresorptive drugs with their associated risks of ONJ and the current understanding of the pathogenesis ONJ, and summarizes current clinical guidelines.

A wide range of human papillomavirus (HPV) genotypes have been detected in oral mucosa. Clinical infections with low-risk genotypes manifest as squamous papilloma, condyloma acuminatum, verruca vulgaris, or multifocal epithelial hyperplasia. Clinical infections with high-risk genotypes have been associated with malignant lesions. The most common genotype isolated from subclinical infection is HPV-16. A causal role for HPV in carcinogenesis of oral squamous carcinoma is minimal. Ongoing vaccination against HPV types 6, 11, 16, and 18 is expected to decrease the spread of infection and decrease the carcinogenic potential of HPV-16 in the oropharynx and oral cavity.

The purpose of this article is to review the common neoplasms, infections, and inflammatory dermatoses that may present around or near the mouth. Dental professionals are well positioned to evaluate perioral skin conditions, further contributing to patients' general health. This article includes a review of seborrheic keratosis, warts, actinic keratoses, actinic cheilitis, and squamous cell carcinoma, among several other perioral cutaneous lesions.

This article provides an overview of common color changes and soft tissue oral nodular abnormalities in children and adolescents. The clinical presentation and treatment options to address these conditions are presented in a concise approach, highlighting key features relevant to the oral health care professional.

DENTAL CLINICS OF NORTH AMERICA

FORTHCOMING ISSUES

July 2014
**Cone Beam Computed Tomography
and Dental Imaging**
Dale A. Miles and
Robert A. Danforth, *Editors*

October 2014
Geriatric Dentistry
Lisa Thompson and
Leonard Brennan, *Editors*

RECENT ISSUES

January 2014
Prosthodontics
Lily T. Garcia, *Editor*

October 2013
**Clinical Approaches to Oral Mucosal
Disorders: Part I**
Thomas P. Sollecito and
Eric T. Stoopler, *Editors*

July 2013
Orofacial Pain
Scott S. De Rossi and
David A. Sirois, *Editors*

NOW AVAILABLE FOR YOUR iPhone and iPad

Preface

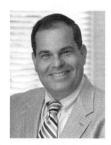
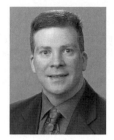

Thomas P. Sollecito, DMD,
FDS RCSEd

Eric T. Stoopler, DMD,
FDS RCSEd, FDS RCSEng

Editors

"Clinical Approaches to Oral Mucosal Disorders Part II" continues the theme of the oral cavity as a functional unit of the whole and as a window to overall health. As in Part I of this series, the articles in this volume are written by internationally renowned scholars, clinicians, and researchers and provide up-to-date information regarding numerous acute and chronic oral mucosal diseases, which are frequently encountered in clinical practice. New insights are provided into several of the most common oral mucosal disorders, such as herpes infections, aphthous stomatitis, and lichen planus/lichenoid mucositis. Oral cancer and the complications of cancer therapies, including chemotherapy and radiation-induced mucositis, graft-versus-host disease, and antiresorptive drug-related osteonecrosis of the jaws, are fully explored in this collection. A comprehensive analysis of human papilloma virus in oral disease as well as perioral skin lesions are contained in this issue. Finally, a concise review of pediatric oral soft tissue lesions provides information for evaluation and management of common oral mucosal disorders in this patient population.

Collectively, "Clinical Approaches to Oral Mucosal Disorders Parts I and II" represent the most current and clinically relevant information regarding a wide variety of conditions affecting the oral cavity and perioral structures. We anticipate these works will provide oral health care providers with indispensable information that will improve the quality of patient care for many years to come.

DEDICATION

We acknowledge and thank all of our mentors, colleagues, residents, students, and patients, who have contributed to our professional development. In addition, we express our sincere appreciation and gratitude to all of the contributing authors of these

Dent Clin N Am 58 (2014) xi–xii
http://dx.doi.org/10.1016/j.cden.2014.01.002
0011-8532/14/$ – see front matter © 2014 Elsevier Inc. All rights reserved.

dental.theclinics.com

works. It has been a truly enjoyable experience and it is extremely rewarding to see our collective efforts reach fruition.

Thomas P. Sollecito, DMD, FDS RCSEd

Eric T. Stoopler, DMD, FDS RCSEd, FDS RCSEng
University of Pennsylvania School of Dental Medicine
240 South 40th Street
Philadelphia, PA 19104, USA

E-mail addresses:
tps@dental.upenn.edu (T.P. Sollecito)
ets@dental.upenn.edu (E.T. Stoopler)

Update on Oral Herpes Virus Infections

Ramesh Balasubramaniam, BDSc, MS[a,b], Arthur S. Kuperstein, DDS[c],
Eric T. Stoopler, DMD, FDS RCSEd, FDS RCSEng[d],*

KEYWORDS

- Herpes virus • Viral infection • Oral cavity • Mouth • Antivirals

KEY POINTS

- Oral herpes virus infections (OHVIs) are commonly encountered in clinical practice.
- OHVIs can resemble other types of oral mucosal diseases.
- Diagnosis of OHVIs is usually based on patient history and clinical examination findings, but adjunctive laboratory tests may be necessary to establish the diagnosis.
- Treatment of OHVIs usually consists of palliative care, but may include use of topical or systemic antiviral medications.
- Immunosuppressed patients with OHVIs are potentially at risk of developing life-threatening complications and may require aggressive treatment.

INTRODUCTION

There are 80 known herpes viruses, and at least 8 of them are known to cause infections in humans. These viruses include herpes simplex virus (HSV) -1 and -2, varicella – zoster virus (VZV) [human herpes virus {HHV} 3], Epstein – Barr virus (EBV) [HHV-4], Cytomegalovirus (CMV) [HHV-5], HHV-6, -7, and -8 [Kaposi's sarcoma herpes virus {KSHV}].[1,2] There are structural and behavioral characteristics that are common to the members of the herpes virus family (ie, they contain 4 layers: an inner core of double-stranded DNA, a protein capsid, the tegument, and a lipid envelope containing glycoproteins derived from the nuclear membrane of host cells).[1,2] Herpes viruses

A version of this article appeared as Stoopler, ET. Oral herpetic infections (HSV 1–8). Dent Clin N Am 2005;49:15–29.
Disclosures for authors: no disclosures.
[a] Orofacial Pain Clinic, School of Dentistry, University of Western Australia, 35 Stirling Highway, Crawley, Western Australia 6009, Australia; [b] Perth Oral Medicine and Dental Sleep Centre, St John of God Hospital, Suite 311, 25 McCourt Street, Subiaco, Western Australia 6008, Australia; [c] Department of Oral Medicine, University of Pennsylvania School of Dental Medicine, 240 South 40th Street, Room 207, Philadelphia, PA 19104, USA; [d] Department of Oral Medicine, University of Pennsylvania School of Dental Medicine, 240 South 40th Street, Room 206, Philadelphia, PA 19104, USA
* Corresponding author.
E-mail address: ets@dental.upenn.edu

cause a primary infection when the person initially contacts the virus, and it remains latent within the nuclei of specific cells for the life of the individual. The site of latency differs among the herpes viruses, with HSV-1, HSV-2, and VZV remaining latent in the sensory nerve ganglia; EBV in B lymphocytes, oropharyngeal epithelial cells, and salivary gland tissue[3]; CMV in monocytes, bone marrow hematopoietic progenitor cells, epithelial cells, endothelial cells,[4] and possibly, salivary gland tissue[5]; and HHV-6 and HHV-7 in CD4 lymphocytes.[1,2] HHV-8 also remains latent in B lymphocytes circulating in the hematopoietic system.[6] After reactivation, herpes viruses can cause localized or disseminated recurrent infections. They are transmitted between hosts by direct contact with saliva or genital secretions. HHV-8 may be transmitted via organ transplantation.[7,8] Viruses are often shed in the saliva of asymptomatic hosts, who act as vectors for new primary infections in previously non-infected individuals.[9] EBV has been associated with malignancies in humans, such as nasopharyngeal carcinoma and B-cell lymphomas. Other malignancies are associated with EBV, including nasal T-cell/natural killer cell lymphoma seen most commonly in Southeast Asia.[10] HHV-8 has been definitively linked to malignant processes, such as KS, as well as several lymphoproliferative disorders and Castleman disease.[7]

HSV

HSV-1 and HSV-2 are the two major types of herpes viruses known to cause most common oral and perioral infections.[11,12] They can be distinguished by the distinct antibodies that are formed against each type of virus or by analysis of the nuclear DNA by restriction endonuclease analysis.[1,2] Classically, HSV-1 causes most cases of oral and pharyngeal infection, meningoencephalitis, and dermatitis above the waist; HSV-2 is implicated in most genital and anal infections.[1,2] Depending on sexual practices, both types can cause primary or recurrent infections in the oral, perioral, or genital area.[1,2] HSV infections of the finger (herpetic whitlow) develop after contact with infected saliva or bronchial secretions. The incidence of herpetic whitlow is 4 cases per 100,000 per year.[13]

PRIMARY HERPES SIMPLEX INFECTIONS

The incidence of primary infections with HSV-1 increases after 6 months of age as a result of loss of anti-HSV antibodies acquired from the mother during gestation. The incidence of primary HSV-1 infection reaches a peak between 2 and 3 years of age.[1,2] Primary HSV-1 infections may still occur in adolescents and adults, with occasional cases being reported in patients older than 60 years.[14] Incidence of primary HSV-2 infection does not increase until sexual activity begins. In a prevalence study between 1999 and 2004, 57.7% of the US population tested had HSV-1 antibodies. Data from the Centers for Disease Control showed that 16.2% of Americans aged between 14 and 49 years had HSV-2 antibodies.[15] This prevalence was higher among women (20.9%) compared with men (11.5%) and higher among Blacks (39.2%) compared with Whites (12.3%).[16]

Many primary herpes infections are subclinical or cause pharyngitis, which is difficult to distinguish from other upper respiratory viral infections. Symptomatic primary HSV disease is preceded or accompanied by systemic symptoms, which may include fever, headache, malaise, nausea, vomiting, and accompanying lymphadenopathy.[17,18] These prodromal symptoms are important to consider when clinically differentiating HSV infections from other vesiculoulcerative diseases of the oral cavity. In the oral cavity, vesicles and ulcers appear on the oral mucosa and generalized acute marginal gingivitis occurs 1 to 2 days after the prodromal symptoms appear (**Fig. 1**).

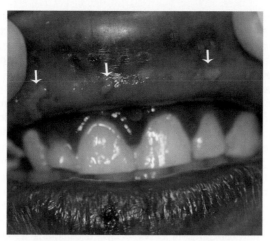

Fig. 1. Primary herpetic gingivostomatitis. Note vesiculoulcerative lesions on the labial mucosa (*arrows*) and the intense erythema of the maxillary gingiva.

Primary HSV in healthy children is a usually a self-limiting disease, with fever disappearing in 3 or 4 days and oral lesions that heal in a week to 10 days.

Treatment of primary HSV infection is usually palliative. Milder cases can be managed by supportive care, including maintenance of fluids, use of acetaminophen to reduce fever, and use of topical anesthetics such as viscous lidocaine or a mixture of liquid benadryl, milk of magnesia, and carafate to decrease oral pain.[11,12] If the patient presents to the clinician within 24 to 48 hours of onset of vesicle eruption, antiviral medication may be helpful to accelerate healing time of the lesions by inhibiting DNA replication in HSV-infected cells.[18] Acyclovir, an antiviral medication, has been shown to decrease symptoms of primary HSV infection in children, including days with fever and viral shedding.[19] Valacyclovir and famciclovir are also common antiviral agents used to treat primary HSV infections; because of their increased bioavailability compared with acyclovir, treatment is effective with fewer daily doses (**Table 1**).[20]

RECURRENT HERPES SIMPLEX INFECTION

After resolution of a primary HSV infection, the virus migrates to the trigeminal nerve ganglion, where it is capable of remaining in a latent state. Reactivation of virus may follow exposure to cold, exposure to sunlight, stress, trauma, or immunosuppression and cause recurrent infection.[1,2] Recurrent herpes labialis (RHL) is the most common

Table 1 Systemic antiviral medications for the treatment of primary HSV infection				
	Acyclovir		**Valacyclovir**	**Famciclovir**
Dose (mg)	200[a]	400[b]	1000[a]	250[b]
Frequency (x/d)	5	3	2	3
Duration (d)	7–10	7–10	7–10	7–10

[a] US Food and Drug Administration treatment recommendations for genital herpes.
[b] Recommendations from the Centers for Disease Control and Prevention for genital herpes.
From Stoopler ET, Balasubramaniam R. Topical and systemic therapies for oral and perioral herpes simplex virus infections. J Calif Dent Assoc 2013;41(4):262.

form of recurrent HSV infection, typically appearing on the mucocutaneous junction of the lip, and is often referred to as a cold sore or fever blister (**Fig. 2**).[1,2] Recurrent herpes infections in healthy patients should be treated on a symptomatic basis. Treatment, as well as chronic suppression, of severe, painful, or deforming recurrent herpes may require systemic antiviral medications.

Studies comparing topical antiviral medications for treating RHL have been published.[21,22] Topical penciclovir reduces the duration and pain of RHL by 1 to 2 days.[23] The recommended dosage of topical penciclovir is application to the area every 2 hours for 4 days while awake.[12] Acyclovir is also available for topical use and has been reported to decrease duration of RHL lesions by 12 hours.[21,24] Studies have investigated the use of 10% n-docosanol cream and found that when applied 5 times a day for 10 days, it significantly accelerates healing time and decreases pain, especially if commenced during the prodrome.[25,26] The US Food and Drug Administration has approved n-docosanol as the only non-prescription medication for treatment of RHL. Overall, the benefit of applying these medications to RHL lesions is limited compared with topical penciclovir.[21] Some clinicians advocate the off-label use of suppressive doses of systemic antivirals to prevent severe, frequent disfiguring recurrences of RHL in immunocompetent patients.

Although most recurrent herpes infections occur on the lips and heavily keratinized mucosa of the palate and gingiva, recurrent intraoral herpes (RIH) can occur on any intraoral mucosal surface and is seen more frequently in immunocompromised patients (**Fig. 3**).[1,2] Patients at high risk for severe recurrences are those receiving cancer chemotherapy or immunosuppressive drugs to prevent graft rejection after transplantation, as well as patients with advanced AIDS.[1,2] Recurrent HSV lesions in immunocompromised patients appear as progressively enlarging ulcers, which may involve large portions of the labial, intraoral, genital, or rectal mucosa if left untreated.[27] These lesions have the potential to disseminate and cause generalized infection (**Fig. 4**); therefore, it is imperative for clinicians to rule out HSV as a cause of oral vesicles or ulcers in immunosuppressed individuals.[1,2]

Immunosuppressed patients with HSV infection generally respond well to acyclovir administered orally or intravenously.[28] Cases of acyclovir-resistant HSV have been reported, and foscarnet, another antiviral drug, has been effective therapy for these patients.[29] Valacyclovir should be used with caution for immunosuppressed patients,

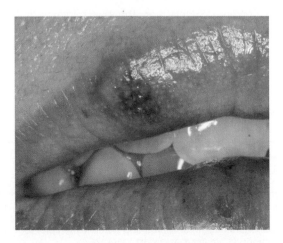

Fig. 2. RHL.

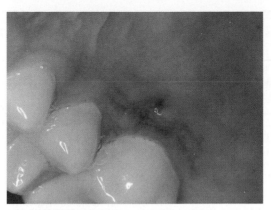

Fig. 3. RIH affecting the palatal mucosa.

because of the potential risk of hemolytic uremic syndrome. A comprehensive listing of medications and recommended dosing regimens used to treat recurrent oral HSV infections are given in **Table 2**.

Recurrent HSV has been known to trigger episodes of erythema multiforme (EM). HSV is believed to be the most common cause of recurring episodes of EM in susceptible individuals who develop an immune response to HSV.[1,2] Patients who experience severe, recurring EM from HSV commonly receive prophylactic doses of antiviral medication to prevent recurrence of EM. Oral acyclovir 400 mg twice daily may be

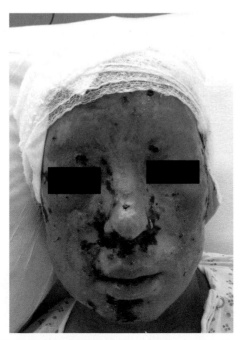

Fig. 4. Disseminated herpes simplex with orofacial lesions. (*Courtesy of* Thamer Musbah, BDS, Philadelphia, PA.)

Table 2
Systemic therapies for treatment of recurrent oral HSV infections

Indication	Therapy
Treatment of RHL in the immunocompetent host	• Oral acyclovir 400 mg 3 times a day for 5–7 d • Oral valacyclovir 500 mg–2000 mg twice a day for 1 d • Oral famciclovir 500 mg 2–3 times a day for 3 d
Prophylaxis of RHL in the immunocompetent host[a]	• Oral acyclovir 400 mg 2–3 times a day • Oral valacyclovir 500 mg–2000 mg twice a day
Treatment of recurrent HSV infections in the immunocompromised host	• Oral acyclovir 400 mg 3 times a day for 10 d or longer as necessary • Oral valacyclovir 500–1000 mg twice a day for 10 d or longer as necessary • Oral famciclovir 500 mg twice a day for up to 1 y
Prophylaxis of recurrent HSV infections in the immunocompromised host	• Oral acyclovir 400–800 mg 3 times a day • Oral valacyclovir 500–1000 mg twice a day • Oral famciclovir 500–1000 mg twice a day

[a] Duration of the prophylaxis is based on the extent and frequency of exposure to triggers of RHL episodes, such as sunlight, dental treatment, and so forth.
From Stoopler ET, Balasubramaniam R. Topical and systemic therapies for oral and perioral herpes simplex virus infections. J Calif Dent Assoc 2013;41(4):262.

effective in suppressing EM, and in cases non-responsive to acyclovir, valacyclovir 500 mg twice daily may be used.[30]

DIAGNOSIS
Differential Diagnosis

Most HSV infections are diagnosed clinically; however, a differential diagnosis should be formulated that includes other vesiculoulcerative diseases. Recurrent aphthous stomatitis (RAS) is commonly misdiagnosed as an HSV infection; however, there are key clinical features that are unique to each disease.[2] HSV infections typically have a prodrome of systemic symptoms before vesicle/ulcer eruption; RAS generally does not have the same prodromal symptoms before ulcer formation. HSV infections usually present with associated gingival erythema; this is uncommon with RAS.

HSV infections may appear clinically similar to coxsackie viral infections, the most common being herpangina and hand-foot-and-mouth disease. Herpangina can be differentiated from HSV infection because lesions associated with herpangina are typically confined to the posterior oropharynx, including the soft palate, uvula, tonsils, and pharyngeal wall. In contrast, HSV lesions may appear throughout the oral cavity. Herpangina infections are usually milder than HSV infections, generally occur in epidemics, and do not cause a generalized acute gingivitis seen with primary HSV infection.[1,2] Hand-foot-and-mouth disease can also present with oral ulcerations and can be differentiated from HSV infection by lesions involving the hands and feet.

EM may also be considered in the differential diagnosis of HSV infections. Distinguishing features of an EM infection include intraoral lesions, with a wide range of clinical presentations and typically associated target lesions on the skin. In contrast, HSV lesions tend to be more uniform and consistent in clinical presentation. In addition, EM lesions do not typically appear on the gingival tissue or cause gingival erythema, which are characteristic features of HSV infections.

Laboratory Diagnosis

Laboratory tests may be necessary to diagnose atypical presentations of HSV infections.[31] These tests should be used when evaluating immunocompromised patients with atypical lesions for definitive diagnosis.

VIROLOGIC TESTS

The classic standard for virus identification and diagnosis is isolation in tissue culture. The goal of virus isolation is to observe cytopathic effects (CPE) of the cells inoculated with virus. CPE are the degenerative changes that cells undergo when infected with virus. The rate at which CPE develops is dependent on the type of host cell, the type of virus, and the concentration of virus.[1,2] When viewed at high power via light microscopy, virally infected cells show multinucleated giant cells, syncytium, and ballooning degeneration of nuclei.

CYTOLOGY SMEARS

A smear taken of epithelial cells at the base of a suspected lesion may be analyzed to determine if these cells show changes consistent with HSV infection. The most common stain used is Giemsa, and virally infected cells have the same characteristics that are shown by virologic testing. When a Papanicolaou stain is performed, eosinophilic intranuclear viral inclusion bodies (Lipschutz or Cowdry type A) can be seen.

IMMUNOMORPHOLOGIC TESTS

The diagnosis of herpes virus infections can be made more quickly and accurately by using immunomorphologic techniques.[32] In the direct fluorescent assay (DFA), the specimen is incubated with fluorescein isothiocyanate–labeled HSV type-specific monoclonal antibody.[33] The positively infected cells are fluorescent green when examined under a fluorescent microscope, and this technique is often used for the rapid diagnosis of a clinical specimen.[34] Studies have concluded that the overall sensitivity when using DFA techniques to detect HSV is 80%, the specificity is 98% to 100%, and the positive predictive value ranges from 90% to 100%.[35,36]

POLYMERASE CHAIN REACTION TEST

Polymerase chain reaction (PCR) is the most sensitive method for HSV diagnosis.[37] PCR does not require viable virus or infected cells for detection, unlike tissue culture and direct assays. Also, real-time detection allows for PCR to be carried out promptly, and it may be used to discriminate HSV types.[38] Detection of viral DNA by PCR is considered the test of choice for HSV diagnosis.

SEROLOGIC TESTS

Serologic tests are conducted to detect antibody formation in a patient's blood sample. If serology is used in the diagnosis of suspected HSV infection, an acute specimen should be obtained within the initial 3 days of the infection and a convalescent specimen approximately 4 weeks later. Because of the delayed humoral response, antibodies are not present in the acute specimen but appear during convalescence; a 4-fold or greater antibody increase in convalescent serum is required for the diagnosis of a primary HSV infection. This factor may provide useful retrospective information but is of little help when managing a patient in the acute phase of illness.

VZV

VZV is responsible for two major clinical infections: the primary type is chickenpox (varicella) and the recurrent type is shingles (herpes zoster [HZ]).

Varicella

Chickenpox is characteristically a benign illness of childhood, spread by direct contact of either skin lesions or nasopharyngeal secretions of an infected individual.[1,2] The incubation period is 10 to 21 days, and patients are infectious for approximately 1 week after symptoms begin. Complications of chicken pox include pneumonitis and Reye syndrome, a progressive encephalopathy that most frequently occurs in children who have been given aspirin during an acute varicella infection.[39]

Skin lesions of chickenpox are characterized by maculopapular lesions, which are intensely pruritic. The lesions rapidly develop into fluid-filled vesicles on an erythematous base. Oral lesions may be present that resemble vesicles/ulcers seen in primary HSV infections, but these lesions are not a particularly important symptomatic, diagnostic, or management problem.[1,2]

HZ

After primary infection, VZV becomes latent in dorsal root or cranial nerve ganglia. In 0.3% to 0.5% of the population, the virus becomes reactivated, causing HZ.[1,2] The nerves most commonly affected with HZ are C-3, T-5, L-1, and L-2. When HZ involves the trigeminal nerve, the first division (ophthalmic branch or V_1) is most commonly involved, and ocular involvement is a potentially serious complication.[1,2] Consultation with an ophthalmologist is necessary in these cases. The live virus HZ vaccine is known to reduce the incidence of HZ by approximately 50%.[40] It is well tolerated and effective in the immunocompetent adult,[41] with mild reactions at the site of injection, including rash, erythema, edema, and pruritus.

The initial symptoms of HZ are pain, tenderness, and paresthesia along the course of the affected nerve. Unilateral vesicles appear 3 to 5 days later on an inflamed base along the involved nerve (**Fig. 5**). When the geniculate ganglion of the facial nerve is affected, characteristic signs include unilateral vesicles of the external ear and oral mucosa as well as unilateral facial paralysis, a group of signs referred to as Ramsay-Hunt syndrome.[1,2] HZ may also occasionally affect motor nerves.

Approximately 15% to 20% of cases of HZ of the trigeminal nerves affect either the maxillary division (V_2) or mandibular division (V_3), leading to pain, unilateral facial

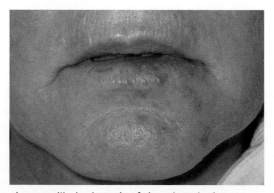

Fig. 5. HZ affecting the mandibular branch of the trigeminal nerve.

lesions, and intraoral lesions along the course of the affected nerve.[1,2] Diagnosis of HZ is usually based on characteristic clinical signs and symptoms. Intraoral lesions caused by HZ usually show a dramatic unilateral distribution associated with intense pain, helping to distinguish it from an HSV recurrence.[42] VZV may cause pain without lesions developing along the course of the nerve; this is referred to as zoster sine herpete or zoster sine eruptione.[1,2] Atypical presentations may require laboratory testing for confirmation of VZV. These methods include viral cultures, cytology smears, immunomorphologic techniques, PCR, and serologic testing, as described earlier.

Immunocompromised patients with HZ are at risk for developing life-threatening infections. In this group, HZ may cause large local lesions or disseminated infection. Oral HZ in immunosuppressed patients has been reported to cause necrosis of alveolar bone and exfoliation of teeth.[1,2] Disseminated infections among immunocompromised individuals may include widespread skin lesions, meningitis, encephalitis, VZV pneumonia, and hepatitis.

Antivirals, such as acyclovir, are effective in shortening the course of HZ, accelerating healing, and reducing acute pain.[1,2,43] Valacyclovir and famciclovir are effective for treating HZ and are dosed less frequently than acyclovir (**Table 3**).[1,2,43]

Postherpetic neuralgia (PHN) is a potential consequence of HZ, resulting from scarring of the involved nerve during infection.[1,2] PHN is a painful, sometimes debilitating condition, which can last months to years after the lesions are healed. The live virus vaccine reduces the incidence of PHN by 66%.[40] The incidence of PHN is increased in patients older than 50 years, and use of acyclovir, valacyclovir, or famciclovir has been advocated to reduce the incidence and duration of PHN.[44-46] The use of a short course of systemic corticosteroids, to decrease the incidence of PHN, is occasionally advocated; however, its efficacy is unknown.[1,2] Other effective therapies for treatment of PHN are gabapentin, topical capsaicin, tricyclic antidepressants, opioids, and topical lidocaine patches.[1,2,47]

EBV

EBV is a herpesvirus that preferentially infects B lymphocytes. Infection of humans with EBV usually occurs by contact with oral secretions, and more than 95% of the world's adult population is seropositive and chronically infected.[3] The virus replicates in epithelial cells of the oropharynx, and nearly all seropositive persons actively shed virus in the saliva.[3,48] Whereas most EBV infections of infants and children are asymptomatic or have non-specific symptoms, infections of adolescents and adults frequently result in infectious mononucleosis.[49,50] Infectious mononucleosis from EBV has an incubation period of up to 8 weeks.[1,2] The initial symptoms consist of a classic triad of symptoms (fever, lymphadenopathy, and pharyngitis) and typically runs a mild, self-remitting course.[51,52] Splenomegaly, hepatomegaly, oral ulcers, and palatal petechiae may also be present and the cervical lymph nodes are involved

Table 3
Antiviral therapy for treatment of HZ

	Acyclovir	Valacyclovir	Famciclovir
Dose (mg)	800	1000	500
Frequency (x/d)	5	3	3
Duration (d)	7–10	7	7

Data from Refs.[1,2,43]

in more than 90% of patients.[1,2] Less common complications include myocarditis, hepatitis, hemolytic anemia, thrombocytopenia, aplastic anemia, splenic rupture, and encephalitis.[49,51,52] In most cases of infectious mononucleosis, supportive therapy is sufficient; however, in immunocompetent patients with complications, the combination of corticosteroids and antivirals is beneficial.[53]

Several malignancies are associated with EBV, including nasopharyngeal carcinoma, Burkitt lymphoma, Hodgkin disease, and lymphoproliferative disease.[1,2] Burkitt lymphoma is a high-grade malignant lymphoma of small, noncleaved B cells. In Africa, tumors of Burkitt lymphoma usually present in the jaw, and more than 90% of these cases are associated with EBV.[48]

Oral hairy leukoplakia is caused by EBV and occurs in a large percentage of HIV-infected patients, as well as in some immunosuppressed transplant recipients.[48] It presents as a raised, white, corrugated lesion of the oral mucosa, which commonly involves the lateral or ventral surfaces of the tongue. It may also appear as a plaque-like lesion and is often seen bilaterally. Histopathologically, it appears as thickened parakeratosis with surface corrugations. It contains patchy bands of balloon cells in the upper spinous layer of the hyperplastic epithelium. Nuclear beading as a result of EBV replication is observed, whereby there is nuclear clearing of scattered cells and peripheral margination of chromatin.[54] Multiple strains of EBV DNA may be present in the lesions.[1,2]

CMV

CMV, also referred to as human CMV, is a frequent cause of asymptomatic infection in humans and may cause significant clinical disease in immunosuppressed patients.[55] The virus is mainly transmitted via contaminated blood and bodily secretions, including breast milk, saliva, and genital fluids.[1,2]

Neonates may develop cytomegalic inclusion disease, an often fatal disease resulting from congenitally acquired CMV infection.[56] In its most severe form, this disease is associated with microcephaly, chorioretinitis, nerve deafness, hepatitis, hepatosplenomegaly, and thrombocytopenia.[55] In immunocompromised adults, salivary gland enlargement is a common finding with this disease.[1,2]

In healthy children and adults, primary CMV infection is usually asymptomatic. This primary CMV infection results from either blood transfusions or sexual contact in a previously seronegative person.[1,2] Clinical symptoms include fever, myalgia, cervical lymphadenopathy, and mild hepatitis. Tonsillopharyngitis is less common than in primary EBV infection, and lymphadenopathy and splenic enlargement are less prominent features.[46] Complications of primary CMV infection may include myocarditis, pneumonitis, gastrointestinal disease, and aseptic meningitis.[56]

CMV infection may produce serious disease and death in immunosuppressed patients who have deficiencies of cell-mediated immunity. Patients at risk for developing life-threatening CMV infections are solid organ and bone marrow transplant recipients, as well as patients with human immunodeficiency virus (HIV) infection. A serious complication of bone marrow transplant recipients is CMV pneumonia, which has a high mortality despite treatment.[57] In advanced HIV, CMV disease may cause retinitis and, less commonly, gastrointestinal disease and encephalitis. CMV retinitis is characterized by hemorrhagic retinal necrosis, spreading along retinal vessels, and threatening sight when disease encroaches on the macula.[58]

The widespread use of antiretroviral therapy has reduced the incidence of complications caused by CMV infection. Incidence of CMV end-organ disease has declined with the use of antiretroviral therapy and is typically seen only in the few who fail to respond to therapy.[59]

There are reports of CMV-related oral lesions in patients with AIDS. These lesions have been described as slowly enlarging ulcers.[1,2,30,60] These ulcers are usually a few millimeters to 2 cm in diameter, painful, punched out, without surrounding edema usually of the palate or gingiva.[61] One study reported that CMV was the sole ulcerogenic viral agent in most oral lesions in a study population of patients with AIDS.[62] Coinfection of oral ulcers with both HSV and CMV has also been reported in patients with AIDS.[62,63] Reports indicate that genomes of CMV are frequently detected in several different types of periodontal disease.[64] Similarly, 1.32% of renal transplant patients present with oral ulcers caused by CMV infection.[65]

The diagnosis of CMV disease is made by histologic evaluation of suspected lesions, viral culture, antigen detection, and CMV DNA detection.[1,2] Biopsy specimens of CMV lesions show characteristic histopathologic changes, including enlarged cells with prominent intranucleolar and intracytoplasmic inclusions, referred to as owl-eye cells.[1,2] Viral culture of suspected lesions is used to detect CMV; however, the major drawback is the prolonged length of time that it takes for a positive culture to develop. PCR techniques are becoming the standard assay for detecting CMV in most laboratories. PCR can detect CMV in body fluids such as urine, blood, and saliva.[1,2] Salivary gland enlargement used to be a major clinical criterion for identifying CMV infection in infants, because of the tendency of CMV to infect salivary glands.[1,2]

One study[66] indicated that there is a relationship between xerostomia and the presence of CMV in saliva of HIV-infected individuals. Prospective studies using viral culture, PCR techniques, and histopathologic examination showed a significant correlation of xerostomia with presence of CMV in the saliva.[67] Similarly, a study[68] assessing frequency of CMV shedding in saliva was associated with occurrence of CMV disease in HIV-infected individuals who were previously without CMV disease. The results of this study suggest a link between CMV in saliva, salivary gland dysfunction, and CMV infection in HIV-infected individuals.[68]

Antiviral agents are used to treat and prevent CMV infections. Drugs such as ganciclovir (and its oral formulation valganciclovir), foscarnet, and cidofivir have been shown to be effective in treating CMV infections.[55,56] Newer drugs are in development for the treatment of CMV infections, including maribavir, CMX001, and AIC246.[56,69]

HHV-6

HHV-6 was discovered in 1986, when it was isolated from peripheral blood lymphocytes of six individuals with lymphoproliferative disorders.[70] Studies showed that CD4 T cells were the major type of cell infected by HHV-6.[71,72] Two variants of HHV-6 have been differentiated: HHV-6A and HHV-6B. Eighty percent to 90% of the population intermittently shed HHV-6 (and HHV-7) in saliva.[73]

Primary infection with HHV-6 can be asymptomatic or cause an unspecified febrile illness or a specific clinical disorder, roseola (exanthema subitum).[74] The virus is commonly isolated from saliva, and respiratory transmission is the major route of primary infection. HHV-6A is the subtype commonly found in skin biopsy specimens from immunocompromised patients[43] and has also been postulated as a cofactor in the progression of HIV disease.[75,76] HHV-6B is the particular subtype implicated as the cause for roseola.[77] Oral lesions are not commonly associated with either HHV-6A or HHV-6B infections.

HHV-7

HHV-7 was discovered in 1990, when the virus was isolated from activated CD4 T cells obtained from a healthy individual. The genomes of HHV-7 and both variants of HHV-6 are closely related, with 20% to 75% nucleic acid homology depending on the genes being compared.[74]

Primary infection with HHV-7 is most often asymptomatic; however, it may cause pityriasis rosea, presenting as a single rose-colored, scaling, and herald patch. Oral lesions involving HHV-7 are rare and may present as punctate hemorrhages, ulcers, bullae, or erythematous plaques.[78] HHV-7 is commonly isolated from saliva, and the mode of transmission is analogous to HHV-6.[1,2]

Reactivation of HHV-7 in immunocompromised patients can lead to widespread multiorgan infection, including encephalitis, pneumonitis, and hepatitis.[74] HHV-6 can be activated from latency by HHV-7 reactivation.[79,80]

HHV-8

HHV-8 was isolated in tumor tissue from a patient with AIDS-associated KS in 1994 and named KS herpesvirus (KSHV).[7] Moritz Kaposi, a Hungarian-born dermatologist, first described idiopathic multiple, pigmented sarcoma of the skin in 1872 and suggested a possible infectious cause for KS.[74]

KSHV is capable of inducing malignant tumors in humans. Of the KSHV-associated malignant diseases, the most prominent is KS.[8] KSHV is believed to stimulate angiogenic and inflammatory cytokines and gene products release found in angiogenesis for the development of KS.[81] In addition, the clinical progression from patch or plaque-like lesions to nodular lesions is associated with the viral load.[82] There is evidence that the risk for developing KS is higher in KSHV-infected solid organ transplant recipients and HIV-seropositive patients, further supporting the etiologic role of KSHV.[83,84]

Oral KS may be an indication of undiagnosed HIV infection.[85] HIV-associated KS can be aggressive, and lesions may become more widespread and prominent, involving oropharyngeal and gastrointestinal mucous membranes.[7] Oral lesions may be solitary, multifocal, or multicentric red-purple macules, plaques, or nodules of varying sizes.[8] The hard palate, gingiva and dorsal tongue are the most frequent sites of oral involvement.[85,86] Treatment strategies for oral KS range from monitoring focal, asymptomatic lesions without intervention to initiating systemic chemotherapy for widespread lesions.[8]

SUMMARY

Oral herpes virus infections are often encountered in clinical practice. An appropriate diagnosis and treatment plan requires advanced knowledge of these diseases. Clinicians should be aware of the potentially critical nature of herpes virus infections, especially in immunocompromised patients, and manage these cases accordingly.

REFERENCES

1. Stoopler ET, Greenberg MS. Update on herpesvirus infections. Dent Clin North Am 2003;47(3):517–32.
2. Stoopler ET. Oral herpetic infections (HSV 1-8). Dent Clin North Am 2005;49(1): 15–29, vii.
3. Jenson HB. Epstein-Barr virus. Pediatr Rev 2011;32(9):375–83 [quiz: 384].
4. Lautenschlager I. CMV infection, diagnosis and antiviral strategies after liver transplantation. Transpl Int 2009;22(11):1031–40.
5. Campbell AE, Cavanaugh VJ, Slater JS. The salivary glands as a privileged site of cytomegalovirus immune evasion and persistence. Med Microbiol Immunol 2008;197(2):205–13.

6. Dittmer DP, Damania B. Kaposi sarcoma associated herpesvirus pathogenesis (KSHV)–an update. Curr Opin Virol 2013;3(3):238–44.
7. Sarid R, Klepfish A, Schattner A. Virology, pathogenetic mechanisms, and associated diseases of Kaposi sarcoma-associated herpesvirus (human herpesvirus 8). Mayo Clin Proc 2002;77(9):941–9.
8. Fatahzadeh M, Schwartz RA. Oral Kaposi's sarcoma: a review and update. Int J Dermatol 2013;52(6):666–72.
9. Miller CS, Danaher RJ. Asymptomatic shedding of herpes simplex virus (HSV) in the oral cavity. Oral Surg Oral Med Oral Pathol Oral Radiol Endod 2008;105(1):43–50.
10. Rickinson A. Epstein-Barr virus. Virus Res 2002;82(1–2):109–13.
11. Stoopler ET, Kuperstein AS, Sollecito TP. How do I manage a patient with recurrent herpes simplex? J Can Dent Assoc 2012;78:c154.
12. Stoopler ET, Balasubramaniam R. Topical and systemic therapies for oral and perioral herpes simplex virus infections. J Calif Dent Assoc 2013;41(4):259–62.
13. Bowling JC, Saha M, Bunker CB. Herpetic whitlow: a forgotten diagnosis. Clin Exp Dermatol 2005;30(5):609–10.
14. MacPhail L, Greenspan D. Herpetic gingivostomatitis in a 70-year-old man. Oral Surg Oral Med Oral Pathol Oral Radiol Endod 1995;79(1):50–2.
15. Xu F, Sternberg MR, Kottiri BJ, et al. Trends in herpes simplex virus type 1 and type 2 seroprevalence in the United States. JAMA 2006;296(8):964–73.
16. Centers for Disease Control and Prevention (CDC). Seroprevalence of herpes simplex virus type 2 among persons aged 14-49 years–United States, 2005-2008. MMWR Morb Mortal Wkly Rep 2010;59(15):456–9.
17. Fatahzadeh M, Schwartz RA. Human herpes simplex labialis. Clin Exp Dermatol 2007;32(6):625–30.
18. Fatahzadeh M, Schwartz RA. Human herpes simplex virus infections: epidemiology, pathogenesis, symptomatology, diagnosis, and management. J Am Acad Dermatol 2007;57(5):737–63 [quiz: 764–6].
19. Amir J, Harel L, Smetana Z, et al. Treatment of herpes simplex gingivostomatitis with aciclovir in children: a randomised double blind placebo controlled study. BMJ 1997;314(7097):1800–3.
20. Balfour HH Jr. Antiviral drugs. N Engl J Med 1999;340(16):1255–68.
21. Vander Straten M, Carrasco D, Lee P, et al. A review of antiviral therapy for herpes labialis. Arch Dermatol 2001;137(9):1232–5.
22. McKeough MB, Spruance SL. Comparison of new topical treatments for herpes labialis: efficacy of penciclovir cream, acyclovir cream, and n-docosanol cream against experimental cutaneous herpes simplex virus type 1 infection. Arch Dermatol 2001;137(9):1153–8.
23. Spruance SL, Rea TL, Thoming C, et al. Penciclovir cream for the treatment of herpes simplex labialis. A randomized, multicenter, double-blind, placebo-controlled trial. Topical Penciclovir Collaborative Study Group. JAMA 1997;277(17):1374–9.
24. Spruance SL, Nett R, Marbury T, et al. Acyclovir cream for treatment of herpes simplex labialis: results of two randomized, double-blind, vehicle-controlled, multicenter clinical trials. Antimicrob Agents Chemother 2002;46(7):2238–43.
25. Habbema L, De Boulle K, Roders GA, et al. n-Docosanol 10% cream in the treatment of recurrent herpes labialis: a randomised, double-blind, placebo-controlled study. Acta Derm Venereol 1996;76(6):479–81.
26. Sacks SL, Thisted RA, Jones TM, et al. Clinical efficacy of topical docosanol 10% cream for herpes simplex labialis: a multicenter, randomized, placebo-controlled trial. J Am Acad Dermatol 2001;45(2):222–30.

27. Greenberg MS, Friedman H, Cohen SG, et al. A comparative study of herpes simplex infections in renal transplant and leukemic patients. J Infect Dis 1987; 156(2):280–7.

28. Redding SW, Montgomery MT. Acyclovir prophylaxis for oral herpes simplex virus infection in patients with bone marrow transplants. Oral Surg Oral Med Oral Pathol 1989;67(6):680–3.

29. MacPhail LA, Greenspan D, Schiodt M, et al. Acyclovir-resistant, foscarnet-sensitive oral herpes simplex type 2 lesion in a patient with AIDS. Oral Surg Oral Med Oral Pathol 1989;67(4):427–32.

30. Tatnall FM, Schofield JK, Leigh IM. A double-blind, placebo-controlled trial of continuous acyclovir therapy in recurrent erythema multiforme. Br J Dermatol 1995;132(2):267–70.

31. Stoopler ET, Pinto A, DeRossi SS, et al. Herpes simplex and varicella-zoster infections: clinical and laboratory diagnosis. Gen Dent 2003;51(3):281–6 [quiz: 287].

32. Meyer MP, Amortegui AJ. Rapid detection of herpes simplex virus using a combination of human fibroblast cell cultures and peroxidase-antiperoxidase staining. Am J Clin Pathol 1984;81(1):43–7.

33. Cohen PR. Tests for detecting herpes simplex virus and varicella-zoster virus infections. Dermatol Clin 1994;12(1):51–68.

34. Erlich KS. Laboratory diagnosis of herpesvirus infections. Clin Lab Med 1987; 7(4):759–76.

35. Chan EL, Brandt K, Horsman GB. Comparison of Chemicon SimulFluor direct fluorescent antibody staining with cell culture and shell vial direct immunoperoxidase staining for detection of herpes simplex virus and with cytospin direct immunofluorescence staining for detection of varicella-zoster virus. Clin Diagn Lab Immunol 2001;8(5):909–12.

36. Sanders C, Nelson C, Hove M, et al. Cytospin-enhanced direct immunofluorescence assay versus cell culture for detection of herpes simplex virus in clinical specimens. Diagn Microbiol Infect Dis 1998;32(2):111–3.

37. Strick LB, Wald A. Diagnostics for herpes simplex virus: is PCR the new gold standard? Mol Diagn Ther 2006;10(1):17–28.

38. Whiley DM, Syrmis MW, Mackay IM, et al. Preliminary comparison of three Light-Cycler PCR assays for the detection of herpes simplex virus in swab specimens. Eur J Clin Microbiol Infect Dis 2003;22(12):764–7.

39. Linnemann CC Jr, Shea L, Partin JC, et al. Reye's syndrome: epidemiologic and viral studies, 1963-1974. Am J Epidemiol 1975;101(6):517–26.

40. Oxman MN, Levin MJ, Johnson GR, et al. A vaccine to prevent herpes zoster and postherpetic neuralgia in older adults. N Engl J Med 2005;352(22): 2271–84.

41. Javed S, Javed SA, Tyring SK. Varicella vaccines. Curr Opin Infect Dis 2012; 25(2):135–40.

42. Huber MA. Herpes simplex type-1 virus infection. Quintessence Int 2003;34(6): 453–67.

43. Cohen JI. Clinical practice: herpes zoster. N Engl J Med 2013;369(3):255–63.

44. Dworkin RH, Nagasako EM, Johnson RW, et al. Acute pain in herpes zoster: the famciclovir database project. Pain 2001;94(1):113–9.

45. Schmader K. Herpes zoster in older adults. Clin Infect Dis 2001;32(10):1481–6.

46. Dwyer DE, Cunningham AL. 10: herpes simplex and varicella-zoster virus infections. Med J Aust 2002;177(5):267–73.

47. Dubinsky RM, Kabbani H, El-Chami Z, et al. Practice parameter: treatment of postherpetic neuralgia: an evidence-based report of the Quality Standards

Subcommittee of the American Academy of Neurology. Neurology 2004;63(6): 959–65.

48. Cohen JI. Epstein-Barr virus infection. N Engl J Med 2000;343(7):481–92.

49. Henke CE, Kurland LT, Elveback LR. Infectious mononucleosis in Rochester, Minnesota, 1950 through 1969. Am J Epidemiol 1973;98(6):483–90.

50. Straus SE, Cohen JI, Tosato G, et al. NIH conference. Epstein-Barr virus infections: biology, pathogenesis, and management. Ann Intern Med 1993;118(1): 45–58.

51. Maakaroun NR, Moanna A, Jacob JT, et al. Viral infections associated with haemophagocytic syndrome. Rev Med Virol 2010;20(2):93–105.

52. Luzuriaga K, Sullivan JL. Infectious mononucleosis. N Engl J Med 2010;362(21): 1993–2000.

53. Rafailidis PI, Mavros MN, Kapaskelis A, et al. Antiviral treatment for severe EBV infections in apparently immunocompetent patients. J Clin Virol 2010;49(3):151–7.

54. Schiodt M, Greenspan D, Daniels TE, et al. Clinical and histologic spectrum of oral hairy leukoplakia. Oral Surg Oral Med Oral Pathol 1987;64(6):716–20.

55. Sissons JG, Carmichael AJ. Clinical aspects and management of cytomegalovirus infection. J Infect 2002;44(2):78–83.

56. Boeckh M, Geballe AP. Cytomegalovirus: pathogen, paradigm, and puzzle. J Clin Invest 2011;121(5):1673–80.

57. Ljungman P, Hakki M, Boeckh M. Cytomegalovirus in hematopoietic stem cell transplant recipients. Infect Dis Clin North Am 2010;24(2):319–37.

58. Jacobson MA. Treatment of cytomegalovirus retinitis in patients with the acquired immunodeficiency syndrome. N Engl J Med 1997;337(2):105–14.

59. Jabs DA, Van Natta ML, Holbrook JT, et al. Longitudinal study of the ocular complications of AIDS: 1. Ocular diagnoses at enrollment. Ophthalmology 2007; 114(4):780–6.

60. Greenberg MS. Herpesvirus infections. Dent Clin North Am 1996;40(2):359–68.

61. Reichart PA. Oral ulcerations in HIV infection. Oral Dis 1997;3(Suppl 1):S180–2.

62. Flaitz CM, Nichols CM, Hicks MJ. Herpesviridae-associated persistent mucocutaneous ulcers in acquired immunodeficiency syndrome. A clinicopathologic study. Oral Surg Oral Med Oral Pathol Oral Radiol Endod 1996;81(4):433–41.

63. Regezi JA, Eversole LR, Barker BF, et al. Herpes simplex and cytomegalovirus coinfected oral ulcers in HIV-positive patients. Oral Surg Oral Med Oral Pathol Oral Radiol Endod 1996;81(1):55–62.

64. Slots J, Contreras A. Herpesviruses: a unifying causative factor in periodontitis? Oral Microbiol Immunol 2000;15(5):277–80.

65. Lopez-Pintor RM, Hernandez G, de Arriba L, et al. Oral ulcers during the course of cytomegalovirus infection in renal transplant recipients. Transplant Proc 2009; 41(6):2419–21.

66. Greenberg MS, Dubin G, Stewart JC, et al. Relationship of oral disease to the presence of cytomegalovirus DNA in the saliva of AIDS patients. Oral Surg Oral Med Oral Pathol Oral Radiol Endod 1995;79(2):175–9.

67. Greenberg MS, Glick M, Nghiem L, et al. Relationship of cytomegalovirus to salivary gland dysfunction in HIV-infected patients. Oral Surg Oral Med Oral Pathol Oral Radiol Endod 1997;83(3):334–9.

68. Fidouh-Houhou N, Duval X, Bissuel F, et al. Salivary cytomegalovirus (CMV) shedding, glycoprotein B genotype distribution, and CMV disease in human immunodeficiency virus-seropositive patients. Clin Infect Dis 2001;33(8):1406–11.

69. Emery VC, Hassan-Walker AF. Focus on new drugs in development against human cytomegalovirus. Drugs 2002;62(13):1853–8.

70. Salahuddin SZ, Ablashi DV, Markham PD, et al. Isolation of a new virus, HBLV, in patients with lymphoproliferative disorders. Science 1986;234(4776):596–601.
71. Lusso P, Markham PD, Tschachler E, et al. In vitro cellular tropism of human B-lymphotropic virus (human herpesvirus-6). J Exp Med 1988;167(5):1659–70.
72. Takahashi K, Sonoda S, Higashi K, et al. Predominant CD4 T-lymphocyte tropism of human herpesvirus 6-related virus. J Virol 1989;63(7):3161–3.
73. Di Luca D, Mirandola P, Ravaioli T, et al. Human herpesviruses 6 and 7 in salivary glands and shedding in saliva of healthy and human immunodeficiency virus positive individuals. J Med Virol 1995;45(4):462–8.
74. Blauvelt A. Skin diseases associated with human herpesvirus 6, 7, and 8 infection. J Investig Dermatol Symp Proc 2001;6(3):197–202.
75. Chen H, Pesce AM, Carbonari M, et al. Absence of antibodies to human herpesvirus-6 in patients with slowly-progressive human immunodeficiency virus type 1 infection. Eur J Epidemiol 1992;8(2):217–21.
76. Lusso P, Gallo RC. Human herpesvirus 6 in AIDS. Immunol Today 1995;16(2):67–71.
77. Schirmer EC, Wyatt LS, Yamanishi K, et al. Differentiation between two distinct classes of viruses now classified as human herpesvirus 6. Proc Natl Acad Sci U S A 1991;88(13):5922–6.
78. Wolz MM, Sciallis GF, Pittelkow MR. Human herpesviruses 6, 7, and 8 from a dermatologic perspective. Mayo Clin Proc 2012;87(10):1004–14.
79. Katsafanas GC, Schirmer EC, Wyatt LS, et al. In vitro activation of human herpesviruses 6 and 7 from latency. Proc Natl Acad Sci U S A 1996;93(18):9788–92.
80. Tanaka-Taya K, Kondo T, Nakagawa N, et al. Reactivation of human herpesvirus 6 by infection of human herpesvirus 7. J Med Virol 2000;60(3):284–9.
81. Kang T, Ye FC, Gao SJ, et al. Angiogenesis, Kaposi's sarcoma and Kaposi's sarcoma-associated herpesvirus. Virol Sin 2008;23(6):449–58.
82. Feller L, Lemmer J. Insights into pathogenic events of HIV-associated Kaposi sarcoma and immune reconstitution syndrome related Kaposi sarcoma. Infect Agent Cancer 2008;3:1. http://dx.doi.org/10.1186/1750-9378-3-1.
83. Iscovich J, Boffetta P, Franceschi S, et al. Classic Kaposi sarcoma: epidemiology and risk factors. Cancer 2000;88(3):500–17.
84. Lebbe C, Legendre C, Frances C. Kaposi sarcoma in transplantation. Transplant Rev (Orlando) 2008;22(4):252–61.
85. Papagatsia Z, Jones J, Morgan P, et al. Oral Kaposi sarcoma: a case of immune reconstitution inflammatory syndrome. Oral Surg Oral Med Oral Pathol Oral Radiol Endod 2009;108(1):70–5.
86. Lager I, Altini M, Coleman H, et al. Oral Kaposi's sarcoma: a clinicopathologic study from South Africa. Oral Surg Oral Med Oral Pathol Oral Radiol Endod 2003;96(6):701–10.

Recurrent Aphthous Stomatitis

Sunday O. Akintoye, BDS, DDS, MS*,
Martin S. Greenberg, DDS, FDSRCS

KEYWORDS

- Aphthous • Immunologic • Crohn disease • Behçet disease • Nutritional deficiency
- Psychological stress • Topical therapy • Systemic therapy

KEY POINTS

- Recurrent aphthous stomatitis (RAS) is the most common ulcerative disease of the oral mucosa.
- Several proposed etiologic theories are reviewed.
- Topical and systemic therapies that are used to manage RAS are presented.

INTRODUCTION

Recurrent aphthous stomatitis (RAS) remains the most common ulcerative disease of the oral mucosa, presenting as painful round, shallow ulcers with well-defined erythematous margin and yellowish-gray pseudomembranous center.[1] RAS has a characteristic prodromal burning sensation that lasts from 2 to 48 hours before an ulcer appears. It occurs in otherwise healthy individuals and is typically located on the buccal and labial mucosa and tongue. Involvement of the heavily keratinized mucosa of the palate and gingiva is less common.

Diseases also causing oral ulcers that may be mistaken for RAS include Behçet disease, cyclic neutropenia, recurring intraoral herpes infections, human immunodeficiency virus (HIV)-related oral ulcers, or gastrointestinal diseases such as Crohn disease and ulcerative colitis. It is incumbent on the clinician managing oral disease to distinguish localized RAS from ulcers caused by an underlying systemic disorder.

Several factors have been proposed as possible causative agents for RAS, including: local factors, such as trauma in individuals who are genetically susceptible to RAS; microbial factors; nutritional factors, such as deficiency of folate and B-complex vitamins; immunologic factors; psychosocial stress; and allergy to dietary constituents.[1] Extensive research has focused predominantly on immunologic factors, but a definitive etiology of RAS has yet to be clearly established.

A version of this article appeared as Akintoye SO, Greenberg MS. Recurrent aphthous stomatitis. Dent Clin N Am 2005;49:31–47.

Department of Oral Medicine, School of Dental Medicine, University of Pennsylvania, 240 South 40th Street, Philadelphia, PA 19104, USA

* Corresponding author.

E-mail address: akintoye@dental.upenn.edu

Dent Clin N Am 58 (2014) 281–297
http://dx.doi.org/10.1016/j.cden.2013.12.002
0011-8532/14/$ – see front matter © 2014 Elsevier Inc. All rights reserved.

dental.theclinics.com

RAS is classified into minor, major, and herpetiform ulcers. More than 85% of RAS presents as minor ulcers that are less than 1 cm in diameter and heal without scars (**Fig. 1**). Ulcers classified as major RAS, also known as Sutton disease or periadenitis mucosa necrotica recurrens, are larger than 1 cm in diameter, persist for weeks to months, and heal with scars (**Fig. 2**). Herpetiform ulcers are clinically distinct because they appear as clusters of multiple ulcers scattered throughout the oral mucosa; despite the name, these lesions have no association with herpes simplex virus. General characteristics of the 3 types of RAS are summarized in **Table 1**.

Management of RAS depends on the frequency and severity of the lesions. Most cases can be adequately managed with topical therapy, but systemic therapy is sometimes indicated for patients with major RAS or for those who experience large numbers of minor lesions that are nonresponsive to topical therapies.

EPIDEMIOLOGY

Approximately 20% of the general population is affected by RAS, but incidence varies from 5% to 50% depending on the ethnic and socioeconomic groups studied.[2,3] The prevalence of RAS is influenced by the population studied, diagnostic criteria, and environmental factors.[1] In children, prevalence of RAS may be as high as 39%, and is influenced by the presence of RAS in one or both parents.[4] Children with RAS-positive parents have a 90% chance of developing RAS, compared with 20% of those with RAS-negative parents.[2] In children of high socioeconomic status, RAS is 5 times more prevalent and represents 50% of oral mucosal lesions in this cohort.[5,6] RAS prevalence was found to be higher (male, 48.3%; female, 57.2%) among professional school students than in the same subjects 12 years later when they had become practicing professionals. This finding led some investigators to theorize that stress during student life is a major factor in RAS, although the differences attributable to age changes should also be considered. The onset of RAS appears to peak between the ages of 10 and 19 years and becomes less frequent with advancing age, geographic location, or gender.[7] If RAS begins or significantly increases in severity after the third decade and well into adult life (see **Table 1**), it should increase suspicion that the cause of the condition may be attributed to an underlying medical disorder such as hematologic or immunologic abnormality, connective tissue disease, or Behçet syndrome.

PREDISPOSING ETIOLOGIC FACTORS

The etiology of RAS lesions is still unknown, but several local, systemic, immunologic, genetic, allergic, nutritional, and microbial factors have been proposed as causative

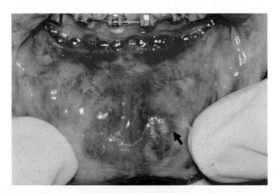

Fig. 1. Minor aphthous ulcer on the lower lip (*black arrow*).

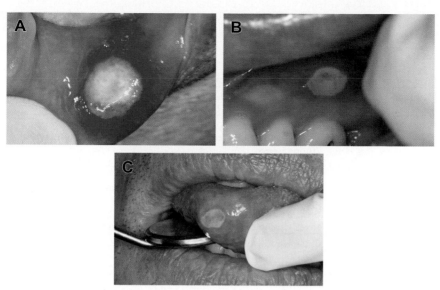

Fig. 2. Major aphthous ulcer on the lower lip (*A*), maxillary unattached gingiva (*B*), and anterior tongue (*C*). The ulcers display characteristic erythematous halo and central yellowish-gray pseudomembrane.

agents. Moreover, some medications including immunosuppressive drugs such calcineurin and mammalian target of rapamycin (mTOR) inhibitors have been associated with severe aphthous-like stomatitis (**Table 2**).[8,9]

Local Factors

Local trauma is regarded as a causative agent for RAS in susceptible individuals.[10,11] Trauma predisposes to RAS by inducing edema and early cellular inflammation associated with an increased viscosity of the oral submucosal extracellular matrix.[12] Not all

Table 1			
Types of recurrent aphthous stomatitis			
	Minor	**Major**	**Herpetiform**
Gender predilection	M = F	M = F	F > M (usually)
Age at onset (y)	5–19	10–19	20–29
Number of ulcers	1–5	1–10	10–100
Size of ulcers (mm)	<10	>10	1–2 (larger if coalesced)
Duration (d)	4–14	>30	<30
Recurrence rate (mo)	1–4	<1	<1
Site predilection	Lips, cheeks, tongue, floor of mouth	Lips, cheeks, tongue, palate, pharynx	Lips, cheeks, tongue, pharynx, palate, gingiva, floor of mouth
Permanent scarring	Unusual	Common	Unusual

Adapted from Porter SR, Scully C, Pedersen A. Recurrent aphthous stomatitis. Crit Rev Oral Biol Med 1998;9(3):306–21.

Table 2
Etiologic factors associated with recurrent aphthous stomatitis

Local	Trauma
	Smoking
	Dysregulated saliva composition
Microbial	Bacterial: streptococci
	Viral: varicella zoster, cytomegalovirus
Systemic	Behçet disease
	Mouth and genital ulcers with inflamed cartilage (MAGIC) syndrome
	Crohn disease
	Ulcerative colitis
	Human immunodeficiency virus infection
	Periodic fever, aphthosis, pharyngitis, and adenitis (PFAPA) or Marshall syndrome
	Cyclic neutropenia
	Stress; psychological imbalance, menstrual cycle
Nutritional	Gluten-sensitive enteropathy
	Iron, folic acid, zinc deficiencies
	Vitamin B_1, B_2, B_6, and B_{12} deficiencies
Genetic	Ethnicity
	Human leukocyte antigen haplotypes
Allergic/immunologic	Local T-lymphocyte cytotoxicity
	Abnormal CD4:CD8 ratio
	Dysregulated cytokine levels
	Microbe-induced hypersensitivity
	Sodium lauryl sulfate sensitivity
	Food sensitivity
Others	Antioxidants
	Nonsteroidal anti-inflammatory drugs
	β-Blockers
	Immunosuppressive drugs

Adapted from Ship II. Socioeconomic status and recurrent aphthous ulcers. J Am Dent Assoc 1966;73(1):120–3.

oral trauma leads to RAS, because denture wearers do not have a high prevalence of RAS despite this cohort being 3 times more susceptible to oral mucosal ulceration.[13] In addition, habitual smokers who constantly expose their oral mucosa to nicotine have demonstrated a negative association between smoking and RAS.[14–16] Therefore, local trauma apparently predisposes to RAS only in those individuals who have a hereditary predilection for the disease.

Some changes in salivary composition that affect the local properties of saliva, such as pH and a stress-induced increase in salivary cortisol, have been correlated with RAS.[17,18] Although direct association of salivary gland dysfunction with RAS has not been demonstrated,[19] patients with a combination of RAS and xerostomia may experience increased symptoms resulting from the increased oral dryness.

Microbial Factors

Despite RAS having not been etiologically associated with herpes simplex virus based on several well-designed studies, both laymen and clinicians often confuse RAS with herpes simplex virus (HSV) infection. HSV virions and antigens have neither been identified in aphthous lesions nor successfully isolated in RAS biopsy tissues.[20,21]

Although it has been suggested that reactivation of varicella zoster virus (VZV) or human cytomegalovirus (CMV) is associated with frequent recurrence of aphthous ulcers,[22] evaluation of RAS biopsy tissue using polymerase chain reaction (PCR) for possible involvement of herpes virus 6, CMV, VZV, or Epstein-Barr virus (EBV) as causative factors did not find evidence to support the role of these viruses in RAS pathogenesis.[20,23] Thus, it is the clinician's responsibility to distinguish RAS from herpes infections and to reassure RAS patients that they do not have an infectious disease, and that antiviral therapy is neither necessary nor effective.

Helicobacter pylori, a common risk factor for gastric and duodenal ulcers, has been proposed to have a causative role in RAS. Despite the fact that stomach ulcers and RAS are linked to dysregulated immune functions, molecular studies that identified *H pylori* in both affected and nonaffected mucosa of RAS patients found no association with RAS.[24,25] Of note, another study[26] reported that eradication of *H pylori* in RAS patients positively correlated with increased Vitamin B_{12} levels and decreased the number of aphthous lesions.[26–29] There has been considerable speculation regarding the possible involvement of *Streptococcus* species in the etiology of RAS, especially *Streptococcus sanguis* 2A. The proposed hypothesis is that oral streptococci act as antigenic stimulants that cross-react with mitochondrial heat-shock proteins of oral keratinocytes. This reaction purportedly induces a T-cell–mediated immune response that causes oral mucosal damage,[30] but this theory remains unproven. EBV and *Lactobacillus* are other organisms that have been studied in RAS patients. A study of the possible role of *Lactobacillus* in RAS has yielded no significant finding; but in a small study sample, EBV was associated with epithelial cells of preulcerative RAS.[31,32] Using PCR techniques, 39% of preulcerative RAS lesions were positive for EBV DNA. Their peripheral blood lymphocytes and serum were also positive for EBV DNA. The report theorized that lymphocytes may serve as a reservoir for latent EBV infection and promote viral shedding into the plasma. However, a causal relationship between Epstein-Barr viral load and RAS was not evaluated.

Underlying Disease

The most prominent medical disorder associated with RAS is Behçet syndrome, characterized by recurring oral and genital ulcers, and eye lesions (see **Table 2**). Behçet syndrome is a multisystem disorder resulting from vasculitis of small and medium-sized vessels and inflammation of epithelium. The abnormal inflammatory response in Behçet syndrome is caused by immune complexes induced by T lymphocytes and plasma cells. Although Behçet syndrome usually affects adults, several cases have been reported in children.[33–35]

Because distinguishing RAS from Behçet disease now depends on clinical criteria, investigators have sought an effective laboratory test. A high titer of anti–*Saccharomyces cerevisiae* antibodies (ASCA) has been detected in Behçet patients relative to RAS patients and apparently healthy individuals.[36] This report suggested that the ASCA test might be a method to distinguish between these 2 patient populations. This distinction may not be as simple as reported, because up to 70% of patients with Crohn disease and 15% of patients with ulcerative colitis are ASCA positive, and both diseases are associated with recurring oral ulcers. The use of the human leukocyte antigen (HLA) system to distinguish RAS from Behçet disease showed significant differences in the frequency of certain HLA antigens, but the distinction between the 2 disorders is still not clearly defined.[37]

Another variant of Behçet syndrome that includes relapsing polychondritis, a disorder characterized by mouth and genital ulcers with inflamed cartilage, has been labeled MAGIC syndrome (see **Table 2**).[38,39]

Inflammatory bowel diseases such as Crohn disease and ulcerative colitis have been associated with oral ulcers that may resemble RAS, but Crohn lesions often have indurated borders and are histologically different because of the granulomatous nature of the lesion (**Fig. 3**). Approximately 10% of patients with Crohn disease have oral mucosal ulcers, and the oral manifestations occasionally precede intestinal symptoms. Some researchers believe that inflammation of minor salivary glands is a possible cause of the oral ulcers.[40]

Celiac disease, an autoimmune sensitivity to gluten, is another medical disorder often associated with RAS, but the causal relationship between these 2 disorders is not completely clear. Prevalence of RAS in patients with celiac disease has been reported to range from 4% to 40%, but oral ulceration in such patients also varies from 3% to 61%.[41] In addition, oral ulcerations in celiac disease do not have the distinctive features of RAS, and often resolve when celiac disease patients are placed on gluten-free diet. Therefore, oral ulceration in patients with celiac disease may not be the typical RAS.[42]

In HIV-positive individuals, RAS occurs more frequently, lasts longer, and causes more painful symptoms than in healthy individuals (**Fig. 4**). It is also a common finding in HIV-positive children.[43,44] RAS is usually a late finding in AIDS patients with CD4$^+$ lymphocyte counts of fewer than 100 cells/mm^3, and it may occasionally be a presenting sign of HIV infection.[4]

Cyclic neutropenia, a rare disorder that presents in childhood, is also associated with recurring oral ulcers during periods when the neutrophil count is severely depressed.[45] Another condition, described as periodic fever, aphthous stomatitis, pharyngitis, and cervical adenitis (PFAPA) or Marshall syndrome, has a presentation similar to that of cyclic neutropenia and is commonly associated with oral ulcers that cannot be distinguished from RAS.[46]

Hereditary and Genetic Factors

The role of heredity is the best-defined underlying cause of RAS. Susceptibility to RAS is significantly increased by its presence in one or both parents. Studies of identical twins have also demonstrated the hereditary nature of this disorder.[4] Individuals with a positive family history of RAS tend to develop RAS at an early age. Specifically, children with two RAS-positive parents have a 90% chance of developing RAS that presents with more severe symptoms and recurs more frequently.[2]

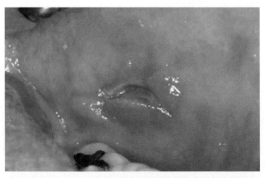

Fig. 3. Ulcer with indurated margin on the buccal mucosa of a patient with Crohn disease. (*From* Akintoye SO, Greenberg MS. Recurrent aphthous stomatitis. Dent Clin N Am 2005;49:36.)

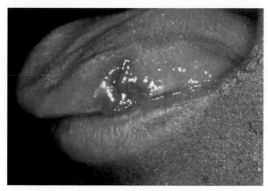

Fig. 4. Aphthous-like lesion in a patient with advanced human immunodeficiency virus disease. (*From* Akintoye SO, Greenberg MS. Recurrent aphthous stomatitis. Dent Clin N Am 2005;49:37.)

Certain genetically specific HLAs have been identified in RAS patients: HLA-A2, HLA-B5, HLA-B12, HLA-B44, HLA-B51, HLA-B52, HLA-DR2, HLA-DR7, and HLA-DQ series.[47] A confounding finding is that certain ethnic groups have been associated with different HLA alleles or haplotypes, with no HLA being consistently associated with RAS.[47] Additional studies are therefore needed to clarify the variability of RAS in host susceptibility.

Allergic Factors

Allergy has been suspected as a cause of RAS. Hypersensitivity to certain food substances, oral microbes such as *S sanguis*, and microbial heat-shock protein have been suggested as possible causative factors, but there is still no conclusive evidence to support allergy as a major cause of RAS.[48,49] Although some studies reported that RAS patients tend to have hypersensitivity to environmental allergens, other reports did not find a significant correlation between hypersensitivity and RAS. In one report, patients wearing nickel-based orthodontic appliances developed RAS that coincided with fitting of the appliance. When the appliance was replaced with a nickel-free type, the mucosal lesion regressed. RAS in this population was attributed to the systemic effect of ingested nickel rather than direct contact, because a patch test to nickel sulfate did not reactivate the mucosal ulceration.[50] In patients presenting with refractory cases of RAS and known allergy to food items such as milk, cheese, and wheat, sequential elimination of these dietary items was found to be beneficial in a small subset of RAS patients, thereby suggesting a possible link between food allergy and some cases of RAS.[51]

The denaturing effect of sodium lauryl sulfate (SLS), commonly found in toothpastes, has also been discussed as a cause of RAS. It was proposed that SLS might erode the oral mucin layer, exposing the underlying epithelium, thereby making the individual more susceptible to RAS. This theory still needs further clarification, because it has also been demonstrated that the use of SLS-free toothpastes did not affect the development of new lesions in RAS patients.[52,53]

Immunologic Factors

There has been significant research on the cause of RAS, focusing on detecting an abnormality in the immunologic response. Early work suggested a relationship between several immune-mediated reactions and the development of RAS. These reactions include cytotoxicity of T lymphocytes to oral epithelium, antibody-dependent cell-mediated cytotoxicity, and defects in lymphocyte subpopulations.[49,54,55] One theory is that multiple immune reactions cause damage induced by deposition of immune complexes within the oral epithelium. In some patients, an elevated level of salivary immunoglobulin A has been reported during acute and remission phases of minor RAS.[56] Some other studies have shown an association between RAS severity and abnormal proportions of $CD4^+$ and $CD8^+$ cells, alteration of the $CD4^+$:$CD8^+$ ratio,[57,58] and increased levels of several cytokines including interleukin-2, interferon-γ, and tumor necrosis factor-α (TNF-α) mRNA in RAS lesions.[59,60] Immunohistochemical studies of RAS biopsy tissues demonstrated numerous inflammatory cells with variable ratios of $CD4^+$:$CD8^+$ T lymphocytes depending on the ulcer duration. $CD4^+$ cells were more numerous during the preulcerative and healing stages, whereas $CD8^+$ cells tended to be more numerous during the ulcerative state of the ulcer. It is interesting that studies on nonaffected sites were negative, making researchers focus more on the theory that RAS may be caused by an antigen-triggering effect. Because levels of serum immunoglobulins and natural killer cells are essentially within normal limits in RAS patients, the focus is still on a dysregulated local cell-mediated immune response conducive to accumulation of subsets of T cells, mostly $CD8^+$ cells. This local immune response is thought to cause tissue breakdown that eventually manifests as RAS.

Nutritional Factors

The role of nutritional deficiency as a cause of RAS has been highlighted by the association of a subset of 5% to 10% of RAS patients with low serum levels of iron, folate, zinc, or vitamins B_1, B_2, B_6, and B_{12}, which indicates that nutritional deficiency is an etiologic factor for RAS.[61,62] Some of these nutritional deficiencies may be secondary to other diseases such as malabsorption syndrome or gluten sensitivity associated with (or without) enteropathy. Hematologic screening of RAS patients for anemia or deficiency of iron, folate, and B vitamins is appropriate for patients with major RAS or cases of minor RAS that worsen during adult life. A deficiency of calcium and vitamin C has also been proposed in patients with RAS, but these findings were in association with vitamin B_1 deficiency, supporting the idea of combined nutritional deficiency in RAS patients.[63] The recovery of some RAS patients after treatment of the nutritional deficiency has further corroborated the causative role of nutritional deficiency in a subset of RAS patients.[64,65]

Psychological Stress

Stress and psychological imbalance have been associated with RAS.[6,10,66] Stressful life events can increase the chances that a RAS-susceptible patient will develop a new lesion. One study reported that mental stress is more strongly associated with episodes of RAS than is physical stress, and that these stressful events tend to correlate more with onset of RAS than with duration of the lesions.[10] In women, appearance of RAS may coincide with menses. Stress of academic load may be the precipitating factor for the higher prevalence of RAS in professional school students.[63] Clinicians should consider questioning patients with worsening episodes of RAS regarding psychosocial, physical, or environmental stress.

Other Factors

The role of antioxidants in RAS is still attracting attention because blood and salivary levels of antioxidants, such as erythrocyte superoxide dismutase and catalase, seem to be higher in patients with RAS and Behçet syndrome than in normal controls,[67–69] but their causative roles in RAS are yet to be clearly defined. There have also been several reported cases of drug-induced RAS. A case-control study associated a higher risk of RAS with drug exposure, and found a significant association with nonsteroidal anti-inflammatory drugs and β-blockers.[70] Nicorandil, a vasodilator used extensively outside the United States to manage angina, as well as calcineurin and mTOR inhibitors used as immunosuppressors, have been associated with severe aphthous-like ulcers.[8,9,71] Therefore, it is imperative to closely scrutinize the medication history and current medications of RAS patients to identify any pattern associated with the frequency and duration of RAS lesions.

CLINICAL MANIFESTATION AND PATHOGENESIS

RAS patients usually experience prodromal burning sensations that last from 2 to 48 hours before an ulcer appears. Ulcers are round with well-defined erythematous margins and a shallow ulcerated center, covered with yellowish-gray fibrinous pseudomembrane. RAS ulcers usually develop on nonkeratinized oral mucosa, with the buccal and labial mucosa being the most common sites, and last approximately 10 to 14 days without scar formation (see **Table 1**). The oral ulcers seen in Behçet disease are clinically similar, but are more likely to be major aphthae.[72] Microscopic characteristics of RAS are nonspecific. The preulcerative lesion demonstrates subepithelial inflammatory mononuclear cells with abundant mast cells, connective tissue edema, and lining of the margins with neutrophils.[73] Damage to the epithelium usually begins in the basal layer and progresses through the superficial layers, leading eventually to ulceration and surface exudate. The presence of extravasated erythrocytes around the ulcer margin, subepithelial extravascular neutrophils, numerous macrophages loaded with phagolysosomes, and the nonspecific binding of stratum spinosum cells to immunoglobulins and complements may be a result of vascular leakage and passive diffusion of serum proteins. These findings suggest that the pathogenesis of RAS may be mediated by immune-complex vasculitis.[74] The onset of a RAS lesion is associated with cell-mediated immune response, generation of T cells, and production of TNF-α. Peripheral blood mononuclear cells of RAS patients have been shown to secrete high amounts of TNF-α, an indication that TNF-α plays a key role in RAS pathogenesis.[54,74–76] Consequently, TNF-α-mediated endothelial cell adhesion and neutrophil chemotaxis initiate the cascade of inflammatory processes that lead to ulceration.[77] Most TNF-α is produced in response to activation of toll-like receptors (TLRs), a set of functional membrane receptors associated with immune response and protection of the epithelial barrier. TLRs have both proinflammatory and anti-inflammatory properties. Whereas proinflammatory TLRs were found to be greatly increased in the epithelium and lamina propria of RAS lesions in some patients,[78] a decrease in expression levels of TLRs with anti-inflammatory activities was also found in another cohort of RAS patients.[79] Therefore the role of TLRs in RAS pathogenesis still needs to be better defined, but it is possible that an imbalance in proinflammatory and anti-inflammatory activities of TLRs could increase susceptibility to RAS in some individuals.

MANAGEMENT

The proper treatment of RAS depends on the severity of symptoms and the frequency, size, and number of ulcers. Patients who experience occasional episodes of minor aphthous ulcers experience significant relief with appropriate topical therapy. Symptoms resulting from occasional small lesions are often adequately controlled with the use of a protective emollient such as Zilactin (Zila Pharmaceuticals, Phoenix, AZ) or

Orabase (Bristol Myers Squibb, Princeton, NJ), either alone or mixed with a topical anesthetic such as benzocaine. Other topical agents that can minimize patient discomfort include diclofenac, a nonsteroidal anti-inflammatory drug, or amlexanox paste, which has been shown to decrease the healing time of minor aphthae.[80,81] Patients can also obtain some pain relief by swishing 3 to 4 times a day with Magic Mouth Wash (MMW), which can be custom-mixed by the pharmacy. Several formulations of MMW are available, the most common being a mixture of equal parts of viscous lidocaine, diphenhydramine, and Maalox or similar antacid.

In patients with more frequent or more severe disease, use of a topical glucocorticoid is an effective therapy to decrease both the size and healing time of the ulcers, especially when the medication is used early in the development stage.[82,83] Patients should be counseled regarding the proper use of high-potency topical steroids, and instructed to apply medication sparingly on the mucosal areas involved. This precaution will significantly decrease the risk of developing local and systemic side effects. Some clinicians advocate mixing high-potency steroids with an adhesive such as Orabase to promote contact between the lesion and medication. When patients have large, slowly healing lesions of major RAS, topical steroids may not be effective, so the use of intralesional steroid injections may help decrease the healing time.

Topical antibiotics have been advocated as therapy for RAS.[84] Tetracycline mouth rinses have been reported to decrease both the healing time and the pain of the lesions in several trials, but the association of these rinses with oral candidiasis and reports of allergic reactions have limited the use of this form of therapy. The effectiveness of topical tetracycline may result from a combination of the antibacterial and the anti-inflammatory effects of this group of antibiotics. A placebo-controlled study of the topical use of penicillin G troches to treat minor RAS showed efficacy in reducing both pain and healing time of RAS.[85] The risk of allergic reactions from this potentially useful form of therapy has not been reported, even in studies involving large numbers of RAS patients.

Topical therapy is effective for the treatment of most patients with RAS; however, topical therapy alone does not decrease the formation of new lesions and may not be adequate for patients with major RAS or those who experience frequent episodes of multiple minor RAS. Systemic therapy should be considered for this relatively small group of patients, but the potential benefit of the drug should always be carefully weighed against potential side effects, and systemic therapies should be used only by clinicians trained in their use.

A short course of systemic corticosteroids such as prednisone may occasionally be used to treat a particularly severe episode of major RAS, but long-term use of systemic steroids is rarely indicated for RAS because the serious side effects of long-term steroid therapy outweigh the benefits for RAS patients.[86]

Clinicians who treat patients with major RAS have been searching for a substitute for systemic corticosteroids that will prevent formation of new RAS lesions and lower the incidence of serious side effects. Medications that have been reported to have potential effectiveness in reducing the formation of new RAS lesions include pentoxifylline (PTX), colchicine, dapsone, and thalidomide.[87]

PTX, a methylxanthine related to caffeine, has been used for many years to treat intermittent leg cramps in patients with peripheral vascular disease. PTX improves the circulation of blood to the extremities by increasing the flexibility of red blood cells, making it easier for them to physically pass through atherosclerotic vessels. PTX has also been shown to decrease inflammation by its effect on white blood cell function and inflammatory cytokines, making it a useful therapy for inflammatory diseases such as rheumatoid arthritis, vasculitis, and diabetic leg ulcers. There have been several clinical reports on the successful use of PTX, 400 mg 3 times daily, to manage RAS. Patients with major RAS treated with PTX tend to have fewer and smaller ulcers and significant pain reduction, without major side effects (**Fig. 5**).[87,88]

Another drug that has been advocated for management of major RAS is colchicine, which has been used for decades to manage gouty arthritis. Because colchicine has anti-inflammatory activity and inhibits the cell-mediated response, it has proved useful in the management of several dermatologic diseases including psoriasis, Behçet syndrome, dermatitis herpetiformis, and leukocytoclastic vasculitis.[89] There are still no controlled clinical trials of colchicine therapy for RAS, but open trials have shown encouraging results.[87,90] Low doses of colchicine (0.6–1.2 mg/d) have been shown to reduce the number and duration of aphthous lesions, so long-term therapy with 1.2 to 1.8 mg/d is often recommended.[91] Colchicine has a low therapeutic-toxicity window because of myelosuppression, hepatotoxicity, decreased sperm count, and adverse drug interactions.[8] Before starting colchicine therapy, baseline liver function tests and hematology screening of RAS patients should be performed and monitored frequently. Careful medication history should also be obtained to avoid adverse drug interactions. Colchicine has been associated with teratogenicity in animal studies, but limited adverse fetal and maternal effects reported in human studies were not significantly higher than normal.[9] However, some clinicians still recommend that RAS patients use appropriate contraceptive methods before colchicine therapy.[91]

The medication that has been most carefully studied for the management of major RAS is thalidomide, a drug with a long history of major side effects, including severe life-threatening and crippling birth defects.[92] Thalidomide was originally marketed in Europe in the 1950s as a nonaddicting sedative, but was withdrawn from the market when the risk of major teratogenic defects, including phocomelia and neural tube abnormalities, were discovered. Later, investigators discovered its potent anti-inflammatory and immunomodulatory properties, by its ability to inhibit angiogenesis and reduce the activity of TNF-α. Owing to its effectiveness, limited use of the drug was permitted for patients with recalcitrant diseases such as erythema nodosum leprosum, lupus, and Behçet syndrome.[93]

Controlled clinical trials have demonstrated the effectiveness of thalidomide in treating major RAS in HIV-infected patients and in otherwise normal individuals. Thalidomide therapy results in either complete remission or substantial improvement in most patients with major RAS.[94,95] To minimize the risk of birth defects resulting from thalidomide therapy, clinicians prescribing the drug must register in the program

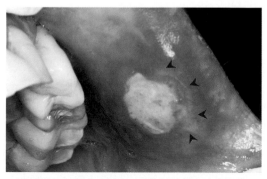

Fig. 5. Major recurrent aphthous stomatitis on left buccal mucosa responding to pentoxifylline therapy. Note the progressive healing and absence of pseudomembrane in a section of the ulcer (*black arrowheads*).

for Risk Evaluation and Mitigation Strategy (REMS), formerly known as the STEPS program.[96] This program educates physicians and dentists on the proper use of the drug, provides counseling for patients, and closely monitors thalidomide use. For example, the program mandates that women in childbearing years must use 2 forms of birth control and have a monthly pregnancy test. Both women and men taking thalidomide must be evaluated every 4 weeks, and both the patient and the prescribing clinician must complete a questionnaire before thalidomide can be prescribed for another 28 days. In addition to birth defects, thalidomide can also cause peripheral neuropathy, neutropenia, and drowsiness.[97]

Other drugs that have been advocated for the management of major RAS not responding adequately to topical therapy include dapsone, a sulfone derivative used to manage several mucocutaneous disorders; azathioprine, an immunosuppressive drug; and etanercept, a recombinant TNF-soluble receptor that binds to TNF-α to limit the amount of active TNF-α. Etanercept has been used successfully to manage rheumatoid arthritis and psoriasis.[87,98,99]

SUMMARY

RAS is the most common ulcerative disease affecting the oral mucosa, whose etiology remains unknown. RAS occurs mostly in healthy individuals and has a more severe clinical presentation in immunocompromised persons. Several local, systemic, immunologic, genetic, allergic, nutritional, and microbial factors, as well as immunosuppressive drugs, have been proposed as causative agents. Clinical management of RAS is aimed at improving the function and quality of life of patients using topical and systemic therapies. The goals of therapy are to decrease pain and ulcer size, promote healing, and decrease the frequency of recurrence.

REFERENCES

1. Porter SR, Scully C, Pedersen A. Recurrent aphthous stomatitis. Crit Rev Oral Biol Med 1998;9(3):306–21.
2. Ship II. Epidemiologic aspects of recurrent aphthous ulcerations. Oral Surg Oral Med Oral Pathol 1972;33(3):400–6.
3. Rogers RS 3rd. Recurrent aphthous stomatitis: clinical characteristics and associated systemic disorders. Semin Cutan Med Surg 1997;16(4):278–83.
4. Miller MF, Garfunkel AA, Ram CA, et al. The inheritance of recurrent aphthous stomatitis. Observations on susceptibility. Oral Surg Oral Med Oral Pathol 1980;49(5):409–12.
5. Crivelli MR, Aguas S, Adler I, et al. Influence of socioeconomic status on oral mucosa lesion prevalence in schoolchildren. Community Dent Oral Epidemiol 1988;16(1):58–60.
6. Gallo Cde B, Mimura MA, Sugaya NN. Psychological stress and recurrent aphthous stomatitis. Clinics (Sao Paulo) 2009;64(7):645–8.
7. Ship JA, Chavez EM, Doerr PA, et al. Recurrent aphthous stomatitis. Quintessence Int 2000;31(2):95–112.
8. Terkeltaub RA. Colchicine update: 2008. Semin Arthritis Rheum 2009;38(6):411–9.
9. Berkenstadt M, Weisz B, Cuckle H, et al. Chromosomal abnormalities and birth defects among couples with colchicine treated familial Mediterranean fever. Am J Obstet Gynecol 2005;193(4):1513–6.
10. Huling LB, Baccaglini L, Choquette L, et al. Effect of stressful life events on the onset and duration of recurrent aphthous stomatitis. J Oral Pathol Med 2012; 41(2):149–52.

11. Wray D, Graykowski EA, Notkins AL. Role of mucosal injury in initiating recurrent aphthous stomatitis. Br Med J (Clin Res Ed) 1981;283(6306):1569–70.
12. Stone OJ. Aphthous stomatitis (canker sores): a consequence of high oral submucosal viscosity (the role of extracellular matrix and the possible role of lectins). Med Hypotheses 1991;36(4):341–4.
13. Espinoza I, Rojas R, Aranda W, et al. Prevalence of oral mucosal lesions in elderly people in Santiago, Chile. J Oral Pathol Med 2003;32(10):571–5.
14. Sawair FA. Does smoking really protect from recurrent aphthous stomatitis? Ther Clin Risk Manag 2010;6:573–7.
15. Marakoglu K, Sezer RE, Toker HC, et al. The recurrent aphthous stomatitis frequency in the smoking cessation people. Clin Oral Investig 2007;11(2):149–53.
16. Atkin PA, Xu X, Thornhill MH. Minor recurrent aphthous stomatitis and smoking: an epidemiological study measuring plasma cotinine. Oral Dis 2002;8(3):173–6.
17. Albanidou-Farmaki E, Poulopoulos AK, Epivatianos A, et al. Increased anxiety level and high salivary and serum cortisol concentrations in patients with recurrent aphthous stomatitis. Tohoku J Exp Med 2008;214(4):291–6.
18. McCartan BE, Lamey PJ, Wallace AM. Salivary cortisol and anxiety in recurrent aphthous stomatitis. J Oral Pathol Med 1996;25(7):357–9.
19. Maurice M, Mikhail W, Aziz M, et al. Aetiology of recurrent aphthous ulcers (RAU). J Laryngol Otol 1987;101(9):917–20.
20. Lin SS, Chou MY, Ho CC, et al. Study of the viral infections and cytokines associated with recurrent aphthous ulceration. Microbes Infect 2005;7(4):635–44.
21. Woo SB, Sonis ST. Recurrent aphthous ulcers: a review of diagnosis and treatment. J Am Dent Assoc 1996;127(8):1202–13.
22. Pedersen A, Hornsleth A. Recurrent aphthous ulceration: a possible clinical manifestation of reactivation of varicella zoster or cytomegalovirus infection. J Oral Pathol Med 1993;22(2):64–8.
23. Sun A, Chang JG, Chu CT, et al. Preliminary evidence for an association of Epstein-Barr virus with pre-ulcerative oral lesions in patients with recurrent aphthous ulcers or Behcet's disease. J Oral Pathol Med 1998;27(4):168–75.
24. Victoria JM, Kalapothakis E, Silva Jde F, et al. *Helicobacter pylori* DNA in recurrent aphthous stomatitis. J Oral Pathol Med 2003;32(4):219–23.
25. Birek C, Grandhi R, McNeill K, et al. Detection of *Helicobacter pylori* in oral aphthous ulcers. J Oral Pathol Med 1999;28(5):197–203.
26. Tas DA, Yakar T, Sakalli H, et al. Impact of *Helicobacter pylori* on the clinical course of recurrent aphthous stomatitis. J Oral Pathol Med 2013;42(1):89–94.
27. Maleki Z, Sayyari AA, Alavi K, et al. A study of the relationship between *Helicobacter pylori* and recurrent aphthous stomatitis using a urea breath test. J Contemp Dent Pract 2009;10(1):9–16.
28. Gisbert JP, Castro-Fernandez M, Perez-Aisa A, et al. Fourth-line rescue therapy with rifabutin in patients with three *Helicobacter pylori* eradication failures. Aliment Pharmacol Ther 2012;35(8):941–7.
29. Albanidou-Farmaki E, Giannoulis L, Markopoulos A, et al. Outcome following treatment for *Helicobacter pylori* in patients with recurrent aphthous stomatitis. Oral Dis 2005;11(1):22–6.
30. Scully C, Gorsky M, Lozada-Nur F. The diagnosis and management of recurrent aphthous stomatitis: a consensus approach. J Am Dent Assoc 2003;134(2):200–7.
31. Acar S, Yetkiner AA, Ersin N, et al. Oral findings and salivary parameters in children with celiac disease: a preliminary study. Med Princ Pract 2012;21(2):129–33.

32. Stevenson G. Evidence for a negative correlation of recurrent aphthous ulcers with lactobacillus activity. J La Dent Assoc 1967;25(2):5–7.
33. Keogan MT. Clinical Immunology Review Series: an approach to the patient with recurrent orogenital ulceration, including Behcet's syndrome. Clin Exp Immunol 2009;156(1):1–11.
34. Krause I, Uziel Y, Guedj D, et al. Mode of presentation and multisystem involvement in Behcet's disease: the influence of sex and age of disease onset. J Rheumatol 1998;25(8):1566–9.
35. Krause I, Rosen Y, Kaplan I, et al. Recurrent aphthous stomatitis in Behcet's disease: clinical features and correlation with systemic disease expression and severity. J Oral Pathol Med 1999;28(5):193–6.
36. Krause I, Monselise Y, Milo G, et al. Anti-*Saccharomyces cerevisiae* antibodies—a novel serologic marker for Behcet's disease. Clin Exp Rheumatol 2002;20(4 Suppl 26):S21–4.
37. Pekiner FN, Aytugar E, Demirel GY, et al. HLA-A, B (Class I) and HLA-DR, DQ (Class II) Antigens in Turkish patients with recurrent aphthous ulceration and Behcet's disease. Med Princ Pract 2013;22(5):464–8.
38. Imai H, Motegi M, Mizuki N, et al. Mouth and genital ulcers with inflamed cartilage (MAGIC syndrome): a case report and literature review. Am J Med Sci 1997;314(5):330–2.
39. Orme RL, Nordlund JJ, Barich L, et al. The MAGIC syndrome (mouth and genital ulcers with inflamed cartilage). Arch Dermatol 1990;126(7):940–4.
40. Greenberg MS, Pinto A. Etiology and management of recurrent aphthous stomatitis. Curr Infect Dis Rep 2003;5(3):194–8.
41. Cheng J, Malahias T, Brar P, et al. The association between celiac disease, dental enamel defects, and aphthous ulcers in a United States cohort. J Clin Gastroenterol 2010;44(3):191–4.
42. Baccaglini L, Lalla RV, Bruce AJ, et al. Urban legends: recurrent aphthous stomatitis. Oral Dis 2011;17(8):755–70.
43. Kerr AR, Ship JA. Management strategies for HIV-associated aphthous stomatitis. Am J Clin Dermatol 2003;4(10):669–80.
44. Ramos-Gomez F. Dental considerations for the paediatric AIDS/HIV patient. Oral Dis 2002;8(Suppl 2):49–54.
45. Rodenas JM, Ortego N, Herranz MT, et al. Cyclic neutropenia: a cause of recurrent aphthous stomatitis not to be missed. Dermatology 1992;184(3):205–7.
46. Vigo G, Zulian F. Periodic fevers with aphthous stomatitis, pharyngitis, and adenitis (PFAPA). Autoimmun Rev 2012;12(1):52–5.
47. Albanidou-Farmaki E, Deligiannidis A, Markopoulos AK, et al. HLA haplotypes in recurrent aphthous stomatitis: a mode of inheritance? Int J Immunogenet 2008; 35(6):427–32.
48. Wray D, Vlagopoulos TP, Siraganian RP. Food allergens and basophil histamine release in recurrent aphthous stomatitis. Oral Surg Oral Med Oral Pathol 1982; 54(4):388–95.
49. Hasan A, Shinnick T, Mizushima Y, et al. Defining a T-cell epitope within HSP 65 in recurrent aphthous stomatitis. Clin Exp Immunol 2002;128(2):318–25.
50. Pacor ML, Di Lorenzo G, Martinelli N, et al. Results of double-blind placebo-controlled challenge with nickel salts in patients affected by recurrent aphthous stomatitis. Int Arch Allergy Immunol 2003;131(4):296–300.
51. Hay KD, Reade PC. The use of an elimination diet in the treatment of recurrent aphthous ulceration of the oral cavity. Oral Surg Oral Med Oral Pathol 1984; 57(5):504–7.

52. Shim YJ, Choi JH, Ahn HJ, et al. Effect of sodium lauryl sulfate on recurrent aphthous stomatitis: a randomized controlled clinical trial. Oral Dis 2012;18(7):655–60.
53. Healy CM, Paterson M, Joyston-Bechal S, et al. The effect of a sodium lauryl sulfate-free dentifrice on patients with recurrent oral ulceration. Oral Dis 1999; 5(1):39–43.
54. Lewkowicz N, Lewkowicz P, Dzitko K, et al. Dysfunction of CD4+CD25 high T regulatory cells in patients with recurrent aphthous stomatitis. J Oral Pathol Med 2008;37(8):454–61.
55. Savage NW, Seymour GJ, Kruger BJ. T-lymphocyte subset changes in recurrent aphthous stomatitis. Oral Surg Oral Med Oral Pathol 1985;60(2):175–81.
56. Mohammad R, Halboub E, Mashlah A, et al. Levels of salivary IgA in patients with minor recurrent aphthous stomatitis: a matched case-control study. Clin Oral Investig 2013;17(3):975–80.
57. Sun A, Chu CT, Liu BY, et al. Expression of interleukin-2 receptor by activated peripheral blood lymphocytes upregulated by the plasma level of interleukin-2 in patients with recurrent aphthous ulcers. Proc Natl Sci Counc Repub China B 2000;24(3):116–22.
58. Bachtiar EW, Cornain S, Siregar B, et al. Decreased CD4+/CD8+ ratio in major type of recurrent aphthous ulcers: comparing major to minor types of ulcers. Asian Pac J Allergy Immunol 1998;16(2–3):75–9.
59. Pekiner FN, Aytugar E, Demirel GY, et al. Interleukin-2, interleukin-6 and T regulatory cells in peripheral blood of patients with Behcet's disease and recurrent aphthous ulcerations. J Oral Pathol Med 2012;41(1):73–9.
60. Boras VV, Lukac J, Brailo V, et al. Salivary interleukin-6 and tumor necrosis factor-alpha in patients with recurrent aphthous ulceration. J Oral Pathol Med 2006;35(4):241–3.
61. Dar-Odeh NS, Alsmadi OM, Bakri F, et al. Predicting recurrent aphthous ulceration using genetic algorithms—optimized neural networks. Adv Appl Bioinform Chem 2010;3:7–13.
62. Kozlak ST, Walsh SJ, Lalla RV. Reduced dietary intake of vitamin B12 and folate in patients with recurrent aphthous stomatitis. J Oral Pathol Med 2010;39(5): 420–3.
63. McCann AL, Bonci L. Maintaining women's oral health. Dent Clin North Am 2001; 45(3):571–601.
64. Volkov I, Rudoy I, Freud T, et al. Effectiveness of vitamin B12 in treating recurrent aphthous stomatitis: a randomized, double-blind, placebo-controlled trial. J Am Board Fam Med 2009;22(1):9–16.
65. Gulcan E, Toker S, Hatipoglu H, et al. Cyanocobalamin may be beneficial in the treatment of recurrent aphthous ulcers even when vitamin B12 levels are normal. Am J Med Sci 2008;336(5):379–82.
66. Keenan AV, Spivakovksy S. Stress associated with onset of recurrent aphthous stomatitis. Evid Based Dent 2013;14(1):25.
67. Arikan S, Durusoy C, Akalin N, et al. Oxidant/antioxidant status in recurrent aphthous stomatitis. Oral Dis 2009;15(7):512–5.
68. Karincaoglu Y, Batcioglu K, Erdem T, et al. The levels of plasma and salivary antioxidants in the patient with recurrent aphthous stomatitis. J Oral Pathol Med 2005;34(1):7–12.
69. Cimen MY, Kaya TI, Eskandari G, et al. Oxidant/antioxidant status in patients with recurrent aphthous stomatitis. Clin Exp Dermatol 2003;28(6):647–50.
70. Boulinguez S, Reix S, Bedane C, et al. Role of drug exposure in aphthous ulcers: a case-control study. Br J Dermatol 2000;143(6):1261–5.

71. Boulinguez S, Sommet A, Bedane C, et al. Oral nicorandil-induced lesions are not aphthous ulcers. J Oral Pathol Med 2003;32(8):482–5.
72. Oh SH, Han EC, Lee JH, et al. Comparison of the clinical features of recurrent aphthous stomatitis and Behcet's disease. Clin Exp Dermatol 2009;34(6): e208–12.
73. Woo SB, Greenberg MS. Ulcerative, vesicular and bullous lesions. In: Greenberg MS, Glick M, Ship JA, editors. Burket's oral medicine. 11th edition. Hamilton (Canada): BC Decker; 2008. p. 41–76.
74. Jurge S, Kuffer R, Scully C, et al. Mucosal disease series. Number VI. Recurrent aphthous stomatitis. Oral Dis 2006;12(1):1–21.
75. Lewkowicz N, Kur B, Kurnatowska A, et al. Expression of Th1/Th2/Th3/Th17-related genes in recurrent aphthous ulcers. Arch Immunol Ther Exp (Warsz) 2011;59(5):399–406.
76. Lewkowicz N, Lewkowicz P, Banasik M, et al. Predominance of Type 1 cytokines and decreased number of CD4(+)CD25(+high) T regulatory cells in peripheral blood of patients with recurrent aphthous ulcerations. Immunol Lett 2005;99(1): 57–62.
77. Natah SS, Hayrinen-Immonen R, Hietanen J, et al. Increased density of lymphocytes bearing gamma/delta T-cell receptors in recurrent aphthous ulceration (RAU). Int J Oral Maxillofac Surg 2000;29(5):375–80.
78. Hietanen J, Hayrinen-Immonen R, Al-Samadi A, et al. Recurrent aphthous ulcers—a Toll-like receptor-mediated disease? J Oral Pathol Med 2012;41(2): 158–64.
79. Gallo C, Barros F, Sugaya N, et al. Differential expression of toll-like receptor mRNAs in recurrent aphthous ulceration. J Oral Pathol Med 2012;41(1): 80–5.
80. Saxen MA, Ambrosius WT, Rehemtula al-KF, et al. Sustained relief of oral aphthous ulcer pain from topical diclofenac in hyaluronan: a randomized, double-blind clinical trial. Oral Surg Oral Med Oral Pathol Oral Radiol Endod 1997; 84(4):356–61.
81. Khandwala A, Van Inwegen RG, Alfano MC. 5% amlexanox oral paste, a new treatment for recurrent minor aphthous ulcers: I. Clinical demonstration of acceleration of healing and resolution of pain. Oral Surg Oral Med Oral Pathol Oral Radiol Endod 1997;83(2):222–30.
82. Liu C, Zhou Z, Liu G, et al. Efficacy and safety of dexamethasone ointment on recurrent aphthous ulceration. Am J Med 2012;125(3):292–301.
83. Pilotte AP, Hohos MB, Polson KM, et al. Managing stomatitis in patients treated with mammalian target of rapamycin inhibitors. Clin J Oncol Nurs 2011;15(5): E83–9.
84. Gorsky M, Epstein J, Rabenstein S, et al. Topical minocycline and tetracycline rinses in treatment of recurrent aphthous stomatitis: a randomized cross-over study. Dermatol Online J 2007;13(2):1.
85. Kerr AR, Drexel CA, Spielman AI. The efficacy and safety of 50 mg penicillin G potassium troches for recurrent aphthous ulcers. Oral Surg Oral Med Oral Pathol Oral Radiol Endod 2003;96(6):685–94.
86. Silverman S Jr, Lozada-Nur F, Migliorati C. Clinical efficacy of prednisone in the treatment of patients with oral inflammatory ulcerative diseases: a study of fifty-five patients. Oral Surg Oral Med Oral Pathol 1985;59(4):360–3.
87. Mimura MA, Hirota SK, Sugaya NN, et al. Systemic treatment in severe cases of recurrent aphthous stomatitis: an open trial. Clinics (Sao Paulo) 2009;64(3): 193–8.

88. Thornhill MH, Baccaglini L, Theaker E, et al. A randomized, double-blind, placebo-controlled trial of pentoxifylline for the treatment of recurrent aphthous stomatitis. Arch Dermatol 2007;143(4):463–70.
89. Tasher D, Stein M, Dalal I, et al. Colchicine prophylaxis for frequent periodic fever, aphthous stomatitis, pharyngitis and adenitis episodes. Acta Paediatr 2008; 97(8):1090–2.
90. Fontes V, Machet L, Huttenberger B, et al. Recurrent aphthous stomatitis: treatment with colchicine. An open trial of 54 cases. Ann Dermatol Venereol 2002; 129(12):1365–9 [in French].
91. Altenburg A, Zouboulis CC. Current concepts in the treatment of recurrent aphthous stomatitis. Skin Therapy Lett 2008;13(7):1–4.
92. Michael O, Goldman RD, Koren G. Safety of colchicine therapy during pregnancy. Can Fam Physician 2003;49:967–9.
93. Calabrese L, Fleischer AB. Thalidomide: current and potential clinical applications. Am J Med 2000;108(6):487–95.
94. Cheng S, Murphy R. Refractory aphthous ulceration treated with thalidomide: a report of 10 years' clinical experience. Clin Exp Dermatol 2012;37(2):132–5.
95. Hello M, Barbarot S, Bastuji-Garin S, et al. Use of thalidomide for severe recurrent aphthous stomatitis: a multicenter cohort analysis. Medicine (Baltimore) 2010;89(3):176–82.
96. Shetty K. Thalidomide in the management of recurrent aphthous ulcerations in patients who are HIV-positive: a review and case reports. Spec Care Dentist 2005;25(5):236–41.
97. Jacobson JM, Greenspan JS, Spritzler J, et al. Thalidomide in low intermittent doses does not prevent recurrence of human immunodeficiency virus-associated aphthous ulcers. J Infect Dis 2001;183(2):343–6.
98. Altenburg A, Abdel-Naser MB, Seeber H, et al. Practical aspects of management of recurrent aphthous stomatitis. J Eur Acad Dermatol Venereol 2007; 21(8):1019–26.
99. O'Neill ID. Efficacy of tumour necrosis factor-alpha antagonists in aphthous ulceration: review of published individual patient data. J Eur Acad Dermatol Venereol 2012;26(2):231–5.

Oral Lichen Planus and Lichenoid Mucositis

Scott S. De Rossi, DMD[a,b,c,*], Katharine Ciarrocca, DMD, MSEd[d]

KEYWORDS

- Lichen planus • Lichenoid mucositis • Lichenoid drug reaction • Oral lichen planus

KEY POINTS

- Oral lichen planus and lichenoid reaction are a common oral mucosal disease process encountered in clinical practice.
- This mucocutaneous disease can manifest as desquamative gingivitis, asymptomatic Wickham striae or plaques, or severe, painful erosions or ulcerations anywhere in the oral cavity.
- Although the cause initiating lichen planus is unknown, current research points to several complex immunologic events and cells that are responsible for the inflammatory destruction and chronicity of these lesions.
- The mainstay of treatment remains topical corticosteroids; however, newer therapies such as tacrolimus are available for recalcitrant lesions. In cases of lichenoid mucositis or reactions, treatment should always be directed at identifying and removing the presumed cause.
- Given the apparent risk of squamous cell carcinoma in these patients, frequent follow-up and repeat biopsy when indicated are vital.

INTRODUCTION

Nature of Problem and Definition

Lichen planus (LP) is a common mucocutaneous disease affecting 1% to 2% of the population. Lesions most commonly occur on both oral and cutaneous surfaces (40%), followed by cutaneous alone (35%) and mucosa alone (25%). Oral LP (OLP)

A version of this article appeared as DeRossi SS, Ciarrocca KN. Lichen planus, lichenoid drug reactions, and lichenoid mucositis. Dent Clin North Am 2005;49:77–89.

[a] Department of Oral Health and Diagnostic Sciences, College of Dental Medicine, Georgia Regents University, 1120 15th Street, Augusta, GA 30912, USA; [b] Department of Otolaryngology/Head & Neck Surgery, Medical College of Georgia, Georgia Regents University, 1120 15th Street, Augusta, GA 30912, USA; [c] Department of Dermatology, Medical College of Georgia, Georgia Regents University, 1120 15th Street, Augusta, GA 30912, USA; [d] Department of Oral Rehabilitation, College of Dental Medicine, Georgia Regents University, 1120 15th Street, Augusta, GA 30912, USA
* Corresponding author. Department of Oral Health and Diagnostic Sciences, College of Dental Medicine, Georgia Regents University, 1120 15th Street, Augusta, GA 30912.
E-mail address: SDEROSSI@gru.edu

occurs in men and women, usually between the ages of 30 and 70 years. Children and adolescents are rarely affected.

Varying in its clinic appearance, OLP can appear keratotic (reticular or plaquelike) or erythematous and ulcerative, and is often accompanied by skin lesions (**Box 1**).[1–3] Spontaneous remission of cutaneous LP after 1 year occurs in approximately 70% of cases. On the other hand, spontaneous remission of OLP is less common, occurring in less than 5% of patients over a 7.5-year follow-up. The reticular form of OLP has the best prognosis, because spontaneous remission occurs in 40% of cases. The reported mean duration of OLP is 5 years, but the erosive form of the disease can persist for up to 15 to 20 years.[4,5]

Prevalence/Incidence

In the literature, different prevalence figures for OLP have been reported and vary from 0.5% to 2.2%.[1–6] These figures may represent an underestimation, because minor lesions may easily be overlooked. The proportion of women is higher than men among referred patients, but this may not be accurate in the general population. The mean age of the time of diagnosis is 55 years.

Cause and Pathogenesis

The cause of LP remains unclear. Research exploring the pathogenesis of LP has yielded many data suggesting that immunologic mechanisms are fundamental to the initiation and perpetuation of LP (**Box 2**).[6] Primarily, focus has been given to the role of the epithelial antigenic processing macrophage, the Langerhans cell,[7] the mast cell,[8–14] and their interactions with the abundant T-cell population accumulated in the underlying connective tissue.[15–18]

Current evidence suggests that LP is a T-cell–mediated process.[15–18] Lesional LP tissue shows massive local activated T-cell populations, with increased local expression of cytokines and altered adhesion molecule expression.[7,11,15,19] In addition, therapies that suppress cell-mediated immune responses reduce the lymphocyte infiltrate and cause clinical improvement of LP lesions.[20] Other evidence supporting the immunologic pathogenesis of LP includes the deposition of fibrinogen along the basement membrane and the cell-mediated autoimmune destruction of basal keratinocytes.[21,22]

Antigenic challenge may come from the external environment or may be the result of keratinocyte autoantigen expression. Dendritic Langerhans cells and antigen-bearing class II molecules on keratinocytes relay molecular information to reactive CD4 cells in the regional lymph nodes, which engender an effector T helper cell (Th1) pathway response, leading to a mucosal or cutaneous eruption. The cellular response is similar to that seen in a contact allergic reaction or delayed-type hypersensitivity reaction (**Fig. 1**).

The chronicity of OLP is significantly greater than its cutaneous counterpart. Although the precise nature of this discrepancy has not been elucidated, some evidence supports the role of T-cell RANTES (regulated upon activation, normal T-cell

Box 1	
Mucosal and cutaneous LP	
Percentage of Cases	Area Affected
40	Mucosal and skin lesions
35	Skin lesions only
25	Mucosal lesions only

Box 2
Immunopathology of LP

- Immunomarker studies have disclosed that the lymphocyte population is exclusively T cell in nature, with a mixture of CD4 and CD8 lymphocytes that express integrin molecules of the α_1 class

  ○ These integrin ligands bind to other adhesion molecules that are upregulated on endothelial cells (vascular cell adhesion molecule) and (intercellular adhesion molecule)

- Lower strata keratinocytes are able to present antigens to cells bearing the CD4-associated T-cell receptor

- CD8 lymphocytes are able to bind to antigen-complexed major histocompatibility complex I molecules on keratinoctyes

- Fibronectin, laminin, and types IV and VII collagens are upregulated in the basement membrane

- Angiogenesis and vasodilation are increased in lesional submucosa

- In the inflamed epithelium, lower strata keratinocytes express and secrete chemokines that are chemotactic to lymphocytes

- Reactive T cells leave submucosal vessels and enter the connective tissues

- Chemokines from keratinocytes direct lymphocyte traffic along extracellular matrix (ECM) using cell-matrix adhesion molecules

- Cytotoxic T cells release perforin and other enzymes, which lyse basal cells, particularly in the erosive form of the disease

- After antigenic challenge, lymphocytes adhering to vascular endothelia emigrate into the submucosa, migrating under the influence of the epithelial secreted chemoattractant molecules

- Lymphocytes are then able to adhere to ECM molecules, which are overproduced along the basement membrane

- On crossing the epithelial-mesenchymal interface, ECM molecules are able to bind, via integrins, to cell-surface adhesion molecules pathologically expressed on keratinocytes

---

expressed and secreted) and mast cell degranulation, leading to the release of tumor necrosis factor α and a cyclical process, where interleukin 4 and interferon γ may predict the chronicity of the disease process in some cases (**Fig. 2**).

Symptoms

The red, inflamed lesions and open sores of OLP can cause a burning sensation or pain. The white, lacy patches may not cause discomfort when they appear on the buccal mucosa but may be painful when they involve the tongue. Most lacy white lesions cause patients to describe a rough sensation of the affected surfaces. Lesions most commonly occur on both oral and cutaneous surfaces (40%), followed by cutaneous alone (35%) and mucosa alone (25%).

The most common presenting symptoms are:

- Erythematous and desquamative gingivae
- Oral pain and soreness, exacerbated with acidic and spicy foods
- Ulceration
- Bleeding and irritation with tooth brushing
- Change in taste or a blunted taste sensation if the tongue is affected
- Sensitivity to hot, acidic, or spicy foods

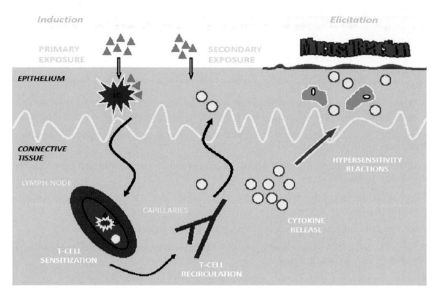

Fig. 1. T-cell–mediated hypersensitivity.

CLINICAL FINDINGS
Physical Examination

A thorough history is vital in arriving at a definitive diagnosis and should include a thorough history of present illness with previous treatments listed, a detailed past medical history, a complete list of current medications, and a thorough review of systems. An exhaustive extraoral and intraoral examination should be performed after a detailed history.

LP has a wide range of clinical appearances, which correlate well with disease severity.[1,23,24] Four distinct clinical presentations are most often described: reticular, erosive, plaquelike, and bullous. Often, patients have a combination of the reticular and erosive forms, whereas plaquelike LP usually occurs as a solitary white plaque resembling leukoplakia and not in combination with other forms (**Fig. 3, Table 1**).

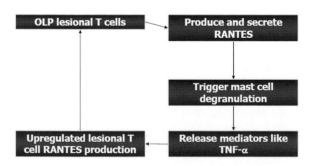

The mast cell IL-4 and T cell INF-γ balance may determine lesion chronicity

Fig. 2. Cyclic mechanisms promote disease chronicity.

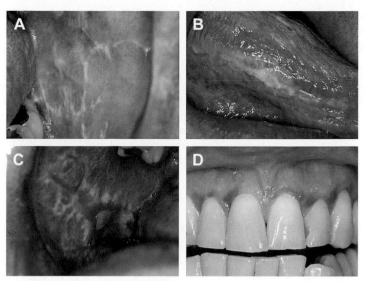

Fig. 3. Clinical presentation of LP. (*A*) Wickham striae/reticular LP. (*B*) Plaquelike. (*C*) Ulcerative/erosive. (*D*) Desquamative gingivitis.

Table 1 Clinical appearances of OLP	
Type	**Clinical Appearance and Most Common Location**
Reticular LP	Thin, slightly raised, white lines that connect in a pattern resembling lacework or reticular, annular appearance
	Arcuate pattern of white lines can be on erythematous or nonerythematous mucosa, and is referred to as Wickham striae
	Rarely experience symptoms and only become aware of their condition when noticed by a dental health professional
	Most common locale for reticular LP is the buccal mucosa, followed by the buccal vestibule, tongue, and gingiva. A common feature of reticular LP is that it occurs bilaterally
Erosive LP	Appears as a mixture of intensely erythematous mucosa with large areas of irregularly shaped ulceration with a whitish-yellow pseudomembrane[25–28]
	Degree of atrophy, erythema, and central ulceration can vary from lesion to lesion
	Junction of the red and normal mucosa shows faint, white, radiating striae
	In some patients, the atrophy and ulceration are confined to the gingival mucosa producing a pattern called desquamative gingivitis (may represent mucous membrane pemphigoid or pemphigus vulgaris, making histopathologic evaluation essential)
Plaquelike LP	A slightly raised or flat white area on the oral mucous membranes
	Cannot be rubbed off, and is indistinguishable from other focal leukoplakias
	Most common location is the tongue
Bullous LP	Rare form of LP characterized by large bullae ranging in size from 4 mm to 2 cm
	The bullae, like pemphigus vulgaris, rupture almost immediately in the oral cavity, leaving an ulceration on a bed of inflamed mucosa
	Seems to most commonly affect the posterior buccal mucosa

Cutaneous lesions of LP do not necessarily resemble their oral counterpart and are often referred to by the 6 Ps: pruritic, polygonal, planar (flat-topped), purple papules, and plaques, as seen in **Fig. 4**.

Diagnostic Modalities

Given the fact that other mucocutaneous diseases, including pemphigus, pemphigoid, lichenoid reactions, premalignant dysplastic lesions, and contact allergy, are included in a differential diagnosis of LP, it is important that a biopsy be performed to confirm a diagnosis. Often, 2 distinct specimens are obtained, one for hematoxylin-eosin–stained sections and the other for direct immunofluorescent (DIF) study. Each specimen should be submitted and transported in specific media for routine histology and immunofluorescent study (**Fig. 5**).

PATHOLOGY

The histopathologic features of LP vary slightly among the various clinical types. However, 3 hallmark features are considered necessary for an LP diagnosis[1]:

1. Hyperorthokeratosis or hyperparakeratosis, usually with a thickening of the spinous cell layer (acanthosis) and shortened, pointed, saw-toothed appearance of the rete ridges. These thickened areas are clinically seen as Wickham striae. Between these areas, the epithelium is often atrophic, with loss of rete ridge formation.
2. Necrosis of the basal cell layer, often referred to as liquefaction degeneration.
3. A dense subepithelial band of chronic inflammatory cells, usually T lymphocytes in the subjacent connective tissue, which can transgress the basement membrane and can be seen in the basilar or parabasilar layers of the epithelium.

Scattered within the epithelium and superficial connective tissue, Civatte bodies are isolated epithelial cells, shrunken with eosinophilic cytoplasm and 1 or multiple pyknotic nuclear fragments. These Civatte bodies are believed to represent apoptotic keratinocytes and other necrotic epithelial components, which are transported to the connective tissue for phagocytosis.[29]

The tissue diagnosis of LP can be difficult but may be greatly aided by the use of immunofluorescence. Immunofluorescent studies of biopsy specimens from lesions of LP show features that suggest the pathogenesis of these lesions and aid in the

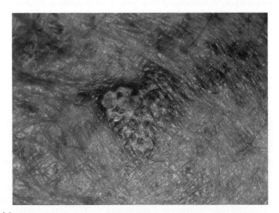

Fig. 4. LP of the skin.

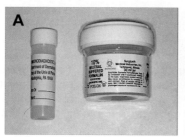
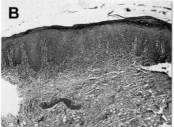

Fig. 5. (*A*) Michel medium and 10% neutral buffered formalin for DIF and routine hematoxylin-eosin, respectively. (*B*) Routine hematoxylin-eosin of OLP.

differentiation of LP from other mucocutaneous diseases.[12] Specifically, DIF study shows a ragged band of fibrinogen in the basement membrane in nearly 100% of cases (**Fig. 6**).

DIAGNOSTIC DILEMMA: A PREMALIGNANT LESION

The possible premalignant character of OLP is the subject of ongoing and controversial discussion in the literature.[30–38] The first identifiable case of carcinoma arising in LP of the oral mucosa was described by Hallapeau in 1910. Since that time, numerous retrospective studies and case reports have been published linking the development of carcinoma with LP. The range of malignant transformation of OLP per year, as described in the literature, is between 0.04% and 1.74%.[30–38] Controversy exists as to the true malignant potential of OLP, primarily because of lack of adequate data in the initial diagnosis of OLP, lack of documentation as to the historical exposure to carcinogens, and the development of carcinomas at anatomic sites remote from the OLP in many of these retrospective studies and case reports. A study using strict diagnostic criteria as outlined by the World Health Organization for OLP and lichenoid lesions reported the development of squamous cell carcinoma in 3 of 173 patients (1.7%).[38]

It is generally accepted that the malignant transformation or development of malignancy in the presence of OLP is more likely to occur in atrophic, erosive, or ulcerative lesions. It had been postulated that these atrophic, erosive, and ulcerative lesions

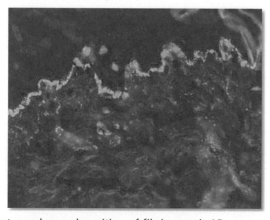

Fig. 6. Subbasement membrane deposition of fibrinogen in LP.

predispose the mucosa to damage from carcinogenic agents. However, many patients who develop carcinoma lack a positive history for tobacco or alcohol use, suggesting that malignancy may be part of the natural course of the disease process or that other unknown extrinsic factors may be involved. Because *Candida* is a natural inhabitant of the oral mucosa in many patients and because it often develops secondary to topical corticosteroid therapy, the role of *Candida* may represent another extrinsic factor involved in the development of malignancy. It has been hypothesized that strains of *Candida albicans* are able to catalyze the formation of the known carcinogen *N*-nitrosobenzylmethylamine.

Other debates have revolved around the use of immunomodulating agents in the treatment of LP as a cause of the development of malignancy. Theoretically, the ability of these medications to depress local cell immunity could promote the progression of LP to malignancy, and given their potent antiinflammatory effects, malignant progression would advance with reduced symptoms. Before a definitive, consensus statement regarding the malignant potential of LP can be made, longitudinal studies with more patients should be performed. Clinically, it is important that patients with OLP undergo biannual follow-up evaluations. This strategy seems most important with patients who have erosive and ulcerative disease (**Fig. 7**).

COMORBIDITIES
Lichenoid Drug Reactions

Lichenoid drug reactions and LP show similar clinical and histologic findings.[39–54] The former is distinguished from the latter based on 2 factors: (1) the association with the administration of a drug, contact with a metal, foodstuff, or systemic disease; and (2) their resolution when the offending agent is eliminated.[40] The prevalence of oral lichenoid drug reactions seems to be increasing, most likely because of the realization that the entity has a cause that is distinct from idiopathic LP.[41,42] The increased occurrence may, in part, be caused by the introduction of numerous new categories of medications that have a greater tendency for lichenoid reactions as a side effect. Most often, antibiotics, antihypertensives, gold compounds, diuretics, antimalarials, and nonsteroidal antiinflammatory agents are responsible for lichenoid reactions (**Table 2**).

Clinically, lesions are indistinguishable from OLP showing erythematous erosions and ulceration with focal areas of radiating striae. Because the histology is

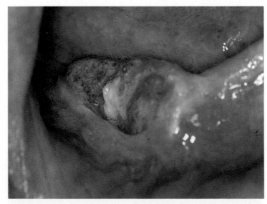

Fig. 7. Oral squamous cell carcinoma of the mandible arising in a patient with long-standing LP and desquamative gingivitis.

Table 2 Histopathology of OLP	
Type	**Histopathologic Description**
Reticular LP	Orthokeratosis and parakeratosis are seen in combination with acanthosis Intermittent areas of epithelial atrophy Basement membrane is thickened, with a dense band of T lymphocytes
Erosive LP	Thinning and ulceration of the epithelium with complete loss of rete ridge formation Dense T-cell infiltrate extending well into the middle and upper levels of the epithelium Liquefaction of the basement membrane and vacuolization and destruction of the basal cell are seen in most areas Epithelium is often lost, showing underlying connective tissue
Plaquelike LP	Similar to the striae of the reticular form, without the intermittent areas of epithelial atrophy Orthokeratosis and parakeratosis are seen in combination with acanthosis Basement membrane is thickened, with a band of T lymphocytes less dense than in the reticular form
Bullous LP	Subepidermal bulla showing degeneration of the epidermal basal layer Other features of LP

indistinguishable from OLP, diagnosis is often dependent on establishing a temporal relationship between lesion onset and use of offending agent along with resolution of symptoms on withdrawal of the offending agent. A drug history can be one of the most important aspects of the assessment of a patient with oral lichenoid lesions. Occasionally, drug-induced lesions may show a deep and superficial perivascular lymphocytic infiltrate with the presence of eosinophils, plasma cells, and neutrophils. Treatment of lichenoid reactions, in addition to cessation or reduction in the dose of the offending medication, is usually restricted to topical corticosteroids. The resolution of lesions after removal of an offending agent may be prompt or may take months to clear.

Hepatitis C and OLP

Reports of hepatitis C infection associated with OLP have frequently appeared in the literature.[55–57] Although most of these reports come from Asian or Mediterranean countries, anecdotal evidence suggests that an association exists in both the United States and Great Britain. The relationship of hepatitis C to dermatologic diseases is not limited to OLP and seems to be related to the upregulation of the immune response by the virus.

MANAGEMENT
Goals

Management strategies for effective outcome:

- Establishing a definitive diagnosis with biopsy
- Understanding of the local, systemic, and psychological factors that may be responsible for disease progression
- Establishing a treatment plan based on the presenting symptoms and clinical presentations in the initial visit and treatment modifications based on investigations and previous treatment outcomes in the following visits

---

Box 3
Treatment of LP

- Medications can be applied to the lesions with cotton swabs or gauze pads impregnated with medication and left on affected areas for 10 minutes 2 or 3 times daily
- Extensive erosive lesions on the gingiva can be treated 2 or 3 times daily with occlusive splints that hold the steroid medication on the affected areas
- Occlusive splint therapy can lead to systemic absorption of steroid (**Fig. 8**)
- Candidal overgrowth with clinical thrush is an occasional side effect, requiring concomitant topical or systemic antifungal therapy
- In lesions recalcitrant to topical therapy, intralesional injections of steroid can be effective (**Fig. 9**)

Pharmacologic Strategies: Topical Medications

No cure for OLP or its dermal counterpart exists. The treatment goal is always 2-fold:

1. Alleviation of symptoms
2. Monitoring for dysplastic changes[58]

Small areas of the reticular or plaquelike form of OLP are rarely treated unless they become symptomatic, persist, or become widespread. For cases of lichenoid reaction, identification and elimination of the offending agent are important but often not possible.

Topical corticosteroids have been shown to be the most predictable and effective medications for controlling the signs and symptoms of OLP. Various applications techniques and precautions need to be recommended when prescribing these agents (**Box 3**).

Other topical agents have shown to be beneficial in both primary treatment as well as adjuvant therapy with topical corticosteroids. Agents and indications are listed in **Tables 3** and **4**.

Pharmacologic Strategies: Systemic Therapies

There are no controlled studies that have evaluated the efficacy of systemic corticosteroids in OLP. Occasionally, systemic steroids are indicated for brief treatment of

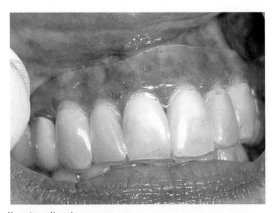

Fig. 8. Occlusive splints/medication trays.

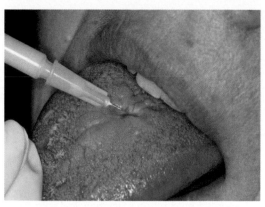

Fig. 9. Intralesional injections.

severe exacerbations or for short periods of treating recalcitrant lesions that fail to respond to topical therapy. Prednisone, 0.50 to 0.75 mg/kg per day for less than 10 days without tapering, is recommended by many clinicians.[3] Often, combination topical and systemic therapy may prove more beneficial than any single modality.

Systemic and topically administered β all-trans retinoic acid, vitamin A, systemic etretinate, and systemic and topical isotretinoin all have shown some measure of efficacy in open studies or anecdotal case reports.[3] Topical retinoids are usually favored over their systemic counterparts, because the latter may be associated with adverse side effects such as liver dysfunction and teratogenicity.

Other treatments for OLP have been reported to be useful; however, additional research data are necessary. Oral PUVA (psoralen combined with UV-A) therapy with low-dose UV-A has been shown to be effective in treating OLP in several open studies.[65] Additional medications, including griseofulvin, levamisole, dapsone, and

Table 3
Diseases, drugs, and materials commonly implicated in lichenoid reactions

Category	Drug or Material
Antiarthritics	Aurothioglucose, gold salts
Antihypertensives	Angiotensin-converting enzyme inhibitors, thiazide diuretics, mercurial diuretics, labetolol, practolol, methyldopa
Antimicrobials	Dapsone, ketoconazole, streptomycin, sulfamethoxazole, tetracycline
Antiparasitics	Chloroquine, quinacrine, pyramethamine, organic arsenicals
Anxiolytics	Lorazepam
Nonsteroidal antiinflammatory drugs	Ibuprofen, fenclofenac, naproxen, phenylbutazone
Oral hypoglycemic agents	Chlorpropamide, tolazamide, tolbutamide
Uricosuric agents	Allopurinol
Dental restorative materials/foodstuffs	Amalgam components, acrylic, casting alloys, betel quid, peppermint and cinnamon
Systemic disease	Graft-versus-host disease, hepatitis C, thymoma, lupus erythematosus

Table 4
Topical treatment in OLP

Medication	Indications and Special Precautions
Flucinonide 0.05% (Lidex)	Prescribed as gel and applied daily according to disease severity[59,60]
Clobetasol 0.05% (Temovate)	Prescribed as gel and applied daily according to disease severity[59,60]
Retinoic acid	Used in combination with topical corticosteroids as an adjuvant therapy Useful in the more plaquelike and reticular lesions that are persistent or widespread After withdrawal of these medications, lesions frequently recur
Cyclosporine	Beneficial in treating recalcitrant cases of OLP[20] Use is limited because of its hydrophobicity, high cost, and poor taste Concerns over its role in promoting viral reproduction and malignant change have restricted its use to patients with severe disease and otherwise intractable lesions
Tacrolimus or pimeocrolimus	Solution or cream form of these agents can be helpful in OLP resistant to topical or systemic therapies[61–64] These immunosuppressives are used in dermatology primarily to treat atopic dermatitis Mode of action is unclear, but seem to inhibit T-cell activation and proliferation[61–64] Side effects include carcinogenicity, mutagenicity, and infertility

thalidomide, have been reported to be effective in the treatment of OLP in various case reports throughout the literature.[3,66]

SUMMARY

OLP and lichenoid reaction are a relatively common oral mucosal disease process encountered in clinical practice. This mucocutaneous disease can manifest as desquamative gingivitis, asymptomatic Wickham striae or plaques, or severe, painful erosions or ulcerations anywhere in the oral cavity. Although the cause initiating LP is unknown, current research points to several complex immunologic events and cells that are responsible for the inflammatory destruction and chronicity of these lesions. The mainstay of treatment remains topical corticosteroids; however, newer therapies such a tacrolimus are available for recalcitrant lesions. In cases of lichenoid mucositis or reactions, treatment should always be directed at identifying and removing the presumed cause. Given the apparent risk of squamous cell carcinoma in these patients, frequent follow-up and repeat biopsy when indicated are vital.

REFERENCES

1. Stoopler ET, Sollecito TP, De Rossi SS. Oral lichen planus. Update for the general practitioner. N Y State Dent J 2003;69(6):26–8.
2. Mollaoglu N. Oral lichen planus: a review. Br J Oral Maxillofac Surg 2000;38(4): 370–7.
3. Eisen D. The clinical manifestations and treatment of oral lichen planus. Dermatol Clin 2003;21(1):79–89.
4. Goldblum OM. Lichen planus. Skinmed 2002;1(1):52–3.
5. Edwards PC, Kelsch R. Oral lichen planus: clinical presentation and management. J Can Dent Assoc 2002;68(8):494–9.

6. Thornhill MH. Immune mechanisms in oral lichen planus. Acta Odontol Scand 2001;59(3):174–7.
7. Hasseus B, Jontell M, Brune M, et al. Langerhans cells and T cells in oral graft versus host disease and oral lichen planus. Scand J Immunol 2001;54(5): 516–24.
8. Sugerman PB, Savage NW, Walsh LJ, et al. The pathogenesis of oral lichen planus. Crit Rev Oral Biol Med 2002;13(4):350–65.
9. Zhao ZZ, Savage NW, Sugerman PB, et al. Mast cell/T cell interactions in oral lichen planus. J Oral Pathol Med 2002;31(4):189–95.
10. Gandara Rey J, Garcia Garcia A, Blanco Carrion A, et al. Cellular immune alterations in fifty-two patients with oral lichen planus. Med Oral 2001;6(4):246–62.
11. Femiano F, Cozzolino F, Gaeta GM, et al. Recent advances on the pathogenesis of oral lichen planus (OLP). The adhesion molecules. Minerva Stomatol 1999; 48(4):151–9.
12. Villarroel Dorrego M, Correnti M, Delgado R, et al. Oral lichen planus: immunohistology of mucosal lesions. J Oral Pathol Med 2002;31(7):410–4.
13. Neppelberg E, Johannessen AC, Jonsson R. Apoptosis in oral lichen planus. Eur J Oral Sci 2001;109(5):361–4.
14. Jose M, Raghu AR, Rao NN. Evaluation of mast cells in oral lichen planus and oral lichenoid reaction. Indian J Dent Res 2001;12(3):175–9.
15. Kawamura E, Nakamura S, Sasaki M, et al. Accumulation of oligoclonal T cells in the infiltrating lymphocytes in oral lichen planus. J Oral Pathol Med 2003;32(5): 282–9.
16. Iijima W, Ohtani H, Nakayama T, et al. Infiltrating CD8+ T cells in oral lichen planus predominantly express CCR5 and CXCR3 and carry respective chemokine ligands RANTES/CCL5 and IP-10/CXCL10 in their cytolytic granules: a potential self-recruiting mechanism. Am J Pathol 2003;163(1):261–8.
17. da Silva Fonseca LM, do Carmo MA. Identification of the AgNORs, PCNA and ck16 proteins in oral lichen planus lesions. Oral Dis 2001;7(6):344–8.
18. Yamamoto T, Nakane T, Osaki T. The mechanism of mononuclear cell infiltration in oral lichen planus: the role of cytokines released from keratinocytes. J Clin Immunol 2000;20(4):294–305.
19. Little MC, Griffiths CE, Watson RE, et al. Oral mucosal keratinocytes express RANTES and ICAM-1, but not interleukin-8, in oral lichen planus and oral lichenoid reactions induced by amalgam fillings. Clin Exp Dermatol 2003;28(1):64–9.
20. Demitsu T, Sato T, Inoue T, et al. Corticosteroid-resistant erosive oral lichen planus successfully treated with topical cyclosporine therapy. Int J Dermatol 2000; 39(1):79–80.
21. Raghu AR, Nirmala NR, Sreekumaran N. Direct immunofluorescence in oral lichen planus and oral lichenoid reactions. Quintessence Int 2002;33(3):234–9.
22. Sklavounou A, Chrysomali E, Scorilas A, et al. TNF-alpha expression and apoptosis-regulating proteins in oral lichen planus: a comparative immunohistochemical evaluation. J Oral Pathol Med 2000;29(8):370–5.
23. Eisen D. The clinical features, malignant potential, and systemic associations of oral lichen planus: a study of 723 patients. J Am Acad Dermatol 2002;46(2):207–14.
24. Rhodus NL, Myers S, Kaimal S. Diagnosis and management of oral lichen planus. Northwest Dent 2003;82(2):17–9, 22–5.
25. Kuffer R, Lombardi T. Erosion and ulceration occurring on oral lichen planus. Dermatology 2003;207(3):340.
26. Rebora A. Erosive lichen planus: what is this? Dermatology 2002;205(3):226–8 [discussion: 227].

27. Myers SL, Rhodus NL, Parsons HM, et al. A retrospective survey of oral lichenoid lesions: revisiting the diagnostic process for oral lichen planus. Oral Surg Oral Med Oral Pathol Oral Radiol Endod 2002;93(6):676–81.

28. de Moura Castro Jacques C, Cardozo Pereira AL, Cabral MG, et al. Oral lichen planus part I: epidemiology, clinics, etiology, immunopathogeny, and diagnosis. Skinmed 2003;2(6):342–7 [quiz: 348–9].

29. Bloor BK, Malik FK, Odell EW, et al. Quantitative assessment of apoptosis in oral lichen planus. Oral Surg Oral Med Oral Pathol Oral Radiol Endod 1999;88(2): 187–95.

30. Rode M, Kogoj-Rode M. Malignant potential of the reticular form of oral lichen planus over a 25-year observation period in 55 patients from Slovenia. J Oral Sci 2002;44(2):109–11.

31. Vescovi P, Manfredi M, Savi A, et al. Neoplastic transformation of oral lichen planus. I: review of the literature. Minerva Stomatol 2000;49(5):249–55.

32. Warshaw EM, Templeton SF, Washington CV. Verrucous carcinoma occurring in a lesion of oral lichen planus. Cutis 2000;65(4):219–22.

33. Bruno E, Alessandrini M, Russo S, et al. Malignant degeneration of oral lichen planus: our clinical experience and review of the literature. An Otorrinolaringol Ibero Am 2002;29(4):349–57.

34. Manuel Gandara Rey J, Diniz Freitas M. High rate of malignant transformation in atypical oral lichen planus lesions. Med Oral 2003;8(5):309 [author reply: 310].

35. Larsson A, Warfvinge G. Malignant transformation of oral lichen planus. Oral Oncol 2003;39(6):630–1.

36. Lanfranchi-Tizeira HE, Aguas SC, Sano SM. Malignant transformation of atypical oral lichen planus: a review of 32 cases. Med Oral 2003;8(1):2–9.

37. Cardozo Pereira AL, de Moura Castro Jacques C, Cabral MG, et al. Oral lichen planus part II: therapy and malignant transformation. Skinmed 2004;3(1):19–22.

38. Epstein JB, Wan LS, Gorsky M, et al. Oral lichen planus: progress in understanding its malignant potential and the implications for clinical management. Oral Surg Oral Med Oral Pathol Oral Radiol Endod 2003;96(1):32–7.

39. Kato Y, Hayakawa R, Shiraki R, et al. A case of lichen planus caused by mercury allergy. Br J Dermatol 2003;148(6):1268–9.

40. Rice PJ, Hamburger J. Oral lichenoid drug eruptions: their recognition and management. Dent Update 2002;29(9):442–7.

41. Agarwal R, Saraswat A. Oral lichen planus: an update. Drugs Today (Barc) 2002;38(8):533–47.

42. Giunta JL. Oral lichenoid reactions versus lichen planus. J Mass Dent Soc 2001; 50(2):22–5.

43. Kragelund C, Thomsen CE, Bardow A, et al. Oral lichen planus and intake of drugs metabolized by polymorphic cytochrome P450 enzymes. Oral Dis 2003;9(4):177–87.

44. Thornhill MH, Pemberton MN, Simmons RK, et al. Amalgam-contact hypersensitivity lesions and oral lichen planus. Oral Surg Oral Med Oral Pathol Oral Radiol Endod 2003;95(3):291–9.

45. Lavanya N, Jayanthi P, Rao UK, et al. Oral lichen planus: an update on pathogenesis and treatment. J Oral Maxillofac Pathol 2011;15(2):127–32.

46. Payeras MR, Cherubini K, Figueiredo MA, et al. Oral lichen planus: focus on etiopathogenesis. Arch Oral Biol 2013;58(9):1057–69.

47. Ismail SB, Kumar SK, Zain RB. Oral lichen planus and lichenoid reactions: etiopathogenesis, diagnosis, management and malignant transformation. J Oral Sci 2007;49:89–106.

48. Carrozzo M, Thorpe R. Oral lichen planus–a review. Minerva Stomatol 2009;58: 519–37.
49. Roopashree MR, Gondhalekar RV, Shashikanth MC, et al. Pathogenesis of oral lichen planus–a review. J Oral Pathol Med 2010;39:729–34.
50. Cafaro A, Albanese G, Arduino PG, et al. Effect of low-level laser irradiation on unresponsive oral lichen planus: early preliminary results in 13 patients. Photomed Laser Surg 2010;28(Suppl 2):S99–103.
51. Farhi D, Dupin N. Pathophysiology, etiologic factors, and clinical management of oral lichen planus, Part I: facts and controversies. Clin Dermatol 2010; 28(1):100–8.
52. Bagan J, Compilato D, Paderni C, et al. Topical therapies for oral lichen planus management and their efficacy: a narrative review. Curr Pharm Des 2012; 18(34):5470–80.
53. Schlosser BJ. Lichen planus and lichenoid reactions of the oral mucosa. Dermatol Ther 2010;23(3):251–67.
54. DeRossi SS, Ciarrocca KN. Lichen planus, lichenoid drug reactions, and lichenoid mucositis. Dent Clin North Am 2005;49(1):77–89, viii.
55. Nagao Y, Tomonari R, Kage M, et al. The possible intraspousal transmission of HCV in terms of lichen planus. Int J Mol Med 2002;10(5):569–73.
56. Pilli M, Penna A, Zerbini A, et al. Oral lichen planus pathogenesis: a role for the HCV-specific cellular immune response. Hepatology 2002;36(6):1446–52.
57. Engin B, Oguz O, Mert A, et al. Prevalence of oral lichen planus in a group of hepatitis C patients. J Dermatol 2002;29(7):459–60.
58. McCreary CE, McCartan BE. Clinical management of oral lichen planus. Br J Oral Maxillofac Surg 1999;37(5):338–43.
59. Gonzalez-Moles MA, Morales P, Rodriguez-Archilla A. The treatment of oral aphthous ulceration or erosive lichen planus with topical clobetasol propionate in three preparations. A clinical study on 54 patients. J Oral Pathol Med 2002; 31(5):284–5.
60. Buajeeb W, Pobrurksa C, Kraivaphan P. Efficacy of fluocinoloneacetonide gel in the treatment of oral lichen planus. Oral Surg Oral Med Oral Pathol Oral Radiol Endod 2000;89(1):42–5.
61. Hodgson TA, Sahni N, Kaliakatsou F, et al. Long-term efficacy and safety of topical tacrolimus in the management of ulcerative/erosive oral lichen planus. Eur J Dermatol 2003;13(5):466–70.
62. Nazzaro G, Cestari R. Topical tacrolimus ointment in ulcerative lichen planus: an alternative therapeutic approach. Eur J Dermatol 2002;12(4):321.
63. Kaliakatsou F, Hodgson TA, Lewsey JD, et al. Management of recalcitrant ulcerative oral lichen planus with topical tacrolimus. J Am Acad Dermatol 2002;46(1): 35–41.
64. Morrison L, Kratochvil FJ, Gorman A. An open trial of topical tacrolimus for erosive oral lichen planus. J Am Acad Dermatol 2002;47(4):617–20.
65. Taneja A, Taylor CR. Narrow-band UVB for lichen planus treatment. Int J Dermatol 2002;41(5):282–3.
66. Verma KK, Mittal R, Manchanda Y. Azathioprine for the treatment of severe erosive oral and generalized lichen planus. Acta Derm Venereol 2001;81(5): 378–9.

Oral Cancer

Leukoplakia, Premalignancy, and Squamous Cell Carcinoma

Nelson L. Rhodus, DMD, MPH, FICD[a],*, A. Ross Kerr, DDS, MSD[b],
Ketan Patel, DDS, PhD[c]

KEYWORDS

- Cancer • Carcinogenesis • Oral cancer • Diagnosis • Adjunctive techniques

KEY POINTS

- Review the epidemiology, etiologic risk factors, clinical presentation, recognition, and diagnosis of oral precancer and cancer.
- Recommendations on clinical examination and early diagnostic techniques (including adjuncts) are presented.
- Treatment and complications from treatment of oral cancer are only briefly discussed.

Cancer is the second leading cause of death in the United States. In 2013, more than 580,000 people died of cancer, from almost 1.7 million new cases.[1] Oral and pharyngeal cancers account for nearly 40,000 cases of cancer (incidence of 10 per 100,000) and approximately 8000 deaths per year in the United States and is the sixth most common cancer worldwide (**Table 1**).[1–6] Oral and pharyngeal cancer is more common than cervical or liver cancer, Hodgkin lymphoma, and brain, stomach, or ovarian cancer. More than 90% of these oral and pharyngeal cancers are squamous cell carcinomas (SCCs). The other 10% comprise salivary gland tumors, lymphoma, sarcoma, and others. The 5-year survival rate from these cancers has improved only modestly in the past 30 years and remains at approximately 55% to 60%. Head and neck cancer is staged by the TNM classification system and directly related to survival. The incidence and survival are also dependent on the anatomic site based on TNM staging (**Table 2**).

A version of this article appeared as Rhodus NL. Oral cance: leukoplakia and squamous cell carcinoma. Dent Clin N Amer 2005;49:143–65.

[a] Division of Oral Medicine, University of Minnesota, 515 Delaware Street SE, Minneapolis, MN 55455, USA; [b] Department of Oral & Maxillofacial Pathology, Radiology and Medicine, New York University, New York, NY, USA; [c] Division of Oral and Maxillofacial Surgery, University of Minnesota, 515 Delaware Street SE, Minneapolis, MN 55455, USA

* Corresponding author.

E-mail address: rhodu001@umn.edu

http://dx.doi.org/10.1016/j.cden.2013.12.004
0011-8532/14/$ – see front matter © 2014 Elsevier Inc. All rights reserved.

dental.theclinics.com

Table 1
Incidence of head and neck cancer in 2011–2012 (40,000/y)

Location	Incidence	%	% of All Cancer
Oral	17,900	48	2.4
Oropharynx	3500	10	0.8
Nasopharynx	2500	9	0.5
Larynx	9800	25	1.4
Maxillary sinus	1100	3	0.2
Nose	400	1	0.1
Esophagus	800	2	0.2
Ear	300	1	0.2

Data from Siegel R, Ward E, Brawley O, et al. Cancer statistics, 2011. CA Cancer J Clin 2011;61(4):212–5.

The 5-year survival rate for Whites is approximately 58%, whereas that for Blacks is only 31%.[1–6]

The ratio of males to females diagnosed with oral and pharyngeal cancer is 2:1 over a lifetime, although the ratio comes closer to 1:1 with advancing age. Human papillomavirus (HPV)-associated oropharyngeal cancers (ie, cancers predominantly involving the palatine and lingual tonsils/base of tongue) are occurring at the most rapid rate of all head and neck cancers.[7–10] Approximately 90% of oral and pharyngeal cancer is diagnosed in persons older than 40 years, and more than 50% of all cancers occur in persons older than 65 years. The average age at the time of diagnosis is 63 years.[1–6] However, evidence indicates that both oral cavity and oropharyngeal cancers are occurring more frequently in younger persons (<40 years).[4] The overall incidence of oral and pharyngeal cancers has remained stable, relative to the occurrence of newly diagnosed cancers of all sites, with absolute numbers only slightly increasing each year.[1–6]

The observation that oral and pharyngeal cancer generally occurs with advancing age indicates that over time, certain sequenced alterations in the biochemical-biophysical processes (nuclear, enzymatic, metabolic, immunologic) of aging cells that have a particular genetic predisposition undergo and accumulate mutations, resulting in carcinogenic transformation.[11–16] These carcinogenic changes may be influenced by oncogenes, carcinogens, and mutations caused by chemicals, viruses, irradiation, drugs, hormones, nutrients, or physical irritants.[11–16]

An imbalance between abnormal cell proliferation or apoptosis (programmed cell death) may be modified by factors that alter cellular production of growth and suppressor proteins.[11–15]

Table 2
The 5-year survival rate (%) of oral cancer based on TNM staging

Site	Localized	Nodal Involvement	Distant Metastasis	Total
Lip	89	57	40	86
Floor of mouth	65	31	14	44
Others	61	29	18	44
Tongue	52	22	7	33

Data from Refs.[22–24]

Malignancies of the oral cavity often begin as preneoplastic lesions in the form of lesions such as leukoplakia, erythroplakias, and erythroleukoplakia. Leukoplakia is associated with tobacco and alcohol use and chronic inflammation with the risk of malignant transformation to SCC of approximately 5% to 17% (**Fig. 1**).[16–22] Alterations in host immunity, inflammation, angiogenesis, and metabolism have been noted to be prominent clinical features in oral cancer. These tumor-induced T-lymphocyte, granulocyte, and neoangiogenesis responses in the local tumor microenvironment have been associated with increased tumor growth and metastasis and decreased survival rates.[16–22] Pathologic changes in systemic responses have also been observed, including induction of antibody and other acute phase inflammatory protein responses.[16–24]

This article reviews the epidemiology, etiologic risk factors, clinical presentation, recognition, and diagnosis of oral precancer and cancer. The treatment and complications from treatment of oral cancer are only briefly discussed, because complications of therapy are discussed elsewhere in this issue in the article on chemotherapy or radiation-induced oral mucositis by Lalla and colleagues (**Box 1**).

ANATOMIC SITES

The tongue is the most common site for oral cancer in both American men and women (**Table 3**). Recent data (2011) indicate that about 46% (12,000:26,100) of all oral cavity cancers (excluding the pharynx) occur on the tongue.[1–6] There are some differences in the most common oral and pharyngeal sites in other areas of the world, such as Southeast Asia, where nasopharyngeal cancer is more common, and in India, where buccal mucosa carcinomas are the most common oral sites. Data from the SEER (Surveillance Epidemiology and End Results) program show that more than 37% of all oral cancers diagnosed in the United States between 1985 and 2011 occurred in the tongue, followed by the lip and floor of the mouth.[1–6] More recently, the incidence of tongue malignancies has increased to account for 46% of oral cancers.[5,6] The other oral anatomic sites in decreasing order are: lip (18%), floor of mouth (12%), salivary glands (10%), buccal mucosa (5%), gingival (5%), and palate (4%).[1–6]

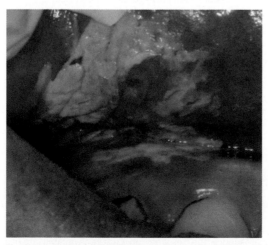

Fig. 1. Leukoplakia in the anterior labial vestibule associated with smokeless tobacco use. (*Courtesy of* Dr Eric Stoopler, DMD, Philadelphia, PA.)

Box 1
TNM classification of carcinomas of the oral cavity

T: primary tumor[a,b]

TNM	FIGO (International Federation of Gynecology and Obstetrics)
TX	Primary tumor cannot be assessed
T0	No evidence of primary tumor
Tis	Carcinoma in situ
T1	Tumor ≤2 cm in greatest dimension
T2	Tumor >2 cm but not >4 cm in greatest dimension
T3	Tumor >4 cm in greatest dimension
T4a (lip)	Tumor invades through cortical bone, inferior alveolar nerve, floor of mouth, or skin (chin or nose)
T4a (oral cavity)	Tumor invades through cortical bone, into deep/extrinsic muscle of tongue (genioglossus, hyoglossus, palatoglossus, and styloglossus), maxillary sinus, or skin of face
T4b (lip and oral cavity)	Tumor invades masticator space, pterygoid plates, or skull base; or encases internal carotid artery

Note: superficial erosion alone of bone/tooth socket by gingival primary is not sufficient to classify a tumor as T4

N: regional lymph nodes[c]

NX	Regional lymph nodes cannot be assessed
N0	No regional lymph node metastasis
N1	Metastasis in a single ipsilateral lymph node, ≤3 cm in greatest dimension
N2	Metastasis as specified in N2a, 2b, 2c below
N2a	Metastasis in a single ipsilateral lymph node, >3 cm but not >6 cm in greatest dimension
N2b	Metastasis in multiple ipsilateral lymph nodes, none >6 cm in greatest dimension
N2c	Metastasis in bilateral or contralateral lymph nodes, none >6 cm in greatest dimension
N3	Metastasis in a lymph node >6 cm in greatest dimension

Note: midline nodes are considered ipsilateral nodes

M: distant metastasis

MX	Distant metastasis cannot be assessed
M0	No distant metastasis
M1	Distant metastasis

Stage grouping

Stage 0	Tis	N0	M0
Stage I	T1	N0	M0
Stage II	T2	N0	M0
Stage III	T1, T2	N1	M0
	T3	N0, N1	M0
Stage IVA	T1, T2, T3	N2	M0
	T4a	N0, N1, N2	M0
Stage IVB	Any T	N3	M0
	T4b	Any N	M0
Stage IVC	Any T	Any N	M1

[a] 947,2418.
[b] A help desk for specific questions about the TNM classification is available at http://www.uicc.org/index.php?id=508.
[c] The regional lymph nodes are the cervical nodes.
From International Agency for Research on Cancer. Available at: http://screening.iarc.fr/atlasoralclassiftnm.php. Accessed February 23, 2013.

Table 3 The incidence of oral cancer ranked by anatomic location		
Oral Location	Incidence	%
Tongue	12,000	46
Lip	4200	18
Floor of mouth	2300	12
Salivary	2000	10
Buccal	1100	5
Gingiva	1100	5
Palatal	800	4

Data from Siegel R, Ward E, Brawley O, et al. Cancer statistics, 2011. CA Cancer J Clin 2011;61(4):212–5.

STAGE AT DIAGNOSIS AND SURVIVAL

Approximately half of all patients with oral and pharyngeal cancers survive their disease 5 years after treatment. Theses figures are less favorable for SCC of the tongue (33%).[4–6,15,25]

In the United States, the outcomes are more favorable for Whites than for Blacks (58% vs 31%; 5-year survival rates). Genetics is significantly involved in the predisposition to cancer, but socioeconomic status, education, and access to the health care system also have an influence.[4–6,15,26] The survival rates for advanced tumors are lower compared with earlier detected, localized cancers. At the time of diagnosis, nearly 50% of all carcinomas of the tongue have already metastasized. An additional 35% to 40% metastasize within 5 years. If all cases of oral cancer were diagnosed and treated early as localized tumors, almost 80% of all patients would survive 5 years.[4–6,15,26] Little progress has been made during the past 40 years in regard to early diagnosis. In addition, based on more than 25,000 SEER program oral/pharyngeal cases for which there was adequate information, localized/early oral cancers were outnumbered by advanced tumors 59% to 41%.

The lip was the only major site at which localized cancers were more frequently found than more advanced cancers.[1–6] Advances in the treatment of oral and pharyngeal cancer have not led to significantly improved survival, and therefore, earlier diagnosis is the most important factor in improving oral and pharyngeal cancer control and reducing morbidity and mortality.[1–6]

TNM STAGING

Head and neck cancer is staged by the TNM classification (see **Table 2**). The TNM classification is based on tumor size, regional lymph node involvement, and distant metastasis. The classification is based on imaging, including computed tomography (CT), magnetic resonance imaging (MRI), and sometimes positron emission tomography (PET) scans are used to facilitate staging, particularly of advanced disease. Most often, a chest radiograph is used to determine metastasis to the lungs. A PET scan is also useful for the identification of metastases.[26–32] As an example, a patient who presents with a suspicious oral lesion, which is 2.5 cm with ipsilateral lymphadenopathy of 2 cm and a negative chest radiograph. is classified as T2N1M0. This classification is useful not only for determining the severity and prognosis of the cancer but the choice of therapy (excisional surgery, modified or radical lymph node dissection, radiation, or chemotherapy).[26–32]

CAUSE AND RISK FACTORS

The cause of oral cancer is multifactorial and involves many alterations in host immunity and metabolism, angiogenesis, exposure to chronic inflammation, in a genetically susceptible individual. The carcinogenic changes may be influenced by oncogenes, carcinogens and mutations caused by chemicals, viruses, irradiation, drugs (tobacco and alcohol), hormones, nutrients, or physical irritants.[9,14–20]

IMMUNE SYSTEM

Multiple studies have shown that the risks of cancer increase in individuals whose immune systems are either congenitally defective or have been suppressed or altered by disease or medications. Furthermore, immune competence and immune cell surveillance diminish with age. This factor likely contributes to the association between age and malignancy.[9,14–20]

TOBACCO

Smoking tobacco is a worldwide epidemic, contributing to serious health problems and systemic diseases of immense proportions. Reports from the US Surgeon General and others conclude that cigarette smoking is the main cause of cancer mortality in the United States, contributing to an estimated 30% of all cancer deaths and substantially to cancers of the head and neck.[10–16]

The association between cigarette use and oral carcinoma has been firmly established from epidemiologic studies, showing that there are more than twice as many smokers among patients who have oral cancer as among control populations.

One study found that 72% of more than 400 patients with oral cancer were smokers and 58% smoked more than 1 pack daily, showing the high risk for tobacco users.[17]

Tobacco use also increases the already high risk for developing recurrences of oral cancer as well as second primary oral and pharyngeal cancers.[18–20] Smoking tobacco is the leading contributor to oral and pharyngeal cancer, but the use of smokeless tobacco has been associated as well (see **Fig. 1**).[16,17]

Certain hydrocarbons isolated from tobacco products have been shown to induce carcinomas in animals under certain experimental conditions.[16,17]

Benzo[a]pyrene, one of the most potent of these carcinogens, binds to nucleoproteins and is mutagenic as well as carcinogenic. The association between tobacco use and oral malignancies also seems to include cigars, pipes, and smokeless preparations.[16,17]

Alcohol intake has also been associated with the incidence of oral cancer, especially with long-term excessive use. One group of investigators found that 44% of 108 patients with cancer of the tongue and 59% of 68 patients with cancer of the floor of the mouth, palate, or tonsillar fossa had unequivocal evidence of alcoholic cirrhosis. **Fig. 2** shows a leukoplakia on the lateral ventral tongue of a patient with a history of heavy tobacco and alcohol use. Approximately 75% drank alcohol excessively.[18] The combined effects of tobacco and alcohol are shown in another study of more than 350 patients who had oral cancer and a mortality of 31% within 5 years.[18]

However, definitive associations between alcohol-containing mouth rinses and the development of oral cancer have not been established.[19] Areca nut products are another established risk factor for oral cancer.

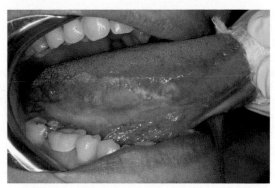

Fig. 2. Leukoplakia of the right lateral tongue. The lesion is soft to palpation, predominantly smooth, homogeneous, and almost translucent except for some thicker whiter changes superiorly and anteriorly. Two biopsies both revealed mild epithelial dysplasia.

ORAL LICHEN PLANUS

Oral lichen planus (OLP) is a complex, chronic, inflammatory disease. The cause of OLP is unknown, but it is believed to be an immunopathologic disease. OLP can occur in any oral site, with the buccal mucosa as the most common location. OLP can usually be recognized by the unique clinical features of reticular, annular, or punctate keratotic (white) patterns on the mucosal surface.[15,20–22] Diagnosis should always be confirmed by biopsy.

A summary of the results from several studies performed in 7 different countries since 1981 indicates that from 0.4% to 5.6% of OLP lesions transformed to SCC.[15,20–22]

NUTRITION

Although some studies indicate a potential association with dietary factors and cancer in general, no clear dietary characteristics (deficiencies or excesses of nutrients) have been recognized that directly correlate with cancer of the oral cavity. Some recent meta-analyses have indicated a positive protective effect with a diet high in fresh fruits and vegetables.[15,23,33,34]

VIRUSES

The role of viruses in development of oral cancer has been a matter of investigation for a long time. Those having oncogenic potential are from 2 groups: the herpesviruses and the Human papilloma viruses.[7–9,33]

One of the most common virus groups in the world affecting the skin and mucosal areas of the body is HPV. More than 120 different subtypes of HPV have been identified, and different types are known to infect different parts of the body.[7–9] The most visible forms of the virus produce warts (verruca vulgaris) on the hands, arms, legs, and other areas of the skin. Most HPVs of this type are common, harmless, nononcogenic, and easily treatable. There are other forms of HPV, which are sexually transmitted, and some of these can cause cancer. The most common of these oncogenic subtypes is HPV-16, and less common subtypes are HPV-18, HPV-31, and HPV-45.[7–9]

HPV-16 causes oropharyngeal cancer. In the oral environment, HPV-16 manifests itself primarily in the oropharynx, including the base of the tongue (lingual tonsils) and palatine tonsils. These oncogenic or cancer-causing versions of HPV are also responsible for other SCCs, particularly of the cervix, anus, and penis.[7–10]

HPV is covered in more detail in another article elsewhere in this issue.

A study conducted by the Johns Hopkins Oncology Center by Dr Maura Gillison furthered the premise that HPV might be associated with oropharyngeal maligancies.[7] This study evaluated 253 patients diagnosed with head and neck cancers. In 25% of these cases, the tissue taken from tumors was HPV positive. HPV-16 was present in 90% of the HPV-positive tissues.[7] We now know that there is a survival advantage that patients with HPV-positive oropharyngeal cancer have over patients who develop cancer from other causes (ie, tobacco). HPV-positive tumors are more susceptible and vulnerable to the radiation treatments than their tobacco-induced counterparts. It is possible that in the future, clinical trials will be conducted that will establish some different treatment protocol for HPV-positive oral cancers (see article elsewhere in this issue by Pringle).[7–10]

CLINICAL ASSESSMENT

Clinicians must perform a comprehensive history and physical examination on every patient. The standard of care examination includes not only thorough examination of every intraoral mucosal surface but the extraoral head and neck tissues, including lymph nodes, as well[15] (described in detail later; also see http://www.dentalce.umn.edu/OralCancerVideo/home.html).

The detection of any abnormal finding requires further investigation contingent on the nature of the abnormality and the experience of the clinician. Regardless of ability, the clinician has an obligation to inform the patient, in terms they understand, about the nature of an abnormal examination finding and management recommendations. Any persistent and progressive epithelial lesion without any identifiable cause should raise suspicion and must be evaluated to rule out premalignant or malignant changes.[11–15]

SIGNS AND SYMPTOMS

Oral cancers and premalignant oral lesions can have variable clinical presentations.[11–15] At one end of the disease spectrum, the signs and symptoms of advanced cancers are generally ominous. Such cancers are often large, grossly exophytic, or deeply ulcerated, they show induration, they bleed easily on slight provocation, and have metastasized to regional lymph nodes, which is associated with palpable lymphadenopathy (**Fig. 3**: advanced oral cancer). Because the cancer has infiltrated deeper structures, including nerves, muscles, and even bone, patients may experience

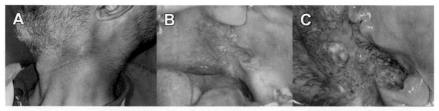

Fig. 3. Stage IV (T2N2bM0) squamous cell carcinoma of the left retromolar trigone. (*A*) shows left sided lymphadenopathy (palpation reveals no tenderness and the nodes are firm and non-moveable (fixed)). (*B* and *C*) show the primary site. The area is painful to touch, palpably firm (induration), appears as a friable mixed red and white lesion with ulceration and a rolled border anteriorly.

significant pain, have difficulty chewing, swallowing, or even speaking. At the other end of the disease spectrum, early cancers and premalignant oral lesions have more subtle signs and often do not elicit any detectable symptoms.[11–15] Their early detection is contingent on a careful visual and tactile examination, in which the clinician must interpret the features of an abnormal examination finding(s), such as lesion color, lesion number and size, lesion topography or morphology, or evidence of induration suggesting submucosal infiltration (in the case of a malignancy), to assess the risk of suspicion for lesions with malignant potential.[6,11–15,26]

Most epithelial lesions are benign, and many may be diagnosed based on their clinical features alone, without the need for further investigation. Frictional keratoses (white lesions caused by chronic low-grade friction to the mucosa) are commonly encountered, and if the putative frictional source is removed (eg, smoothing off a sharp tooth), such lesions should show signs of resolution in 2 to 3 weeks.[35,36]

For those epithelial lesions for which the clinician cannot ascertain the cause, and there is suspicion for malignancy, further investigation is warranted, such as a biopsy with histopathologic examination. The decision of referring a patient to a specialist for biopsy of a lesion that turns out to be benign versus not referring a patient with a lesion that turns out to be an early cancer can be difficult, particularly for clinicians with minimal experience in mucosal pathology.[6,10–15,26,27,31–35,37,38]

The term potentially malignant disorders (PMDs) has been ascribed to epithelial lesions for which there is no apparent cause and therefore should undergo further evaluation to rule out malignancy or precancer.[11,12,14,15,28,39–46] The terms leukoplakia (see **Fig. 2**), erythroplakia, and erythroleukoplakia (see **Fig. 3**; **Fig. 4**) are attributed to PMDs as clinical diagnoses for white patches that cannot be wiped off, red patches, or mixed red/white patches (respectively) for which there is no apparent cause and for which histopathologic examination is required to rule out malignancy or precancer.[11,12,14,15,28,39–46]

Lesions with a red component (ie, erythroplakia and erythroleukoplakia: **Fig. 4**) are more likely to represent malignancy or precancer than a white-only lesion (leukoplakia), although there are exceptions. In addition to lesion color, other clinical features are important. Large lesions (>2 cm in diameter) or multifocal lesions should heighten suspicion. Proliferative verrucous leukoplakia (PVL) is a clinical term describing patients with multifocal PMDs who have a high risk for malignant transformation.[15,47] In terms of topography and morphology, PMDs can present as homogeneous and relatively

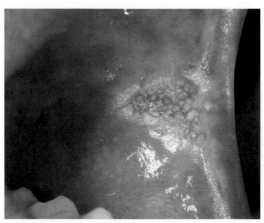

Fig. 4. Erythroleukoplakia of the left anterior buccal mucosa. The lesion is soft to palpation and has a specked appearance. Biopsy revealed moderate epithelial dysplasia.

flat, plaquelike lesions (generally these are white), to nonhomogeneous and thicker lesions with variable topography described as fissured, granular, nodular, or even verrucous or wartlike (such lesions may be white or mixed red-white lesions).[14,28,39–43] Ulceration is defined as a loss of epithelium and may be commensurate with PMDs as a sign of malignancy or in conjunction with high-grade dysplastic lesions (see section on dysplasia), in which the epithelium is lost after local trauma. Ulcers may present alone, or with mixed red-white PMDs. Other clinical features include the presence of induration, an ominous feature associated with palpable firmness associated with submucosal extension, and friability, a feature associated with abnormal bleeding on slight provocation, suggestive of increased angiogenesis.[14,28,39–43]

It is important for clinicians to be aware that although patients with small early stage cancers are often asymptomatic, the presence of pain is not predicated on tumor size and a mass effect on local nerves, but rather likely to be related to sensitization of nerves secondary to the release of pain mediators from the cancer. The pain may be elicited only during oral function (a mechanical allodynia) or when palpating the lesion. Spontaneous pain is also possible and predicts a higher likelihood of metastatic spread.[14,28,39–45]

Clinicians must also recognize that patients can initially present complaining of a swelling in the neck, which represents lymph node metastasis, yet the primary cancer site may be completely asymptomatic. Generally, when there is lymphadenopathy associated with metastatic spread from an oral cavity primary cancer, the cancer is usually visualized during the examination. However, with the recent increase in the number of HPV-associated oropharyngeal cancers, tonsillar primary cancers can be small, asymptomatic, and may not be visualized during the examination or on imaging by CT or MRI (hence the term unknown primary).[48]

The following are clinical diagnoses/common presenting signs of PMDs or oral carcinoma[14,28,39–45]:

- Leukoplakia: white patches of questionable risk having excluded (other) known diseases or disorders that carry no increased risk for cancer; a homogeneous leukoplakia tends to be smooth, uniformly thin and consistent in whiteness, often with shallow fissure; a nonhomogeneous leukoplakia tends to have surface texture and has variable thickness (see **Fig. 2**)
- Erythroplakia: a fiery red patch that cannot be characterized clinically as any other definable disease
- Erythroleukoplakia: a mixed red and white patch that cannot be characterized clinically as any other definable disease (see **Fig. 4**)
- Ulceration or erosion that cannot be characterized clinically as any other definable disease; ulceration may be solitary or part of a white, red or mixed red/white patch
- Induration: mucosal firmness or hardness caused by submucosal infiltration of a carcinoma
- Fixation: invasion of carcinoma into deeper tissues
- Chronicity/persistence: failure of lesions to heal; cancer is not a spontaneously reversible disease; therefore, a malignant lesion normally does not disappear in the absence of definitive antitumor therapy
- Lymphadenopathy: enlargement of regional nodes caused by metastatic spread of neoplastic cells through lymphatic vessels; nodes are usually painless and often become fixed because of capsular erosion and local infiltration; tumors that involve marked induration, fixation, and lymphadenopathy are signs of advanced cancer

It is critical for clinicians to remember that if their clinical impression of a lesion is benign and they treat the lesion empirically (eg, smooth off a sharp cusp in the case of a lesion with possible frictional/traumatic cause), they must closely follow the patient to resolution. Typically, in the early stages, oral carcinomas may appear as small, innocuous, harmless, minor mucosal changes, to which the unsuspecting clinician may not aggressively respond. An extended period beyond 2 to 3 weeks of watching and empirical treatments may allow the lesion to expand and potentially metastasize.[14,28,39–45]

ERYTHROLEUKOPLAKIA AND ERYTHROPLAKIA

Lesions with an erythematous or red component (erythroleukoplakia) are more likely to undergo dysplastic or malignant epithelial changes than leukoplakia.[15,21,22,25,28,43,44] Because red lesions without a white component may also represent either dysplasia or carcinoma, such lesions must be carefully evaluated (see **Fig. 4**). Carcinogenic progression in patients with erythroleukoplakia have been shown to be almost 4-fold that of patients with homogeneous leukoplakia.[6] Therefore, all patients with chronic white or red lesions, whether treated or not, should have periodic diagnostic biopsies. In a representative study of 257 patients, 58% of the patients with leukoplakia had an associated erythematous area, whereas 84% of the patients who developed a carcinoma showed a red component. Other studies have confirmed this association.[15,21,22,25,28,43,44]

Clinicians should take biopsy specimens that include erythematous areas, because of the increased risk of representing dysplasia or neoplasia.[15,21,22,25,28,43,44]

In Mashberg and Samit's prospective study[29] of 222 asymptomatic oral carcinomas, 28% were red only; 62% were red and white; 97% occurred in the mouth floor, oral tongue, and oropharynx; and 84% were less than 2 cm at their largest diameter.

ERYTHROPLAKIA WITH ULCERATION

Another rare but high-risk premalignant lesion is the chronic erythematous change associated with constantly recurring erosive changes. These lesions are often mistaken for recurrent aphthous stomatitis of the herpetiform variety or nonspecific inflammatory immunopathologic vesiculoerosive disease.[15,25,28,29]

PVL

Silverman and colleagues[47] first described a unique form of leukoplakia found in 30 patients. This group of lesions has a high risk of malignant transformation. The name PVL is because of the characteristic appearance: an expanding, exophytic/fissured white lesion (**Fig. 5**):

(1) PVL is a very high-risk precancerous condition with high transformation and mortality, (2) women are affected more than men, (3) less than one-third of PVL patients smoke, and (4) there is usually multisite oral involvement (see **Fig. 5**).[47]

CANDIDIASIS (CANDIDOSIS), LEUKOPLAKIA, AND ERYTHROPLAKIA

Some studies indicate that candidiasis may add a potential risk factor for malignant transformation of leukoplakia. As much as 53% of the patients with leukoplakia who developed carcinomas were *Candida* positive before tumor formation.[14] Other reports have shown a higher prevalence of *Candida* in speckled leukoplakia compared with homogeneous (all-white) leukoplakia.[14,44]

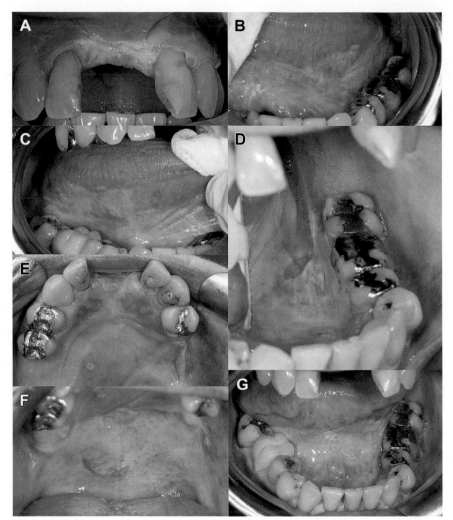

Fig. 5. Proliferative verrucous leukoplakia in a 75 year old female with no classic risk factors and history of a verrucous carcinoma of the left palate. Note the multifocal white and red changes. Biopsy reveals mild to moderate epithelial dysplasia with verrucous hyperplasia.

DELAY IN DIAGNOSIS

The failure of affected patients to seek professional consultation accounts for much of the delay in the diagnosis of oral cancer. However, in many cases, diagnosis has been delayed because a clinician did not suspect the malignant nature of the lesion and failed to further evaluate it.[11,14,15,24,28,39,48]

In a retrospective study, Rhodus and Haws (2003)[49] found that only 14.1% of dentists who had diagnosed a patient with epithelial dysplasia (considered premalignant) followed that lesion with a second biopsy during a 3-year period.

Furthermore, this study indicated that most patients who had been diagnosed with biopsy-proven epithelial dysplasia were not aware that the lesion, although currently benign, could transform into cancer and that they should be monitored.[49]

Most reports show that patients usually delay seeking professional advice for more than 3 months after having become aware of an oral sign or symptom.[12,15,45] Such delays in diagnosis can only lead to local extension of a lesion and increase the risk of metastatic spread of the cancer.[12,15,45]

ORAL CARCINOGENESIS, EPITHELIAL DYSPLASIA, AND MALIGNANT TRANSFORMATION

An insight into carcinogenesis highlighting progression from the earliest cellular changes through to carcinoma in terms of histopathology and genomics may provide the clinician with a deeper understanding of clinical signs and symptoms. Current scientific consensus is that this oral carcinogenesis occurs in a stepwise fashion hallmarked by an accumulation of genetic mutations sufficient for malignant transformation. Such genetic mutations predict changes in the normal maturation of keratinocytes, by affecting the control of the cell cycle, apoptosis, and terminal differentiation.[12,14,15,44,45,50–57]

Such changes are manifested in the epithelial architecture as a transition from normal stratified squamous histology to epithelial dysplasia, and then to invasive SCC. The term epithelial dysplasia is a histopathologic diagnosis rendered when cells with atypical morphology are detected within the epithelium. Dysplastic lesions are graded by severity as mild, moderate, or severe dysplasia or carcinoma in situ. Carcinogenesis is neither linear nor predictable, and it may occur over a variable period; sometimes, malignant transformation can take decades.[12,14,15,44,45,50–57]

In oral epithelial tissues, accumulating mutations (ie, genetic progression), chromosomal damage, and loss of cellular control functions are observed during the course of sequential histologic changes, which culminate in oral cancer.[12,14,15,44,45,50–57] These changes are manifested as the transition from normal histology to early intraepithelial dysplasia and preneoplasia, through increasingly severe intraepithelial neoplasia to superficial cancer and invasive disease.[12,14,15,44,45,50–57] Although the carcinogenic process can be aggressive (eg, in the presence of a DNA repair-deficient genotype or viral transformant such as HPV), these changes generally occur over a long period, usually decades.[7–9,12,14,15,44,45,50–57]

Carcinogenesis is characterized by progressive loss of proliferation and apoptosis controls and increasing cellular disorganization, aneusomy (DNA content), and heterogeneity.[12,14,15,44,45,50–57] The appearance of specific molecular and more general genotypic damage is associated with increasingly severe dysplastic phenotypes. In many cases, crucial early steps include inactivation of tumor suppressor genes (eg, mutation of p53 gene) or activation of oncogenes (eg, *ras*). Carcinogenesis may follow multiple paths and be multifocal; not all cancers in a given tissue nor all cells in a given cancer may contain the same blend of genetic and epigenetic changes. Progression to cancer may also be influenced by factors specific to the host's tissue environment.[12,14,15,44,45,50–57]

Field cancerization refers to the development of tumors at multiple sites in the oral cavity.[52–54] Slaughter and colleagues[52] described this phenomenon on evaluation of dysplastic epithelium adjacent to invasive tumors in head and neck cancers, leading to an increased development of second primary tumors. The tumors were initially believed to develop from independent clonal cells; however, other studies have also shown that these clones would be related to the primary tumors.[52–54] These multifocal clonal cell nests may be a consequence of prolonged exposure to carcinogens, making it challenging to treat SCCs of the head and neck.

MOLECULAR PROGRESSION

The hallmarks of cancer and the novel molecular events that a tumor needs to develop to sustain itself are insensitivity to inhibitors of growth, self-sufficiency in growth signals, unlimited replicative potential, ability to initiate angiogenesis, evasion of programmed cell death, and tissue invasion and metastasis.[6,14,15,26–28] Each of these specific events can lead to transformed cells that have undergone specific genetic alterations in proto-oncogenes or tumor suppressor genes.[6,14,15,26–28] In 1 example, loss of chromosomal region 9p21 is a common genetic change, which occurs early in tumor progression.[14] This situation leads to an inhibition of cyclin-dependent kinase, which is important in cell cycle regulation. In addition, many malignant cells express a mutation of the suppressor p53 gene, which, in turn, diminishes cell senescence and indirectly promotes growth.[6,14,15,55] Activation of proto-oncogenes or loss of tumor suppressor genes can result in the stimulation of cell division.[6,14,15,55] As another phenomenon, telomeres, composed of repeating sequences of 6 nucleotides, are situated at the end of chromosomes. They influence the longevity of cells and regulate their biological clock by progressive shortening. When activated by telomerase, telomere growth may prevent cell senescence by maintaining chromosomal integrity. Thus, telomeres may be a potentially important target in controlling cancer. The complexity and multifactorial aspects of explaining neoplasia are evident.[6,14,15,55]

Once the diagnosis of dysplasia is made, it is difficult to determine which dysplasias will transform into carcinoma. It may be safely assumed that severe epithelial dysplasia will most likely proceed to carcinoma in situ, intraepithelial carcinoma, or frank malignancy over time.[6,14,15,55]

When the dysplasia of the entire epithelium involves disruption of the basal lamina and subsequent invasion of the adjacent connective tissue, the diagnosis of malignancy is certain.[6,14,15,55] There are several investigations under way aimed at identifying reliable and useful biomarkers to aid in detecting this transformation as early as possible.[55–67]

GENOMICS AND PROTEOMICS

Many studies are presently being conducted regarding the role of chromosomes and genes in influencing the development and progression of oral leukoplakia to malignancy. DNA microarray studies of gene expression are being used to determine the differential profile of genes that are expressed in both oral cancer as well as precancerous (leukoplakia) lesions.[6,14,57,58] Ginos and colleagues[57] at the University of Minnesota have found that although there were 2891 genes that were differentially expressed in tissues of patients with oral cancer, there are several categories of genes, including those involved in the host immune response, angiogenesis, apoptosis, and cell differentiation. There have been several subsequent reports reviewing the pathways that are dysregulated in the progression of head and neck SCCs. Over the last decade, epithelial-mesenchymal progression has been another process that has been emerging in the progression of SCCs and provides some insight in the biological behavior of the tumors and resistance to adjuvant therapies.[6,50,51,66–68]

A study by Bradley and colleagues[68] from the University of Toronto showed that there was a direct risk association between chromosome ploidy and progression to malignancy. Abnormal DNA content was a significant predictor of progression to carcinoma, with a hazard ratio of 3.3 (95% confidence interval, 1.5–7.4) in their study. Despite this finding, a total of 8% of epithelial dysplasia progressed to carcinomas after 6 to 131 months.

Over the past few years, proteomics-based identification of biomarkers in SCCs of various specimens like tissue, serum, and saliva has advanced significantly.[59,62,66] A recent study compared oral premalignant leukoplakia with normal controls using both brush biopsy and saliva and found a correlation between both samples, giving light to noninvasive methodology for biomarker identification. Furthermore, the study also showed proteins hnRNPM, IL 1F6, LCN2, S100A8 and NQO1 overexpression compared with controls.[66] Other studies have shown novel proteins like fibrinogen chains, haptoglobin, RSK-2, and leucine-rich α_2 glycoproteins to be overexpressed in tumor specimens compared with controls.[67]

PRECANCEROUS CLASSIFICATION (PMDS)

By the definition that there exists a risk of transforming to carcinoma, oral leukoplakia is a premalignant lesion. This conclusion is based on the following: (1) many oral carcinomas have been associated with leukoplakic changes and (2) in prospective studies, occurrences of malignant transformations in oral leukoplakias exceed the number of oral cancers expected in the general population. The incidence of malignant transformations in oral leukoplakias ranges from approximately 5% to 17%.[12,15,28,33,69] Most longitudinal studies of patients with oral leukoplakia focus on habits, dysplastic and malignant transformations, and classification. However, the possibility of spontaneous regression of oral leukoplakia has been confirmed in several reports.[12,15,28,33,69]

The following conclusions regarding the clinical recognition and diagnosis of oral leukoplakia, the development of epithelial dysplasia, and subsequent malignant transformation, may be made:

1. In oral leukoplakia, the occurrence and time of dysplastic changes are uncertain. De novo transformation from hyperkeratosis to carcinoma may occur without recognizable dysplasia.
2. An erythematous component and discomfort should raise suspicion of dysplastic or malignant transformation.
3. Because epithelial dysplasia increases the risk of development of a malignant tumor, surgical removal (laser therapy or cryotherapy) of moderate or severe dysplastic lesions is usually performed currently. However, this is controversial, because no prospective randomized controlled trial has ever been proved with a control/placebo arm per the Cochrane Database of Systematic Reviews. The investigators concluded that there is no effective treatment in preventing the malignant transformation of leukoplakia.[70]
4. Proliferative verrucous forms of leukoplakia have a high risk of dysplasia and malignant transformation and should be treated aggressively.
5. Although the severity of the degrees of dysplasia has clinical significance regarding neoplasia, patients with mild dysplasia, or even without, should be followed carefully. This advice holds true even after surgical intervention, because recurrences are common.
6. Reproducible interexaminer agreements in diagnosing oral epithelial dysplasia are difficult to achieve, adding to the confusion regarding treatment approaches and aggressiveness.

Therefore, the development of biological markers (eg, monoclonal antibodies, DNA/RNA probes, special stains) emerges as extremely important, and even critical, in producing fundamental advancements in the diagnosis, prognosis, and treatment parameters of precancerous lesions.[12,22,28,49-68]

DIAGNOSIS AND MANAGEMENT

The current gold standard for the diagnosis of PMDs is tissue biopsy followed by his-topathologic diagnosis.[11,15,28,43,49,67]

INCISIONAL AND EXCISIONAL SCALPEL OR PUNCH BIOPSY

An incisional biopsy is one in which a representative sample is taken from within a lesion, leaving residual lesion tissue, in contrast to an excisional biopsy, in which the entire lesion is removed and submitted for histopathologic analysis. The decision to use a punch device or scalpel is based on clinician preference, and it is the selection of biopsy site or sites that requires expertise. Large, heterogeneous-appearing PMDs may have variable histopathology, and it is therefore important to select biopsy sites for representative disease. Patients with multifocal disease (ie, those with PVL or with field cancerization) present a similar challenge. Sites with induration, redness, or ulceration are generally indicated for incisional biopsy. In leukoplakias, areas with heterogeneous surface topography are more likely to show more severe disease. The use of toluidine blue staining can also facilitate biopsy site selection (see later discussion). Depth of biopsy can be important when there is tissue invasion, because depth is an important factor for the management of patients with malignancies.[12,15,28,69]

DIAGNOSTIC ADJUNCTIVE TECHNIQUES

There are simple, reliable, and acceptable noninvasive adjunctive diagnostic techniques (which do not replace the tissue biopsy) available in the marketplace to support the health professional's clinical judgment. The indication for such techniques may also include the monitoring of lesions in high-risk surveillance populations (ie, patients with a history of cancer or epithelial dysplasia).[68,71–82]

CYTOLOGY AND BRUSH BIOPSY

Oral cytology is a diagnostic technique by which epithelial cells (ideally including cells from throughout the layers of the epithelium) are obtained from a lesion and then analyzed by various methods. The entire oral cavity is lined with stratified squamous epithelium, which varies in thickness and keratinization according to anatomic and functional sites.[71] Specially designed brushes are used to obtain representative samples, and various processing and analytical techniques may be used. These techniques include plating and fixing samples on a glass slide followed by different staining techniques (to highlight cytoplasmic or nuclear components) and conventional microscopic examination; liquid-based techniques, in which cell samples are cytospun onto a glass slide as a monolayer, stained and analyzed microscopically using sophisticated image analysis techniques to assess cytomorphologic changes; immunostaining for various biomarkers; and analysis by flow cytometry.[71] Many of these techniques are not approved for clinical use and remain in the purview of research investigation. Two commercially available techniques, the Oral CDX Brush Test (CDX Laboratories, New York, NY), and more recently the Oral Advance System (PMI Labs, Vancouver, Canada) have been compared in clinical studies with the conventional tissue biopsy and histopathologic diagnosis. The Oral CDX Brush Test is based on a sample procured with a brush, the sample plated and fixed on a glass slide by the clinician, sent to the laboratory (along with the brush tip containing residual cells), where the samples are stained with a modified Papanicolaou stain and microscopically analyzed using a neural network software platform, which facilitates the identification of cells with atypical morphology. A cytopathologist renders a diagnosis: negative, atypical, or positive. The accuracy of the Oral CDX brush biopsy test has been reported in several studies with sensitivity and specificity for detecting dysplasia or SCC antigen (SCCA) ranging from 71% to 100% and 27% to 94%, respectively.[71] Several of these studies had flaws in methodology, and in those in which a PMD was brush and tissue biopsied simultaneously, including a recent study,[77] Oral CDX had a sensitivity and specificity higher than 90%. The OralAdvance system is also based on a cell sample procured by a brush, which is then placed into a fixative and sent to a central laboratory, where the sample is cytospun on to a slide and undergoes Feulgen staining (a nuclear stain) and microscopic evaluation of cellular DNA content using a sophisticated image analysis software. A cytopathologist interprets the sample to determine if there is abnormal DNA content (ie cells in which there has been a gross nuclear change [aneuploidy] that deviates from the normal diploid state, and which is consistent with dysplasia or SCCA). The accuracy of this platform has recently been validated in a small trial, showing a sensitivity and specificity for detecting high-grade dysplasia and SCCA of 89% and 97%, respectively, and the presence of aneuploidy may be a predictive marker for malignant transformation.[68,71,77]

Classification of benign oral diseases from cytologic studies is not yet possible, and there is a possibility of false-positive results from benign inflammatory lesions, in which cellular atypia is possible. False-negative results may be minimized if these cyto-pathologic techniques are used on small and relatively flat epithelial lesions, in which a representative sample may be adequately procured by a single brush. It must be emphasized, therefore, that these techniques are not indicated for obvious cancerous or highly suspicious lesions, because they do not yield a histopathologic diagnosis and, therefore, could cause an unnecessary delay in definitive diagnosis and treatment.[71,76]

FINE-NEEDLE ASPIRATION

Fine-needle aspiration (FNA) biopsy is a highly acceptable and accurate technique for differentiating benign from metastatic lymphadenopathy. Use of this minimally invasive technique accelerates diagnosis and treatment and improves overall management. This cytopathologic technique also has greatly aided the evaluation of major salivary gland neoplasms. Thus, FNA biopsy is a safe, quick, and reliable procedure that can immediately differentiate inflammatory, reactive, cystic, and neoplastic processes.[72]

TOLUIDINE BLUE

Vital staining with toluidine blue is an adjunctive technique that can facilitate the diagnostic process by helping to differentiate more severe disease (high-grade dysplastic lesions and SCCA) from benign lesions, and for biopsy site selection in a large hetero-geneous lesion with variable histopathology. Toluidine blue is a metachromatic dye that binds to free anionic groups such as nucleic acids.[73,74] Studies exploring the accuracy of toluidine blue for detection of dysplastic lesions and SCCA show a broad range of 56% to 67% sensitivity and 57% to 81% specificity.[73,74] Its accuracy improves with worsening disease, with a greater than 90% sensitivity in patients with SCCA. Both false-positive and false-negative staining are possible, and clinician experience is important (**Fig. 6**).

VISUALIZATION-BASED ADJUNCTIVE TECHNIQUES

Mucosal tissues undergoing abnormal metabolic or structural changes have different absorbance/reflectance profiles when exposed to various forms of light or

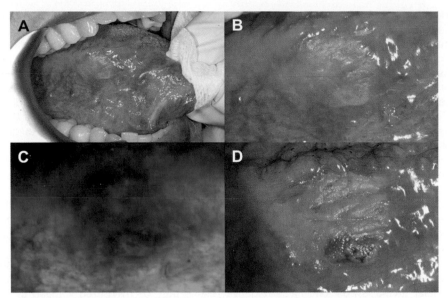

Fig. 6. (*A–D*) Small leukoplakia of the right lateral tongue. The lesion is soft to palpation. The bottom left image shows a loss of tissue autofluorescence. An excisional biopsy revealed a focus of carcinoma in situ (CIS) where the lesion picked up the toluidine blue stain (*D*).

energy.[78–82] Techniques such as optical coherence tomography, narrow-band imaging, high-resolution microendoscopy, and devices to detect changes in tissue autofluorescence have been purported to be able to detect PMDs. Few of these techniques have been tested in clinical trials comparing their performance with histopathologic end points. An autofluorescence device (VELScope system (LED Dental, White Rock, Canada)) showed a range in sensitivity from 50% to 86% (ie, ability to detect a truly positive outcome) and a 15% to 30% specificity (ie, ability to detect a truly negative/benign outcome) for detecting dysplasia or SCCA (see **Fig. 6**).[68,79] Both false-positive and false-negative results are possible, and clinician experience is important.

MONOCLONAL ANTIBODIES

Some monoclonal antibodies for use in the detection of oral cancer have been developed, studied, and reported.[53,56,57,79–82] However, the techniques have not yet been perfected, and there are questions regarding specificity, which have limited large studies and use in diagnostic laboratories. No matter which diagnostic technique is used, the possibility of a false-negative response exists. The development of monoclonal antibodies that have high sensitivity and specificity for epithelial dysplastic and malignant cells would enhance accuracy of diagnosis in some cases, in which the usual or typical cellular characteristics of precancer or cancer are not apparent. Numerous biomarkers now being developed and studied will yield additional information regarding cellular neoplastic potential and even the risks of metastases.[79–82]

IMAGING

Most commonly, neoplasms of the oral cavity and oropharynx are discovered by clinical examination and confirmed by biopsy or FNA. Imaging studies may then be used to map the extent of disease, detect bone invasion and cervical adenopathy, and evaluate adherence of tumor to the carotid artery.[83–85] Occasionally, a patient may present with cervical nodal metastases without a clinically evident primary lesion. In this setting, cross-sectional imaging obtained before panendoscopy and biopsy is useful to locate submucosal tumor and direct biopsies to possible targets. The detection of recurrent disease after therapy may also be facilitated by cross-sectional imaging.[83,85] The advanced imaging techniques presently available include CT, MRI, and PET. Ultrasonography, often in conjunction with FNA biopsy, may also be useful.[83,85]

CHEMOPREVENTION

It has been shown that pharmacologic intervention with agents like retinoids prevents the progression of precancerous lesions to frank carcinoma in primary leukoplakia and in secondary malignancies.[86–96] 13-Cis-retinoic acid has been shown to reverse oral leukoplakia, although relapse rates on discontinuation are high. There is considerable concern over the toxicity of some particular retinoids used in these trials, and patients receiving certain agents have a dropout rate of up to 10%/y secondary to toxicity.[86–96] In addition, patients who have received previous chemotherapy and have hepatic disease have been excluded from these trials. There is a reasonably high likelihood that a patient who has head and neck cancer may have either or both of these exclusion criteria. Because the duration of delivery for chemopreventive agents for head and neck cancer has not been determined, the use of compounds with unacceptable long-term adverse toxicity profiles is questionable.[86–96]

Chemoprevention of Oral Leukoplakia Remains Experimental

However, because of the high potential of effectively treating oral leukoplakia, multiple clinical trials are under way, with several potentially effective chemoprevention agents, such as ketorolac, celecoxib, and pioglitozone.[91–96]

WORKUP FOR PATIENTS WITH ORAL SCCS

The standard workup for patients with biopsy-proven SCCs usually includes imaging of the chest, head and neck CT, and HPV testing is also recommended, according to the National Comprehensive Cancer Network (NCCN) guidelines.[38]

A PET/CT scan from the head to the thighs is not recommended according to the NCCN guidelines; however, it is rapidly becoming a standard of care in the workup for a patient with SCC of the head and neck to rule out distant disease. A skull base to the thoracic inlet CT with contrast or an MRI with gadolinium is recommended to rule out any neck disease.[38,71]

TREATMENT

Long-term survival and functional results of treatment depend on the stage of the tumor, histology, and treatment plan. The treatment plan is often developed by multidisciplinary consultants and subsequent patient/family concurrence. Additional important outcome factors include the patient's nutritional status, general health, tobacco use, alcohol intake, and anticipated compliance with the rigors of therapy.[38,83–85,97–102]

Curative treatment modalities include local surgery with wide margins and radiation or a combination of both. Chemotherapy may be used with these modalities to enhance cure rates and to preserve function, which increasingly has led to organ preservation strategies. If there is high risk of morbidity and mortality, the choice may be to use measures to ensure palliation only, with pain control and quality of life.[38,83–85,97–102]

Head and neck surgeons, radiation oncologists, dentists, and rehabilitation specialists are all involved cooperatively in the treatment process. The side effects of treatment are often permanent and diminish oral function. Treatment planning is based on careful cancer staging and selection of therapies, which allows for prognostication and facilitates the reporting of outcomes. Physical examination, open biopsy, or FNA biopsy, and radiologic imaging studies, which include CT, MRI, and PET, are used to classify and stage the disease and monitor for recurrence.[38,83–85]

Most of the major functional disabilities after treatment are related to the volume of the disease, the degree of radiation or chemotherapy required for treatment, which relates to the postoperative complications, including the extent of mandible (or other tissues) loss, reduction of tongue mobility, caries and loss of dentition, xerostomia, muscle trismus, diminished taste and mastication, risk of osteoradionecrosis, and anesthesia of the oral cavity. To achieve a cure, the treatment plan considers an adequate resection of tumor and surrounding normal tissue and the addition of the lymphatic drainage and attempts to preserve as much normal anatomy and physiology as possible.[38,97,98]

FOLLOW-UP

Because many methods of managing leukoplakia are not always feasible or effective, these patients must be observed periodically.[11,12,15] The follow-up examination should be frequent (<6 months), depending on the diagnosis and clinical scenario. The follow-up examination includes careful clinical observation and biopsy, as indicated (when changes in signs or symptoms occur). These changes may be subtle.[11,12,15] Exfoliative cytology using the brush biopsy technique and vital staining with toluidine blue help supplement clinical judgment and serve as an adjunct to incisional biopsy. Because the gold standard for diagnosis is tissue biopsy with histopathologic examination, the value of adjunctive techniques is to accelerate microscopic evaluation by indicating the need of biopsy in situations in which a biopsy is delayed or not believed to be indicated or necessary. Negative smears or stains must be balanced with good clinical judgment. Therefore, if clinical suspicion persists in a lesion that does not disappear, a standard scalpel biopsy must be considered.[15,28,68,76]

Self-examinations are usually encouraged for patients, and the patients are generally followed up on a 3-month to 6-month basis for early premalignant lesions (mild to severe epithelial dysplasia). More frequent follow-ups are recommended for severe dysplasia and carcinoma in situ.[6,15,26–28,32,33,37]

SCC of the head and neck follow-up guidelines are based on the NCCN recommendations. These guidelines are based on the risk of relapse, second primaries, treatment sequelae, and toxicities. A comprehensive examination is recommended every 1 to 3 months for the first year, every 2 to 6 months for the second year, every 4 to 8 months for years 3 to 5, and every 12 months after 5 years.[6,15,26–28,32,33,37,65] Additional, follow-up management involves obtaining imaging within 6 months of treatment. Further imaging is recommended based on symptoms to rule out any recurrences or second primaries. Smoking cessation education and alcohol counseling are recommended for pertinent patients.[6,15,26–28,32,33,37,65]

REFERENCES

1. American Cancer Society. Cancer facts & figures 2013. Atlanta (GA): American Cancer Society; 2013.

2. Siegel R, Ward E, Brawley O, et al. Cancer statistics, 2011. CA Cancer J Clin 2011;61(4):212–5.
3. Ries LA, Eisner MP, Kosary CL, et al. SEER cancer statistics review, 1975-2000. Bethesda (MD): National Cancer Institute; 2003.
4. Shiboski CH, Shiboski SC, Silverman S Jr. Trends in oral cancer rates in the United States, 1973-1996. Community Dent Oral Epidemiol 2000;28:249–56.
5. Warnakulasuriya S. Global epidemiology of oral and oropharyngeal cancer. Oral Oncol 2009;45:309–16.
6. Forastiere A, Koch W, Trotti A, et al. Head and neck cancer. N Engl J Med 2001; 345:1890–900.
7. Gillison ML, Koch WM, Capone RB, et al. Evidence of a causal association between human papilloma virus and a subset of head and neck cancers. J Natl Cancer Inst 2000;92(9):709–20.
8. Miller CS, Johnstone BM. Human papillomavirus as a risk factor for oral squamous cell carcinoma: a meta-analysis, 1982-1997. Oral Surg Oral Med Oral Pathol Oral Radiol Endod 2001;91:622–35.
9. Lee SY, Cho NH, Choi EC, et al. Relevance of human papilloma virus (HPV) infection to carcinogenesis or oral tongue cancer. Int J Oral Maxillofac Surg 2010;39(7):678–83.
10. Chaturvedi AK, Engels EA, Pfeiffer RM, et al. Human papillomavirus and rising oropharyngeal cancer incidence in the United States. J Clin Oncol 2011;29(32): 4294–301.
11. Silverman S Jr. Demographics and occurrence of oral and pharyngeal cancers: the outcomes, the trends, the challenge. J Am Dent Assoc 2001;132:7S–11S.
12. Silverman S, Gorsky M, Lozada F. Oral leukoplakia and malignant transformation. Cancer 1984;53:563–8.
13. Little JW, Falace DA, Miller CS, et al. Cancer. Dental management of the medically compromised patient. 8th edition. St Louis (MO): Mosby; 2012. p. 394–412.
14. Califano J, van der Riet P, Westra W, et al. Genetic progression model for head and neck cancer: implications for field cancerization. Cancer Res 1996;56(11): 2488–92.
15. Silverman S Jr. Oral cancer. 5th edition. Hamilton (ON), London: BC Decker; 2003. p. 1–128.
16. Ram H, Sarkar J, Kumar H, et al. Oral cancer: risk factors and molecular pathogenesis. J Maxillofac Oral Surg 2011;10(2):132–7.
17. Lewin F, Norell SE, Johansson H, et al. Smoking tobacco, oral snuff, and alcohol in the etiology of squamous cell carcinoma of the head and neck. Cancer 1998; 82:1367–75.
18. Mashberg A, Garfinkel L, Harris S. Alcohol as a primary risk factor in oral squamous cell carcinoma. CA Cancer J Clin 1981;31:146–55.
19. Gandini S, Negri E, Boffetta P, et al. Mouthwash and oral cancer risk–quantitative meta-analysis of epidemiologic studies. Ann Agric Environ Med 2012;19(2): 173–80.
20. Silverman S Jr, Gorsky M, Lozada-Nur F, et al. A prospective study of findings and management in 214 patients with oral lichen planus. Oral Surg Oral Med Oral Pathol 1991;72:665–70.
21. Silverman S Jr, Bahl S. Oral lichen planus update: clinic characteristics, treatment responses and malignant transformation. Am J Dent 1997;10:259–63.
22. Bombeccari GP, Guzzi G, Tettamanti M, et al. Oral lichen planus and malignant transformation: a longitudinal cohort study. Oral Surg Oral Med Oral Pathol Oral Radiol Endod 2011;112:328–34.

23. Petridou E, Zavras AI, Lefatzis D, et al. The role of diet and specific micronutrients in the etiology of oral carcinoma. Cancer 2002;94:2981–8.
24. Shillitoe EJ, Gilchrist E, Pellenz C, et al. Effects of herpes simplex virus on human oral cancer cells, and potential use of mutant viruses in therapy of oral cancer. Oral Oncol 1999;35:326–32.
25. Axell T, Pindborg JJ, Smith CJ, et al. Oral white lesions with special reference to precancerous and tobacco-related lesions: conclusions of an international symposium held in Uppsala, Sweden, May 18–21, 1994. J Oral Pathol Med 1996;25:49–54.
26. Hanahan D, Weinberg RA. Hallmarks of cancer: the next generation. Cell 2011; 144(5):646–74.
27. Hillbertz NS, Hirsch J, Jalouli J, et al. Viral and molecular aspects of oral cancer. Anticancer Res 2012;32:4201–12.
28. van der Waal I. Potentially malignant disorders of the oral and oropharyngeal mucosa; terminology, classification and present concepts of management. Oral Oncol 2009;45(4–5):317–23.
29. Mashberg A, Samit A. Early diagnosis of asymptomatic oral and oropharyngeal squamous cancers. CA Cancer J Clin 1995;45:328–51.
30. Zini A, Czerninski R, Sgan-Cohen HD. Oral cancer over four decades: epidemiology, trends, histology, and survival by anatomical sites. J Oral Pathol Med 2010;39:299–305.
31. Ganly I, Patel S, Shah J. Early stage squamous cell cancer of the oral tongue–clinicopathologic features affecting outcome. Cancer 2012;118(1):101–11.
32. Neville BW, Day TA. Oral cancer and precancerous lesions. CA Cancer J Clin 2002;52:195–215.
33. van der Waal I. Potentially malignant disorders of the oral and oropharyngeal mucosa; present concepts of management. Oral Oncol 2010;46:423–5.
34. Lodi GS, Bez C, Demarosi F, et al. Interventions for treating oral leukoplakia. Cochrane Database Syst Rev 2006;(4):CD001829.
35. Mehanna HM, Rattay T, Smith J, et al. Treatment and follow-up of oral dysplasia–a systematic review and meta-analysis. Head Neck 2008;31:1600–9.
36. Tilakaratne WM, Sherriff M, Morgan PR, et al. Grading oral epithelial dysplasia: analysis of individual features. J Oral Pathol Med 2011;40:533–40.
37. Devita VT Jr, Lawrence TS, Rosenberg SA, editors. Cancer principles and practice of oncology, vol. 1, 8th edition. Philadelphia: Lippincott Williams & Wilkins; 2008. p. 799–808.
38. NCCN clinical practice guidelines in oncology. Head and neck cancers V.I. 2009. National Comprehensive Cancer Network.
39. Warnakulasuriya S, Reibel J, Bouquot J, et al. Oral epithelial dysplasia classification systems: predictive value, utility, weaknesses and scope for improvement. J Oral Pathol Med 2008;37:127–33.
40. Kreimer AR, Clifford GM, Boyle P, et al. Human papillomavirus types in head and neck squamous cell carcinomas worldwide: a systematic review. Cancer Epidemiol Biomarkers Prev 2004;14(2):467–75.
41. Bouquot JE, Gorlin RJ. Leukoplakia, lichen planus, and other oral keratoses in 23,616 white Americans over the age of 35 years. Oral Surg Oral Med Oral Pathol 1986;61(4):373–81.
42. Warnakulasuriya S, Johnson NW, van der Waal I. Nomenclature and classification of potentially malignant disorders of the oral mucosa. J Oral Pathol Med 2007;36(10):575–80.
43. Warnakulasuriya S, Kovacevic T, Madden P, et al. Factors predicting malignant transformation in oral potentially malignant disorders among patients accrued

over a 10-year period in South East England. J Oral Pathol Med 2011;40: 677–83.

44. Lee JJ, Hong WK, Hittelman WN, et al. Predicting cancer development in oral leukoplakia: ten years of translational research. Clin Cancer Res 2000;6: 1702–10.

45. Schepman KP, van der Meij EH, Smeele LE, et al. Malignant transformation of oral leukoplakia: a follow-up study of a hospital-based population of 166 patients with oral leukoplakia from the Netherlands. Oral Oncol 1998;34: 270–5.

46. Lam DK, Schmidt BL. Orofacial pain onset predicts transition to head and neck cancer. Pain 2011;152(5):1206–9.

47. Silverman S Jr, Gorsky M. Proliferative verrucous leukoplakia. A follow-up study of 54 cases. Oral Surg Oral Med Oral Pathol Oral Radiol Endod 1997;84: 154–7.

48. Zengel P, Assmann G, Mollenhauer M, et al. Cancer of unknown primary originating from oropharyngeal carcinomas are strongly correlated to HPV positivity. Virchows Arch 2012;461(3):283–90.

49. Rhodus NL, Haws J, Ondrey F. A follow-up study of 285 oral epithelial dysplastic lesions in Minnesota. Dent Clin North Am 2005;49(1):143–65.

50. Stransky N, Egloff AM, Tward AD, et al. The mutational landscape of head and neck squamous cell carcinoma. Science 2011;333(6046):1157–60.

51. Krisanaprakornkit S, Iamaroon A. Epithelial-mesenchymal transition in oral squamous cell carcinoma. ISRN Oncol 2012;2012:681469, 1–10.

52. Slaughter DP, Southwick HW, Smejkal W. "Field cancerization" in oral stratified squamous epithelium. Cancer 1953;6:963–8.

53. Bedi GC, Westra WH, Gabrielson E, et al. Multiple head and neck cancer tumors: evidence for a common clonal origin. Cancer Res 1996;56:2484–7.

54. Braakhuis BJ, Tabor MP, Kummer JA, et al. A genetic explanation of Slaughter's concept of field cancerization: evidence and clinical implications. Cancer Res 2003;63:1727–30.

55. Boyle JO, Hakim J, Koch W, et al. The incidence of p53 mutations increases with progression of head and neck cancer. Cancer Res 1993;53(19):4477–80.

56. Barnes L, Eveson J, Reichart P, et al. World Health Organization classification of tumors. Pathology and genetics of tumors of the head and neck. Lyon (France): IARC Press; 2008.

57. Ginos MA, Page GP, Michalowicz BS, et al. Identification of a gene expression signature associated with recurrent disease in squamous cell carcinoma of the head and neck. J Canc Res 2003;62(2):111–23.

58. Sudbo J, Kildal W, Risberg B, et al. DNA content as a prognostic marker in patients with oral leukoplakia. N Engl J Med 2001;344:1270–80.

59. Rhodus NL, Ho V, Myers SL, et al. NFkB dependent cytokines in saliva of patients with premalignant lesions and squamous cell carcinoma. Cancer Detect Prev 2005;29(1):42–7.

60. Kelloff GJ, Sigman CC, Johnson KM, et al. Perspectives on surrogate end-points in the development of drugs that reduce the risk of cancer. Cancer Epidemiol Biomarkers Prev 2000;9:127–34.

61. Ondrey FG, Dong G, Van Waes C. Constitutive expression of AP-1 and NF IL-6 in squamous carcinoma of the head and neck. Proc Am Assoc Canc Res 1998; 39:3081.

62. Smith CW, Chen Z, Dong G, et al. The host environment promotes the development of primary and metastatic squamous cell carcinomas that constitutively

express pro-inflammatory cytokines IL-1 alpha, IL-6, GM-CSF, and KC. Clin Exp Metastasis 1998;16(7):655–71.

63. Dong G, Loukinova E, Smith CW, et al. Genes differentially expressed with malignant transformation and metastatic tumor progression of murine squamous cell carcinoma. J Cell Biochem Suppl 1997;28–29:90–100.

64. Van Waes C, Chen Z, Ondrey FG, et al. Cytokines in the immune pathogenesis and therapy of head and neck cancer. Head Neck 1998;20(5):153.

65. Boone CW, Kelloff GJ. Biomarker end-points in cancer chemoprevention trials. In: Toniolo P, Boffetta P, Shuker DE, et al, editors. Application of biomarkers in cancer epidemiology (IARC Scientific Publications No. 142). Lyon (France): IARC; 1997. p. 273–80.

66. Kooren JA, Rhodus NL, Griffin TJ, et al. Evaluating the potential of a novel oral lesion exudate collection method coupled with mass spectrometry-based proteomics for oral cancer biomarker study. Clin Proteomics 2011;8(13):1–11.

67. Tung CL, Lin S, Chou H, et al. Proteomics-based identification of plasma biomarkers in oral squamous cell carcinoma. J Pharm Biomed Anal 2013; 75:7–17.

68. Bradley G, Odell EW, Raphael S, et al. Abnormal DNA content in oral epithelial dysplasia is associated with increased risk of progression to carcinoma. Cancer 2010;103(9):1432–9.

69. Liu W, Bao ZX, Shi LJ, et al. Malignant transformation of oral epithelial dysplasia: clinicopathological risk factors and outcome analysis in a retrospective cohort of 138 cases. Histopathology 2011;59:733–40.

70. Christian DC. Computer-assisted analysis of oral brush biopsies at an oral cancer screening program. J Am Dent Assoc 2002;133:357–62.

71. Mehrotra R, Mishra S, Singh M, et al. The efficacy of oral brush biopsy with computer-assisted analysis in identifying precancerous and cancerous lesions. Head Neck Oncol 2011;3:39.

72. Scher RL, Oostingh PE, Levine PA, et al. Role of fine-needle aspiration biopsy in the diagnosis of lesions of the oral cavity, oropharynx, and nasopharynx. Cancer 1988;62:2602–6.

73. Portugal LC, Wilson KM, Biddinger PW, et al. The role of toluidine blue in assessing margin status after resection of squamous cell carcinomas of the upper aerodigestive tract. Arch Otolaryngol Head Neck Surg 1996;122:517–9.

74. Warnakulasuriya KA, Johnson NW. Sensitivity and specificity of OraScan toluidine blue mouthrinse in the detection of oral cancer and precancer. J Oral Pathol Med 1996;25:97–103.

75. Mehrotra R, Hullmann M, Smeets R, et al. Oral cytology revisited. J Oral Pathol Med 2009;38(2):161–6.

76. Patton LL, Epstein JB, Kerr AR. Adjunctive techniques for oral cancer examination and lesion diagnosis: a systematic review of the literature. J Am Dent Assoc 2008;139(7):896–905 [quiz: 93–4].

77. Ng SP, Mann IS, Zed C, et al. The use of quantitative cytology in identifying high-risk oral lesions in community practice. Oral Surg Oral Med Oral Pathol Oral Radiol 2012;114(3):358–64.

78. Cancela-Rodriguez P, Cerero-Lapiedra R, Esparza-Gomez G, et al. The use of toluidine blue in the detection of pre-malignant and malignant oral lesions. J Oral Pathol Med 2011;40(4):300–4.

79. Rahman F, Tippu SR, Khandelwal S, et al. A study to evaluate the efficacy of toluidine blue and cytology in detecting oral cancer and dysplastic lesions. Quintessence Int 2012;43(1):51–9.

80. Awan KH, Yang YH, Morgan PR, et al. Utility of toluidine blue as a diagnostic adjunct in the detection of potentially malignant disorders of the oral cavity–a clinical and histological assessment. Oral Dis 2012;18(8):728–33.
81. Mehrotra R, Singh M, Thomas S, et al. A cross-sectional study evaluating chemiluminescence and autofluorescence in the detection of clinically innocuous precancerous and cancerous oral lesions. J Am Dent Assoc 2010;141(2):151–6.
82. Awan KH, Morgan PR, Warnakulasuriya S. Evaluation of an autofluorescence based imaging system (VELscopeTM) in the detection of oral potentially malignant disorders and benign keratoses. Oral Oncol 2011;47(4):274–7.
83. Curtin HD, Ishwaran H, Mancuso AA, et al. Comparison of CT and MR imaging in staging of neck metastases. Radiology 1998;207:123–30.
84. Braams JW, Pruim J, Freling NJ, et al. Detection of lymph node metastases of squamous cell cancer of the head and neck with FDG-PET and MRI. J Nucl Med 1995;36:211–6.
85. Schaefer SD, Maravilla KR, Suss RA, et al. Magnetic resonance imaging vs. computed tomography. Comparison in imaging oral cavity and pharyngeal carcinomas. Arch Otolaryngol 1985;111:730–4.
86. Lippman SM, Lee JS, Lotan R, et al. Biomarkers as intermediate end points in chemoprevention trials. J Natl Cancer Inst 1990;82:555–60.
87. Benner SE, Pajak TF, Lippman SM, et al. Prevention of second primary tumors with 13cRA in squamous cell carcinoma of the head and neck: long term follow-up. J Natl Cancer Inst 1994;86:140–1.
88. Kelloff GJ. Perspectives on cancer chemoprevention research and drug development. Adv Cancer Res 2000;278:199–334.
89. Lippman SM, Spitz M, Zoltan T, et al. Epidemiology, biology, and chemoprevention of aerodigestive cancer. Cancer 1994;74:2719–25.
90. Tanaka T, Tanake M, Tanaka T. Oral carcinogenesis and oral cancer chemoprevention: a review. Patholog Res Int 2011;2011:431246, 1–10.
91. Ribeiro AS, Salles PR, da Silva TA, et al. A review of the nonsurgical treatment of oral leukoplakia. Int J Dent 2010;2010:186018.
92. Lippman SM, Benner SE, Hong WK. Cancer chemoprevention. J Clin Oncol 1994;12:851–73.
93. Lippman SM, Batsakis JG, Toth BB, et al. Comparison of low-dose 13cRA with beta carotene to prevent oral carcinogenesis. N Engl J Med 1993;328:15–20.
94. Hong WK, Sporn MB. Recent advances in chemoprevention of cancer. Science 1997;278:1073–7.
95. Sporn MB, Suh N. Chemoprevention of cancer. Carcinogenesis 2000;21:525–30.
96. Rhodus NL, Rohrer M, Pambuccian S, et al. Phase 11A chemoprevention clinical trial of pioglitozone for the treatment of oral leukoplakia. J Dent Res 2011; 91(3):191 [abstract 2241].
97. Krakoff IH. Systemic treatment of cancer. CA Cancer J Clin 1996;46:134–41.
98. Schuchter LM, Hensley ML, Meropol NJ, et al. 2002 update of recommendations for the use of chemotherapy and radiotherapy protectants: clinical practice guidelines of the American Society of Clinical Oncology. J Clin Oncol 2002; 20:2895–903.
99. Puthawala A, Nisar Syed AM, Gamie S, et al. Interstitial low-dose- rate brachytherapy as a salvage treatment for recurrent head-and-neck cancers: long-term results. Int J Radiat Oncol Biol Phys 2001;5:354–62.
100. Fu KK, Pajak TF, Trotti A, et al. A Radiation Therapy Oncology Group (RTOG) phase III randomized study to compare hyperfractionation and two variants of accelerated fractionation to standard fractionation radiotherapy for head and

neck squamous cell carcinomas: first report of RTOG 9003. Int J Radiat Oncol Biol Phys 2000;48:7–16.

101. Kramer AM. The role of chemotherapy in head and neck malignancy. Oral Maxillofac Surg Clin 1993;5:303–17.

102. Merlano M, Vitale V, Rosso R, et al. Treatment of advanced squamous cell carcinoma of the head and neck with alternating chemotherapy and radiotherapy. N Engl J Med 1992;327:1115–7.

Chemotherapy or Radiation-Induced Oral Mucositis

Rajesh V. Lalla, DDS, PhD, CCRP[a],*, Deborah P. Saunders, BSc, DMD[b],
Douglas E. Peterson, DMD, PhD, FDS RCSEd[a]

KEYWORDS

- Oral mucositis • Stomatitis • Cancer • Chemotherapy • Radiation therapy

KEY POINTS

- Oral mucositis is a significant toxicity of systemic chemotherapy and of radiation therapy to the head and neck region.
- The morbidity of oral mucositis can include pain, nutritional compromise, impact on quality of life, alteration in cancer therapy, risk for infection, and economic costs.
- Management includes general symptomatic support and targeted therapeutic interventions for the prevention or treatment of oral mucositis.
- Evidence-based clinical practice guidelines are available to guide clinicians in the selection of effective management strategies.

INTRODUCTION, EPIDEMIOLOGY, AND PATHOGENESIS

An estimated 1.6 million people receive cancer therapy in the United States each year and worldwide numbers are much higher.[1] Although advancements in cancer therapy improved survival rates for many tumor types, these treatments also cause several side-effects, including some in the oral cavity. One of the more significant oral complications of cancer therapy is oral mucositis, which refers to inflamed erosive or ulcerative lesions of the oral mucosa. Oral mucositis can result from systemic chemotherapy, from radiation therapy (RT) to the oral mucosa, or a combination thereof. It affects approximately 20% to 40% of patients receiving conventional chemotherapy regimens for solid tumors, depending on the dose and cytotoxicity of the drug.[2] In patients receiving very high doses of chemotherapy before a hematopoietic stem cell transplant (HSCT), oral mucositis is seen in about 80%.[3] Almost all patients receiving therapeutic radiation for head and neck (H&N) cancer will develop oral

[a] Section of Oral Medicine, University of Connecticut Health Center, 263 Farmington Avenue, Farmington, CT 06030-1605, USA; [b] Department of Dental Oncology, Northeast Cancer Centre, Health Sciences North, Northern Ontario School of Medicine, 41 Ramsey Lake Road, Sudbury, ON P3E 5J1, Canada
* Corresponding author. MC1605 UConn Health Center, 263 Farmington Avenue, Farmington, CT 06030-1605.
E-mail address: Lalla@uchc.edu

Dent Clin N Am 58 (2014) 341–349
http://dx.doi.org/10.1016/j.cden.2013.12.005
0011-8532/14/$ – see front matter © 2014 Elsevier Inc. All rights reserved.

dental.theclinics.com

mucositis.[4] Collectively in the United States, it is estimated that about 400,000 patients suffer from oral mucositis each year.[5]

Historically, mucositis was thought to result only from damage to basal epithelial cells due to chemotherapy or RT. It is now understood that the pathogenesis is much more complex and involves the generation of damaging reactive oxygen species, activation of transcription factors such as nuclear factor-κB and inflammatory pathways such as the cyclooxygenase pathway, and the upregulation of proinflammatory cytokines such as tumor necrosis factor (TNF)-α and interleukin (IL)-1β.[6] The various factors involved have been integrated into a five-step pathogenesis model (**Fig. 1**).[7]

MORBIDITY OF ORAL MUCOSITIS
Pain

The primary morbidity of oral mucositis is the intense pain usually associated with ulcerative lesions. Most patients with ulcerative mucositis need systemic opioids for pain management. In one study, a 1-point increase in peak mucositis scores in patients with HSCT was associated with 2.6 additional days of injectable narcotic therapy.[8] Systemic opioids have several side-effects, including risk of dependence, altered mental state, and constipation.

Nutritional Compromise

Because of the pain, patients with severe oral mucositis may be unable to continue eating by mouth. Therefore, they are fed intravenously via total parenteral nutrition (TPN) or through a gastrostomy tube. A 1-point increase in peak mucositis scores in HSCT patients was associated with 2.7 additional days of TPN.[8] Patients who have H&N cancer with oral mucositis are significantly more likely to have weight loss of 5% or more.[9] Impaired nutrition affects healing and resistance to infection, and leads to a general failure to thrive.

Quality of Life

The pain and nutritional compromise adversely affects quality of life. This is especially prominent in patients receiving H&N RT[10] and in patients receiving high-dose chemotherapy for HSCT.[11] Patients undergoing HSCT report oral mucositis as the most debilitating complication of transplantation.[11]

Impact on Cancer Therapy

Severe mucositis can necessitate undesirable dose reductions or interruptions in cancer therapy. In patients receiving chemotherapy for solid tumors or lymphoma, a reduction in the next dose of chemotherapy was twice as common after cycles with mucositis than after cycles without mucositis.[12] Eleven percent of patients receiving RT for H&N cancer had unplanned breaks in RT because of severe mucositis.[13] Such modifications in cancer therapy can negatively affect cancer prognosis.

Infection

Ulcerative oral mucositis is colonized by oral microflora and is sometimes complicated by local infection such as herpes simplex virus (HSV) infection and candidiasis. In patients who are immunosuppressed due to chemotherapy, these ulcerative lesions can provide a route for systemic sepsis, which is potentially life threatening.[14–16] For example, in patients receiving conventional chemotherapy for solid tumors or lymphoma, the rate of infection during cycles with mucositis was more than twice that of cycles without mucositis and was proportional to its severity.[12] Infection-related

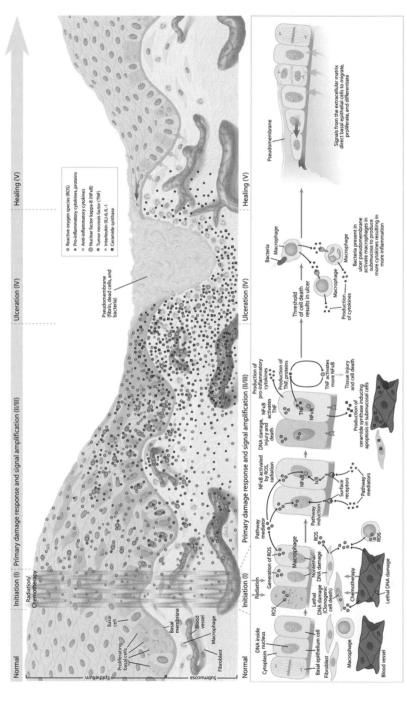

Fig. 1. The five-stage model for the pathobiology of oral mucositis developed by Dr Stephen T. Sonis. The model incorporates a complex interaction among multiple components. These include direct damage to basal epithelial cells from cancer therapy and secondary insult to tissues due to upregulation of proinflammatory factors and products of colonizing microflora. (*From* Sonis ST. Pathobiology of oral mucositis: novel insights and opportunities. J Support Oncol 2007;5:3–11.)

deaths were more common during cycles with mucositis. In patients receiving high-dose chemotherapy for HSCT, moderate to severe oral mucositis has been correlated with systemic infection and transplant-related mortality.[17] Increased severity of oral mucositis has been associated with increased incidence of significant infection, number of days with fever, and a 3.9-fold increase in 100-day mortality risk.[3]

Impact on Oral Health

Patients with painful oral mucositis may have difficulty carrying out routine oral hygiene measures such as brushing and flossing. In addition, transient or permanent hyposalivation is a frequent finding in patients receiving cancer therapy.[18] In combination, these factors can increase the risk of dental caries and periodontal disease. Furthermore, as mentioned above, lesions of oral mucositis can be secondarily infected with oral candidiasis or HSV, in the setting of possible immunosuppression. Thus, oral mucositis has a significant negative impact on oral and dental health.

Economic Impact

Oral mucositis results in increased costs associated with pain management, TPN or gastrostomy tubes with liquid diet supplements, secondary infections, and hospitalizations. In patients receiving H&N RT, oral mucositis was associated with an increase in costs ranging from $1700 to $6000 per patient, depending on severity of mucositis.[9] In patients receiving conventional dose chemotherapy for solid tumors, average duration of hospitalization was significantly longer for cycles with mucositis and cost of hospitalization was 60% higher in cycles with oral mucositis.[12] In patients receiving high-dose chemotherapy for HSCT, increased severity of oral mucositis was associated with increased time in hospital, and increased total inpatient charges.[3] A single-point increase in oral mucositis severity was associated with 2.6 additional days in hospital and more than $25,000 in additional hospital charges.[8]

CLINICAL FINDINGS

Diagnosis of oral mucositis is usually made clinically, based on clinical appearance and a history of cytotoxic cancer therapy within the expected timeframe. It initially presents as erythema of the oral mucosa, which often progresses to erosion and frank ulceration. The ulcerations are typically covered by a pseudomembrane (**Fig. 2**). The nonkeratinized mucosa is more often affected. Chemotherapy-induced oral mucositis

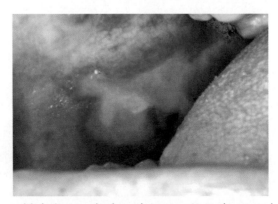

Fig. 2. An oral mucositis lesion on the buccal mucosa. Note the central area of ulceration covered by a white pseudomembrane, surrounded by an erythematous erosive area.

presents 7 to 14 days after initiation of chemotherapy and typically heals within a few weeks after end of chemotherapy. In patients receiving the typical 6 to 7 week regimen of RT for H&N cancer, onset of oral mucositis occurs by the second or third week of RT, and the severity worsens with increasing dose of RT. The areas affected are defined by the field of radiation (**Fig. 3**). The duration typically extends for several weeks after the end of RT, depending on the size of the lesions. In cases in which the clinical appearance or duration is not consistent with mucositis, secondary infection or an alternative diagnosis should be considered. The most common clinically relevant secondary infections of oral mucositis lesions involve *Candida* species fungi[19] and HSV.[20] These are more likely to be seen in patients who are immunosuppressed due to chemotherapy or in patients with hyposalivation due to RT.

Several measurement scales are available for oral mucositis. The most commonly used scales for clinical practice are the World Health Organization (WHO) scale (**Box 1**) and the National Cancer Institute Common Terminology Criteria for Adverse Events (NCI-CTCAE) (**Box 2**).

MANAGEMENT OF ORAL MUCOSITIS

The goals of mucositis management are to prevent or reduce the severity of the toxicity and to manage the associated symptoms. This, in turn, will allow the continued delivery of cancer therapy without interruption or dose reduction, improving the overall prognosis. General symptom management and targeted therapeutic interventions are discussed in the context of evidence-based clinical practice guidelines developed by the Multinational Association of Supportive Care in Cancer/International Society of Oral Oncology (MASCC/ISOO). These guidelines include recommendations (based on higher level evidence), suggestions (based on lower level evidence), or a determination of "no guideline possible" in cases of inadequate or conflicting evidence.[21,22]

Symptom Management

Pain is the most prominent symptom of oral mucositis. Thus, pain control plays a central role in mucositis management. Many centers use a mouth rinse containing a topical anesthetic such as lidocaine, often in combination with other agents such as diphenhydramine, and a coating agent such as Maalox. Due to inadequate evidence, no MASCC/ISOO guideline was possible for such combination rinses. However, the

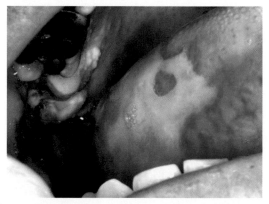

Fig. 3. A large oral mucositis lesion on the lateral tongue of a patient receiving RT for squamous cell carcinoma of the tongue.

Box 1
World Health Organization (WHO) scale for oral mucositis

Grade 0 = No oral mucositis

Grade 1 = Erythema and soreness

Grade 2 = Ulcers; able to eat solids

Grade 3 = Ulcers; requires liquid diet (due to mucositis)

Grade 4 = Ulcers; alimentation not possible (due to mucositis)

---

evidence did support suggestions in favor of 0.5% doxepin mouthwash and 2% morphine mouthwash in patients receiving RT for H&N cancer.[23]

Although such rinses can provide short-term relief, most patients also need systemic opioid analgesics for adequate pain control. In patients receiving conventional or high-dose chemotherapy, a suggestion in favor of transdermal fentanyl was possible. A recommendation in favor of patient-controlled analgesia with morphine was made for treating oral mucositis pain in patients undergoing HSCT.[23]

Several topical coating agents are marketed for oral mucositis, with the rationale that covering the ulcerated area will protect the nerve endings and reduce pain. Although there was inadequate evidence to formulate a guideline on any of the commercial agents, a large number of studies were reviewed related to sucralfate, which is a generically available coating agent. The evidence demonstrated a lack of efficacy for sucralfate and supported recommendations against its use for prevention or treatment of oral mucositis secondary to chemotherapy or RT.[23]

Maintenance of good oral hygiene is considered a good clinical practice and can be helpful in alleviating symptoms of oral mucositis. In addition, there is some evidence that maintaining good oral hygiene may reduce the severity of oral mucositis. Therefore, a suggestion was made in favor of using oral care protocols to prevent oral mucositis across all cancer treatment modalities.[24]

Severe oral mucositis can compromise oral intake. Such patients need nutritional support from a dietician, including advice on the use of a soft diet and/or liquid diet supplements. Hospitalized patients may be fed via TPN. A gastrostomy tube may be necessary in outpatients, such as patients receiving RT for H&N cancer.

Targeted Therapeutic Interventions

Cryotherapy

Oral cryotherapy, or oral cooling, involves the placement of ice chips in the mouth. It has been demonstrated that oral cryotherapy, during the administration of chemotherapy drugs with a short half-life, can reduce the severity of oral mucositis. The oral cooling causes vasoconstriction, which decreases the amount of chemotherapy

---

Box 2
NCI-CTCAE version 4 for oral mucositis

Grade 1: Asymptomatic or mild symptoms; intervention not indicated

Grade 2: Moderate pain not interfering with oral intake; modified diet indicated

Grade 3: Severe pain interfering with oral intake

Grade 4: Life-threatening consequences; urgent intervention indicated

Grade 5: Death

---

drug delivered to the oral mucosa. The MASCC/ISOO includes two guidelines in favor of cryotherapy: (1) a recommendation for 30 minutes of oral cryotherapy to prevent oral mucositis in patients receiving bolus 5-fluorouracil chemotherapy and (2) a suggestion for oral cryotherapy to prevent oral mucositis in patients receiving high-dose melphalan as conditioning for HSCT.[25]

Low-level laser therapy

Treatment of the oral mucosa with low-level laser therapy (LLLT) has been demonstrated to have an antiinflammatory effect and promote healing.[26,27] The MASCC/ISOO mucositis guidelines recommend the use of LLLT with a wavelength at 650 nm, power of 40 mW, and each square centimeter treated with the required time to a tissue energy dose of 2 J/cm^2 to prevent oral mucositis in patients receiving HSCT, conditioned with high-dose chemotherapy. A suggestion was also made for the use of LLLT (wavelength around 632.8 nm) to prevent oral mucositis in patients undergoing radiotherapy, without concomitant chemotherapy, for H&N cancer. No guideline was possible in relation to LLLT in other populations.[28]

Growth factors

Growth factors that promote epithelial proliferation can be beneficial in ulcerative oral mucositis. The only drug approved by the Food and Drug Administration for oral mucositis is palifermin, a recombinant human keratinocyte growth factor-1. The MASCC/ISOO guidelines include a recommendation for the use of intravenous palifermin to prevent oral mucositis in patients receiving high-dose chemotherapy and total body irradiation, followed by autologous stem cell transplantation, for a hematological malignancy.[29] On the other hand, granulocyte-macrophage colony stimulating factor was found not effective. Therefore, a suggestion was made against its use for prevention of oral mucositis in patients receiving high-dose chemotherapy for HSCT.[29]

Antiinflammatory agents

Because the inflammatory response to cancer therapy is thought to play an important role in the pathogenesis of oral mucositis, several antiinflammatory agents have been evaluated. Benzydamine is a nonsteroidal antiinflammatory drug that inhibits the production of proinflammatory cytokines, including TNF-α and IL-1β. Benzydamine also has topical analgesic and anesthetic effects. The MASCC/ISOO guidelines include a recommendation in favor of benzydamine mouthwash to prevent oral mucositis in patients with H&N cancer receiving moderate-dose radiotherapy (up to 50 Gy) without concomitant chemotherapy.[30] Benzydamine mouthwash is not commercially marketed in the United States but can be available from a compounding pharmacy. It is worth noting that most patients receiving definitive RT for H&N cancer receive greater than 50 Gy, often with concomitant chemotherapy. Due to lack of efficacy, a suggestion was developed against the use of misoprostol mouthwash (prostaglandin E1 analog) for prevention of oral mucositis in patients with H&N cancer receiving RT. No guideline was possible for any other antiinflammatory agent.[30]

Antimicrobial agents

Several antimicrobial agents have been tested for oral mucositis based on the rationale that secondary colonization of oral mucositis ulcerations may aggravate their severity. However, results of studies testing antimicrobial agents have been mostly disappointing. The MASCC/ISOO guidelines include a recommendation against the use of polymyxin, tobramycin, amphotericin B (PTA) lozenges and paste; or bacitracin, clotrimazole, and gentamicin (BCoG) lozenges for the prevention of oral mucositis in patients receiving RT for H&N cancer. In addition, a suggestion was made against the use of chlorhexidine mouthwash for mucositis prevention in the same population.[23] It should be noted that this, and all the other MASCC/ISOO mucositis guidelines, apply only to the use of the intervention for the prevention or treatment of mucositis (or mucositis-related pain). Thus, providers may choose to use chlorhexidine for other indications unrelated to mucositis, such as oral decontamination.

SUMMARY

Oral mucositis is a significant toxicity of systemic chemotherapy and of RT to the H&N region. The morbidity of oral mucositis can include pain, nutritional compromise, impact on quality of life, alteration in cancer therapy, risk for infection, and economic costs. Management includes general symptomatic support and targeted therapeutic interventions for the prevention or treatment of oral mucositis. Evidence-based clinical practice guidelines are available to guide clinicians in the selection of effective management strategies.

REFERENCES

1. National Cancer Institute. Surveillance, Epidemiology, and end results program. Online document [cited 4 November, 2013]. 2013. Available at: http://seer.cancer.gov. Accessed November 4, 2013.
2. Jones JA, Avritscher EB, Cooksley CD, et al. Epidemiology of treatment-associated mucosal injury after treatment with newer regimens for lymphoma, breast, lung, or colorectal cancer. Support Care Cancer 2006;14(6):505–15.
3. Vera-Llonch M, Oster G, Ford CM, et al. Oral mucositis and outcomes of allogeneic hematopoietic stem-cell transplantation in patients with hematologic malignancies. Support Care Cancer 2007;15(5):491–6.
4. Vera-Llonch M, Oster G, Hagiwara M, et al. Oral mucositis in patients undergoing radiation treatment for head and neck carcinoma. Cancer 2006;106(2):329–36.
5. Managing oral mucositis in patients with hematologic malignancies. J Support Oncol 2006;4(2):79.
6. Al-Dasooqi N, Sonis ST, Bowen JM, et al. Emerging evidence on the pathobiology of mucositis. Support Care Cancer 2013;21(7):2075–83.
7. Sonis ST. The pathobiology of mucositis. Nat Rev Cancer 2004;4(4):277–84.
8. Sonis ST, Oster G, Fuchs H, et al. Oral mucositis and the clinical and economic outcomes of hematopoietic stem-cell transplantation. J Clin Oncol 2001;19(8):2201–5.
9. Elting LS, Cooksley CD, Chambers MS, et al. Risk, outcomes, and costs of radiation-induced oral mucositis among patients with head-and-neck malignancies. Int J Radiat Oncol Biol Phys 2007;68(4):1110–20.
10. Duncan GG, Epstein JB, Tu D, et al. Quality of life, mucositis, and xerostomia from radiotherapy for head and neck cancers: a report from the NCIC CTG HN2 randomized trial of an antimicrobial lozenge to prevent mucositis. Head Neck 2005;27(5):421–8.
11. Bellm LA, Epstein JB, Rose-Ped A, et al. Patient reports of complications of bone marrow transplantation. Support Care Cancer 2000;8(1):33–9.
12. Elting LS, Cooksley C, Chambers M, et al. The burdens of cancer therapy. Clinical and economic outcomes of chemotherapy-induced mucositis. Cancer 2003;98(7):1531–9.
13. Trotti A, Bellm LA, Epstein JB, et al. Mucositis incidence, severity and associated outcomes in patients with head and neck cancer receiving radiotherapy with or without chemotherapy: a systematic literature review. Radiother Oncol 2003;66(3):253–62.

14. Westbrook SD, Kirkpatrick WR, Freytes CO, et al. *Candida krusei* sepsis secondary to oral colonization in a hemopoietic stem cell transplant recipient. Med Mycol 2007;45(2):187–90.
15. Redding SW, Marr KA, Kirkpatrick WR, et al. *Candida glabrata* sepsis secondary to oral colonization in bone marrow transplantation. Med Mycol 2004;42(5): 479–81.
16. Rapoport AP, Miller Watelet LF, Linder T, et al. Analysis of factors that correlate with mucositis in recipients of autologous and allogeneic stem-cell transplants. J Clin Oncol 1999;17(8):2446–53.
17. Ruescher TJ, Sodeifi A, Scrivani SJ, et al. The impact of mucositis on alpha-hemolytic streptococcal infection in patients undergoing autologous bone marrow transplantation for hematologic malignancies. Cancer 1998;82(11):2275–81.
18. Jensen SB, Pedersen AM, Vissink A, et al. A systematic review of salivary gland hypofunction and xerostomia induced by cancer therapies: prevalence, severity and impact on quality of life. Support Care Cancer 2010;18(8):1039–60.
19. Nicolatou-Galitis O, Velegraki A, Sotiropoulou-Lontou A, et al. Effect of fluconazole antifungal prophylaxis on oral mucositis in head and neck cancer patients receiving radiotherapy. Support Care Cancer 2006;14(1):44–51.
20. Schubert MM. Oral manifestations of viral infections in immunocompromised patients. Curr Opin Dent 1991;1(4):384–97.
21. Bowen JM, Elad S, Hutchins RD, et al. Methodology for the MASCC/ISOO Mucositis Clinical Practice Guidelines Update. Support Care Cancer 2013;21(1): 303–8.
22. Elad S, Bowen J, Zadik Y, et al. Development of the MASCC/ISOO Clinical Practice Guidelines for Mucositis: considerations underlying the process. Support Care Cancer 2013;21(1):309–12.
23. Saunders DP, Epstein JB, Elad S, et al. Systematic review of antimicrobials, mucosal coating agents, anesthetics, and analgesics for the management of oral mucositis in cancer patients. Support Care Cancer 2013;21(11):3191–207.
24. McGuire DB, Fulton JS, Park J, et al. Systematic review of basic oral care for the management of oral mucositis in cancer patients. Support Care Cancer 2013; 21(11):3165–77.
25. Peterson DE, Ohrn K, Bowen J, et al. Systematic review of oral cryotherapy for management of oral mucositis caused by cancer therapy. Support Care Cancer 2013;21(1):327–32.
26. Lopes NN, Plapler H, Chavantes MC, et al. Cyclooxygenase-2 and vascular endothelial growth factor expression in 5-fluorouracil-induced oral mucositis in hamsters: evaluation of two low-intensity laser protocols. Support Care Cancer 2009;17(11):1409–15.
27. Lopes NN, Plapler H, Lalla RV, et al. Effects of low-level laser therapy on collagen expression and neutrophil infiltrate in 5-fluorouracil-induced oral mucositis in hamsters. Lasers Surg Med 2010;42(6):546–52.
28. Migliorati C, Hewson I, Lalla RV, et al. Systematic review of laser and other light therapy for the management of oral mucositis in cancer patients. Support Care Cancer 2013;21(1):333–41.
29. Raber-Durlacher JE, von Bultzingslowen I, Logan RM, et al. Systematic review of cytokines and growth factors for the management of oral mucositis in cancer patients. Support Care Cancer 2013;21(1):343–55.
30. Nicolatou-Galitis O, Sarri T, Bowen J, et al. Systematic review of anti-inflammatory agents for the management of oral mucositis in cancer patients. Support Care Cancer 2013;21(11):3179–89.

Oral Graft-Versus-Host Disease

Michal Kuten-Shorrer, DMD[a], Sook-Bin Woo, DMD, MMSc[b],
Nathaniel S. Treister, DMD, DMSc[b],*

KEYWORDS

- Graft-versus-host disease • GVHD • Allogeneic • Hematopoietic cell transplantation
- Oral mucosal disease

KEY POINTS

- Allogeneic hematopoietic cell transplantation (allo-HCT) is used for the treatment of a variety of disorders, primarily hematologic malignancies.
- Graft-versus-host disease (GVHD) is a significant complication following allo-HCT and a major cause of morbidity and mortality.
- The oral cavity is frequently involved in GVHD, leading to pain, functional impairment, and reduced quality of life.
- Early diagnosis, management, and long-term follow-up of oral GVHD are important components of overall patient care.

INTRODUCTION

Allogeneic hematopoietic cell transplantation (allo-HCT) is considered to be a curative treatment of many hematologic malignancies as well as for a wide range of hematologic and immune deficiency states and immune diseases.[1] Graft-versus-host disease (GVHD, **Box 1**), an immunologically mediated disease, is a major cause of morbidity and mortality after allo-HCT and the most significant barrier to treatment success.[2]

In 1966, Billingham[3] outlined the 3 fundamental requirements for GVHD. First, the graft must contain immunologically competent cells; second, the host must express tissue antigens that seem foreign to the graft; and finally, the host must be incapable of rejecting the donor graft.[3,4] As stipulated in the third precondition, recipients undergo myelosuppressive and immunosuppressive regimens before allo-HCT, reducing the risk of graft rejection.[1,5] After transplantation, donor-derived immunocompetent T lymphocytes may react against histocompatibility antigens on the recipient cells and induce immune responses, resulting in recipient tissue damage.[5,6]

Disclosure: None.
[a] Department of Oral Medicine, Infection, and Immunity, Harvard School of Dental Medicine, 188 Longwood Avenue, Boston, MA 02115, USA; [b] Division of Oral Medicine and Dentistry, Brigham and Women's Hospital, 1620 Tremont Street, 3rd Floor, Boston, MA 02115, USA
* Corresponding author.
E-mail address: ntreister@partners.org

Dent Clin N Am 58 (2014) 351–368
http://dx.doi.org/10.1016/j.cden.2013.12.007
0011-8532/14/$ – see front matter © 2014 Elsevier Inc. All rights reserved.

> **Box 1**
> **What is GVHD?**
>
> A clinical syndrome that results from an immunologic attack by donor immunocompetent T cells on patient tissues, directly or through exaggerated inflammatory responses, following allogeneic HCT

The major risk factor for GVHD development is human leukocyte antigens (HLA) disparity.[4,5] HLAs are expressed on the cell surfaces of all nucleated cells in the body and are encoded by the major histocompatibility complex (MHC) located on the short arm of chromosome 6. If incompatible with the recipient, the donor's immune cells mount an alloimmune response against antigens on the recipient cells leading to GVHD. Careful matching of donor and recipient HLA reduces the risk for GVHD (as in sibling HLA-matched grafts). The current guidelines recommend high-resolution DNA-matching (ie, indicating that the donor and recipient express identical alleles) for the following 4 HLA loci in order to maximize post-HCT survival: HLA-A, -B, -C, and -DRB1 (8/8 match).[7,8] Ideally, unrelated donors should be genotypically identical to the recipients at all HLA loci; however, finding the ideal match is often extremely challenging in light of the millions of potential haplotypes existing.[4] Furthermore, despite selection of an HLA-matched donor, T lymphocyte reaction may still be elicited by minor histocompatibility antigens encoded by non-MHC loci, contributing to GVHD development.[4,9] Other important factors determining GVHD development and severity are listed in **Box 2**.[2]

Along with the increase in morbidity and mortality, GVHD is also associated with a reduced incidence of malignancy relapse due to the graft-versus-tumor (GVT) effect.[1,10] It is thought that this is mediated by donor T lymphocytes that recognize tumor antigens and elicit antitumor responses.[1] Successful transplantation results from carefully balancing GVT effects against chronic GVHD (cGVHD). Overtreatment of cGVHD may adversely impact malignancy relapse rates, whereas too robust a GVT effect, such as that achieved by donor lymphocyte infusion (DLI) for patients who relapse after HCT, may induce severe GVHD with its attendant morbidities.[6,11]

PATHOBIOLOGY AND INCIDENCE OF GVHD

Traditionally, GVHD has been classified as either acute (aGVHD) or chronic according to the time of clinical onset after transplantation.[6,12] Any GVHD manifestations before day +100 after transplantation were defined as aGVHD, and any manifestations present after day +100 were defined as cGVHD.[12,13] Recently, however, it has been accepted that acute and chronic GVHD represent a clinical continuum with distinct clinical features and underlying pathophysiologic mechanisms.[6] aGVHD is

> **Box 2**
> **Factors influencing the risk of GVHD**
>
> - Donor/recipient sex mismatch (especially female donors to male recipients)
> - Increasing recipient age
> - Choice of progenitor cells source
> - Pretransplantation manipulations and graft composition
> - Intensity of conditioning regimen

characterized by strong inflammatory features, whereas cGVHD displays more auto-immune and fibrotic characteristics (**Table 1**).[1] The current consensus, therefore, is that aGVHD and cGVHD should be differentiated according to clinical manifestations and pathologic features rather than merely the time of onset after transplantation.[6,12] The National Institutes of Health (NIH) Consensus Development Project on Criteria for Clinical Trials in cGVHD has further defined 2 subcategories for both aGVHD and cGVHD.[12] Acute GVHD can be classic, occurring within 100 days after HCT, or persistent, recurrent, or late when occurring beyond day +100 after HCT (for example, in cases of nonmyeloablative conditioning).[14] Similarly, cGVHD can be either classic (ie, without concomitant features or characteristics of aGVHD) or can manifest in an overlap syndrome with features of both cGVHD and aGVHD occurring simultaneously as can be seen in patients receiving DLI.[12]

aGVHD

The pathobiology of aGVHD is considered to be a 3-step process, starting with tissue damage induced by the pretransplantation conditioning regimen, followed by donor-derived T lymphocyte activation and clonal expansion, and ultimately tissue destruction induced by immune and inflammatory responses in the effector step.[5] In the first

Table 1
Classic features of aGVHD and cGVHD

Organ or Site	aGVHD[a]	cGVHD[b]
Skin	Erythema Maculopapular rash Pruritus	Poikiloderma Lichen planus–like features Sclerotic and morphealike features
Oral	Gingivitis Mucositis Erythema Pain	Lichen planus features Hyperkeratotic plaques Restriction of mouth opening from sclerosis
GI tract	Anorexia Nausea Vomiting Diarrhea Weight loss	Esophageal web Strictures or stenosis in the upper to mid third of the esophagus
Genitalia		Lichen planus–like features Vaginal scarring or stenosis
Liver	Total bilirubin, alkaline phosphatase >2 times upper limit of normal ALT or AST >2 times upper limit of normal	
Lung		Bronchiolitis obliterans
Muscles, joints		Fasciitis Joint stiffness or contractures secondary to sclerosis

Abbreviations: ALT, alanine aminotransferase; AST, aspartate aminotransferase; GI, gastrointestinal.
  [a] Manifestations that can also be found in cGVHD.
  [b] Diagnostic features. These features are sufficient to establish the diagnosis of cGVHD.
Data from Filipovich AH, Weisdorf D, Pavletic S, et al. National Institutes of Health consensus development project on criteria for clinical trials in chronic graft-versus-host disease: I. Diagnosis and staging working group report. Biol Blood Marrow Transplant 2005;11(12):945–56.

step, the conditioning regimen, comprised of chemotherapy, radiation therapy, and/or immunosuppressive medications, induces tissue damage and subsequent activation of patient antigen presenting cells (APCs). In the second step, APCs present the patients' alloantigens to donor-derived T lymphocytes, leading to their activation characterized by a primarily T-helper 1 (Th1) response. In step 3, the effector T lymphocytes, along with natural killer cells, macrophages, and proinflammatory cytokines, inflict direct tissue damage, as well as indirect damage, through intense inflammatory responses associated with the massive cytokine production, known as the *cytokine storm*.[1,4,5]

The incidence of aGVHD varies with relation to several immunologically based factors, primarily the degree of donor-recipient histocompatibility (**Table 2**).[15] The primary target organs of aGVHD are the skin, the liver, and the gastrointestinal (GI) tract. Other organs may also be involved, including the oral cavity.[16,17] The severity of overall aGVHD is graded from I to IV by combining each of the 3 target organs' clinical stage of involvement.[18] The grade of aGVHD has long been known to correlate with overall survival, with the best survival for patients with grade I disease.[19] This correlation was demonstrated by the Chronic Leukemia Working Party of the European Group for Bone Marrow Transplantation, who reported transplant-related mortality rates for grades I to IV aGVHD to be 27%, 43%, 68%, and 92%, respectively, in 1294 patients after allo-HCT for chronic myeloid leukemia.[20]

cGVHD

The mechanisms underlying cGVHD are not well understood. Two basic theories for the pathobiology of cGVHD have been proposed.[4,21] According to the first theory, cGVHD is simply an end-stage alloreactivity in which donor T lymphocytes have differentiated toward a Th2 phenotype, associated with B-cell activation and autoantibody production.[22] The second theory suggests that cGVHD is the outcome of poor/dysfunctional immunologic recovery after HCT, involving altered peripheral mechanisms of tolerance and decreased negative selection related to impaired thymic function, resulting in an increase in peripheral autoreactive T lymphocytes that generate further activation of effector functions (cytokine secretion, cytolytic activity, and antibody production).[1,2,4] Although the association of cGVHD with altered B-cell homeostasis is well established, the exact role of B lymphocytes in the pathogenesis of GVHD remains unknown.[1,23,24] In the clinical setting, reduction of alloreactive B lymphocytes responses using rituximab, a CD20-specific monoclonal antibody, can be effective in the treatment of cGVHD.[23,25]

Three patterns of cGVHD onset have been identified: (1) de novo onset, without prior aGVHD; (2) quiescent onset, following a recovery period without any GVHD manifestations (postresolution of aGVHD); and (3) progressive onset, with cGVHD directly following aGVHD.[26,27] The manifestations of cGVHD may be limited to one organ or widespread and most frequently involve the skin, eyes, oral cavity, GI tract, liver,

Table 2 Incidence of aGVHD according to histocompatibility		
	Matched (%)	Mismatched (%)
Related	20–50	75–80
Unrelated	70	80–90

Data from Goker H, Haznedaroglu IC, Chao NJ. Acute graft-vs-host disease: pathobiology and management. Exp Hematol 2001;29(3):259–77.

and lungs.[12,28] With reported incidence rates ranging from 25% to 80% in long-term survivors, cGVHD is the most common late complication following allo-HCT and the leading cause of nonrelapse mortality.[2,28,29] The incidence and severity of cGVHD are correlated with multiple factors, including HLA disparity, increasing recipient age, sex mismatch, and source of progenitor cells (see **Box 2**).[12,28] However, the most important risk factor for cGVHD development is the diagnosis of previous aGVHD.[30]

ORAL GVHD
Incidence

Although not a classic target organ of aGVHD, oral manifestations may be encountered, clinically presenting as mucosal erythema, ulcerations, and painful desquamative lesions.[17] Because these manifestations are nonspecific, oral aGVHD may be mistaken for or obscured by several other conditions, including conditioning-induced mucositis and herpes simplex virus (HSV) infection.[11,17] However, because aGVHD typically develops well after engraftment and resolution of mucositis, and acyclovir prophylaxis is highly effective in preventing reactivation of HSV, these entities can be readily differentiated.[31] The incidence of oral aGVHD is unknown but is thought to be exceedingly rare. In contrast, the oral cavity is one of the most frequently affected sites in cGVHD, with more than 70% of patients who develop cGVHD demonstrating oral involvement.[32,33]

Clinical Findings

As mentioned earlier, oral manifestations of aGVHD are predominated by erythema and ulcerations but can also present as lichen planus–like hyperkeratotic lesions, likely in the context of overlap syndrome.[11] Lip involvement with crusting is also a common feature, similar to that seen in patients with erythema multiforme (**Fig. 1**).

The diverse spectrum of oral cGVHD manifestations can be classified into 3 distinct groups, according to the main sites and anatomic structures involved: oral mucosal disease, salivary gland disease, and sclerotic disease.[17,33,34]

Oral mucosal cGVHD is characterized by lichenoid inflammation that frequently involves the tongue and buccal mucosa but can affect any site in the oral cavity and can range from limited disease with only mild changes to more extensive and symptomatic disease. Clinical changes include white papules, plaques, and hyperkeratotic

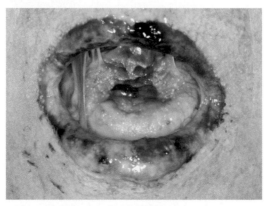

Fig. 1. Oral aGVHD with prominent crusting of lips.

reticulations resembling Wickham striae in oral lichen planus, erythema, and pseudo-membranous ulcerations (**Fig. 2**).[11,33,34] The symptom most often associated with oral mucosal cGVHD is sensitivity to otherwise normally tolerated items, such as spicy, acidic, or rough (crunchy) foods and drinks as well as mint and strongly flavored tooth-paste and mouthwashes.[33] Most patients report little or no oral discomfort at rest, even in the presence of extensive oral ulcerations.

Chronic GVHD of the salivary glands results in both quantitative and qualitative al-terations in saliva, including altered concentrations of electrolytes, epidermal growth factor, and salivary proteins.[35,36] Because of these changes, patients experience increased morbidity from xerostomia, difficulty with speaking, chewing and swallow-ing, as well as recurrent candidiasis.[11,33,37] Patients may present with rampant caries, characterized by cervical and interproximal patterns of decay that develop at a median of less than 2 years after HCT (**Fig. 3**).[38] In addition to the sialochemical and sialomet-ric changes, oral cGVHD is also associated with recurrent superficial mucoceles, pre-senting primarily as asymptomatic 0.2- to 0.5-cm vesicles on the palatal mucosa (**Fig. 4**). Their putative etiopathogenesis is damage to excretory salivary ducts second-ary to cGVHD.[33]

Sclerotic disease affecting the oral cavity is rare but can be a potentially serious complication. Sclerosis can present in the orofacial region as an extension of primary sclerotic cutaneous cGVHD or as a sequela of long-standing mucosal cGVHD and is characterized by sclerodermalike manifestations, including fibrosis and limited mouth opening associated with pain and secondary ulcerations (**Fig. 5**). The decreased mouth opening results in functional impairment (difficulty with speaking, eating, and maintaining oral hygiene), potentially contributing to infection and malnutrition.[33,34,37]

Diagnosis and Assessment

The diagnosis of oral GVHD can typically be made based on history, clinical findings, and context of onset. For standardization purposes, the NIH has introduced criteria for clinical (see **Table 1**) and histologic diagnosis of cGVHD, a scoring system to docu-ment the extent and severity of clinical involvement (**Fig. 6**), and a staging system for assessing the functional impact (**Table 3**).[12,37,39,40] The global scoring of cGVHD can be calculated based on the number of organs involved (eg, oral cavity) and the severity of involvement according to a 4-point scale, resulting in a classification of mild, moderate, or severe.[12]

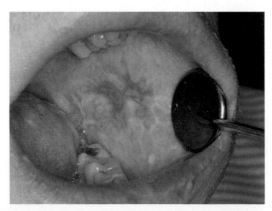

Fig. 2. Oral cGVHD involving the buccal mucosa with pseudomembranous ulceration and li-chenoid hyperkeratosis. Hyperkeratotic changes can also be noted on the lower lip.

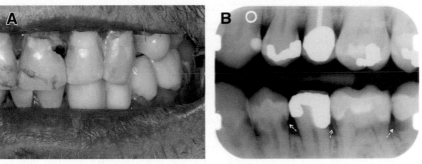

Fig. 3. (*A*) Rampant cervical caries affecting nearly all teeth. (*B*) Bitewing radiograph demonstrating multiple interproximal radiolucent changes (caries, indicated by *arrows*) involving the crown and root surfaces, in some cases at the margins of restorations.

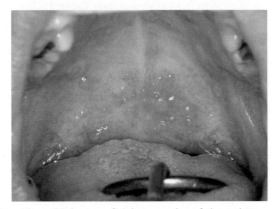

Fig. 4. Oral cGVHD with multiple superficial mucoceles of the palate.

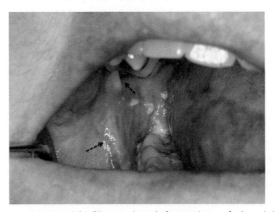

Fig. 5. Oral sclerotic cGVHD with fibrous band formation of the right buccal mucosa (*arrows*) secondary to long-standing mucosal cGVHD, resulting in limited opening and impaired oral hygiene.

Mouth	Mucosal change	No evidence of cGVHD	Mild		Moderate		Severe	
Mouth — Hard Palate, Soft Palate, Pharynx, Uvula, Tongue	Erythema	None 0	Mild erythema or moderate erythema (<25%)	1	Moderate (≥25%) or Severe erythema (<25%)	2	Severe erythema (≥25%)	3
	Lichenoid	None 0	Hyperkeratotic changes(<25%)	1	Hyperkeratotic changes(25-50%)	2	Hyperkeratotic changes (>50%)	3
	Ulcers	None 0	None	0	Ulcers involving (≤20%)	3	Severe ulcerations (>20%)	6
	Mucoceles*	None 0	1-5 mucoceles	1	6-10 scattered mucoceles	2	Over 10 mucoceles	3
			*Mucoceles scored for lower labial and soft palate only				Total score for all mucosal changes	

Fig. 6. The NIH's oral cGVHD clinical scoring instrument. In this 0- to 15-point system, clinical evidence of erythema, lichenoid changes, ulcerations, and mucoceles is assessed globally as to reflect the severity and extent of involvement. (*From* Treister NS, Stevenson K, Kim H. Oral chronic graft-versus-host disease scoring using the NIH consensus criteria. Biol Blood Marrow Transplant 2010;16:108–14; with permission. *Courtesy of* American Society for Blood and Marrow Transplantation, www.asbmt.org.)

Diagnosis of cGVHD can be established by the presence of hallmark diagnostic manifestations, including lichen planus–like changes, hyperkeratotic plaques, and decreased oral range of motion from sclerosis (see **Table 1**). This, however, requires that all other possible diagnoses, such as secondary viral and fungal infections (most frequently, recrudescent HSV, and candidiasis), have been excluded.[12,37,41] When the oral changes are not typical, a biopsy of the oral mucosa or minor salivary glands can provide valuable confirmatory information.[17,40] According to the NIH's minimum histologic criteria for cGVHD, histopathologic features of oral mucosal cGVHD include lichenoid interface inflammation, leukocyte exocytosis, and keratinocyte apoptosis (**Fig. 7**). Salivary gland cGVHD is characterized by intralobular periductal lymphocytic infiltration (often with associated fibrosis) and exocytosis of lymphocytes into intralobular ducts and acini.[31,40] Immunohistochemical studies demonstrate a lymphocytic infiltrate of primarily CD4+ and CD8+ T lymphocytes as well as the presence of Langerhans cells and CD68+ macrophages.[37,42,43]

IMPACT OF GVHD
Overall Survival

GVHD, in its acute and chronic forms, is a main cause of nonrelapse mortality and a leading contributing factor for morbidity associated with prolonged immunosuppressive therapy, impaired functional status, and decreased quality of life.[27,44,45] The impact of GVHD on patients depends on the severity of the disease and its response to treatment.[11,46] Both advanced-grade aGVHD and severe cGVHD constitute a major threat to survival after allo-HCT, with GVHD-related organ failure second only to infection as the leading causes of death.[27] The negative effects of cGVHD are balanced by its positive effect on survival, attributed to a reduced incidence of relapse caused by

Table 3			
The NIH's organ scoring of cGVHD: mouth			
Score 0	Score 1	Score 2	Score 3
No symptoms	Mild symptoms with disease signs but not limiting oral intake significantly	Moderate symptoms with disease signs with partial limitation of oral intake	Severe symptoms with disease signs on examination with major limitation of oral intake

Data from Filipovich AH, Weisdorf D, Pavletic S, et al. National Institutes of Health consensus development project on criteria for clinical trials in chronic graft-versus-host disease: I. Diagnosis and staging working group report. Biol Blood Marrow Transplant 2005;11(12):945–56.

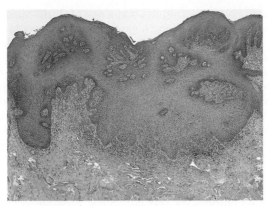

Fig. 7. Oral mucosal cGVHD biopsy specimen obtained from the tongue dorsum demonstrating acanthosis and hyperkeratosis with a dense bandlike lymphocytic infiltrate at the basement membrane interface (Hematoxylin-eosin, original magnification ×100).

the GVT effect. However, with increasing severity of cGVHD there is more treatment-related mortality, explaining the negative correlation between severity of cGVHD and survival.[47]

Quality of Life

Patients who develop aGVHD have been found to report a decrease in their quality of life over the first 6 months after allo-HCT, influenced by infectious complications, intense immunosuppressive regimens, or longer durations of hospitalization.[48] This condition improves significantly at 1 year after HCT in the absence of cGVHD onset. In long-term allo-HCT survivors, cGVHD is associated with compromised quality of life, influenced by multiple factors, including a decrease in general health status, side effects of therapies, reduction in sexual activity, and loss of employment.[27,46,48] However, patients with successfully resolved cGVHD do not seem to have long-term impairment and, moreover, have a similar health status to that of allo-HCT survivors who never had cGVHD, emphasizing the importance of a timely diagnosis and effective therapy protocols.[46]

Oral GVHD

The impact of oral GVHD, as that of GVHD in general, depends on its severity and on the extent of tissue involvement. Severe oral cGVHD results in pain, impaired alimentation and speech, diminished social well-being, and difficulty with maintaining oral and dental health.[11,49,50] Morbidity is more pronounced in patients with concomitant salivary gland involvement compared with mucosal disease only. Although clinically plausible, the data on the association between oral cGVHD and swallowing difficulty, nutrition, and weight loss are lacking.[51–53]

PREVENTION AND MANAGEMENT OF GVHD
Management Principles

Prevention of GVHD focuses primarily on minimizing risk factors, starting with optimal donor selection. Nevertheless, the use of unrelated or related HLA-mismatched donors accounts for most of the allogeneic grafts, and preventive measures are used accordingly. One approach involves pretransplantation graft manipulation by T-cell depletion, aimed not only at reducing the frequency of GVHD but also at reducing the recipient's immune responses, favoring engraftment.[54] All patients receive GVHD prophylaxis, with the most frequently used immunosuppressive regimens consisting of a combination of methotrexate (MTX) and a calcineurin inhibitor (CNI).[55]

Once GVHD has developed, management is largely dependent on the extent and severity of disease, ranging from topical steroid therapy alone to intensive multiagent systemic immunosuppressive therapy. Patients with mild aGVHD or limited forms of cGVHD can be managed using topical immunosuppressive therapies only; in the case of grade I aGVHD, continuation of prophylactic regimens alone may suffice.[11,13] Systemic pharmacologic therapy, including high-dose systemic corticosteroids, is indicated for patients with grade II or worse aGVHD or severe cGVHD, because of their broad immunosuppressive properties.[13]

Because infection is the leading cause of nonrelapse mortality in patients with cGVHD, antimicrobial prophylaxis and supportive care are critical components of disease management. Supportive care is also directed at symptomatic relief and management of the deleterious cGVHD-related effects in the involved organs, with the aim of ameliorating function and quality of life.[56]

Prophylaxis

The mainstay of GVHD prophylaxis is the combination therapy for a CNI (cyclosporine [CsA] or tacrolimus [TAC]) and a short course of MTX. The administration of the CNI begins just before transplantation and extends into the post-HCT period for as long as 6 months thereafter, whereas MTX is administered early after transplantation, usually on days +1, +3, +6, and +11 only. Following studies that demonstrated a reduced incidence of aGVHD (but not cGVHD) with combination regimens containing TAC and short-course MTX, TAC has become more frequently used than CsA.[6,54]

Because of the toxicity associated with MTX, including severe mucositis, delays in neutrophil and platelet engraftment, and pulmonary as well as hepatic toxicity, the effectiveness of other combination regimens is being explored. The use of mycophenolate mofetil (MMF) instead of MTX in a CNI-based regimen seems to provide equivalent rates of GVHD prevention, with the additional benefit of a decrease in the incidence and severity of treatment-related mucositis.[6,57] Similarly, the substitution of MTX with the mammalian target of rapamycin (mTOR) inhibitor sirolimus in a TAC-based regimen was found to be advantageous because of the associated lower incidence of aGVHD and a significantly reduced rate of mucositis.[6,58,59]

Systemic Therapy

Systemic corticosteroids serve as the first-line therapy for GVHD and are indicated for advanced grade aGVHD (grade II or worse) as well as for patients with severe cGVHD involving 3 or more organs or with a score of 2 or greater in any single organ, indicating major disability.[12,13] Treatment of aGVHD with high-dose systemic steroid therapy for 1 to 2 mg/kg/d of methylprednisolone or a prednisone equivalent is associated with a 20% to 70% response rate and a durable response in 20% to 40% of patients.[6,13] In order to improve durable response rates in steroid-refractory cases and to mitigate the adverse effects associated with long-term systemic steroid therapy, such as osteoporosis and avascular necrosis, other agents have been evaluated as steroid sparing second-line therapies with various successes. These agents include MMF, sirolimus, CNIs, monoclonal antibodies (eg, rituximab, alemtuzumab), and extracorporeal photopheresis (ECP).[6,19,60] Because there is currently no standard of care for secondary therapies, these are typically evaluated empirically on an individual basis.[6,61,62]

The initial systemic treatment of cGVHD is with prednisone at a starting dosage of 1 mg/kg/d, often in combination with a CNI.[6,63] For patients with progressive cGVHD who were already on steroid and CNI therapy during the onset of cGVHD, other strategies are considered, such as adding ECP to the existing regimen or the substitution of the CNI with an mTOR inhibitor.[63] Topical therapies based on agents such as corticosteroids or TAC may also be used as an adjunct to systemic therapy for improved local disease control.[63] Overall, clinical resolution of cGVHD is a slow process, with more than 50% of patients requiring systemic immunosuppressive therapy for more than 2 years and 15% of HCT survivors requiring continued treatment for more than 7 years.[64–66]

MANAGEMENT OF ORAL GVHD
Pharmacologic Strategies

Topical management of oral cGVHD may be indicated as complementary therapy to systemic treatment in locally refractory cases or as the sole therapy in cases whereby the oral cavity is the only site involved.[11,37,67] The primary goals of oral GVHD management are to reduce symptoms and maintain oral function. The topical management of both oral aGVHD and cGVHD is essentially the same, with the caveat that cGVHD may require treatment for many years after HCT.

The first-line therapy for oral mucosal GVHD is intensive topical corticosteroid therapy that can be delivered in various formulations (**Table 4**). Solutions and gels are most commonly used because of their ease of use and hydrophilic properties.[11,33,67] The potency of the agent, as well as the delivery formulation and the duration/ frequency of use, can have a significant impact on the treatment effectiveness. In order to ensure maximal efficacy, patients must be given explicit instructions on use (see **Table 4**).[11,33,37,67] It should be noted that most of these agents are not approved by

Table 4
Topical treatment of oral GVHD

Formulation	Treatment (Dosage Per Use)	Instruction for Use
Corticosteroids		
Solutions	Dexamethasone 0.1 mg/mL (5 mL) Budesonide 0.3–0.6 mg/mL (10 mL) Prednisolone 3 mg/mL (5 mL) Triamcinolone 1% (5 mL)	Hold solution and swish in mouth for 4–6 min before expectoration Wait 10–15 min after topical therapy before eating/drinking or brushing teeth Repeat up to 4–6 times per day
Gels, creams, and ointments	Fluocinonide 0.05% gel, cream, ointment Clobetasol 0.05% gel, cream, ointment Betamethasone dipropionate 0.05% gel Triamcinolone 0.1%–0.5% ointment	Apply to lesions 2–4 times per day Gels can be applied with gauze and left in place 10–15 min
Nonsteroidal immunosuppressives		
Solution	Tacrolimus 0.1 mg/mL (5 mL)[a]	Hold and swish in mouth for 4–6 min before expectoration Repeat up to 4–6 times per day
Ointment	Tacrolimus 0.1% ointment	Apply to lesions 2–4 times per day

[a] Typically used concurrently with steroid therapy.

the US Food and Drug Administration for intraoral mucosal therapy, and patients should also be made aware of the risks associated with systemic absorption caused by swallowing or transmucosal penetration.[34,37]

In keeping with the NIH's guidelines for ancillary therapy in cGVHD, the various corticosteroid solutions should be swished in the mouth for 4 to 6 minutes before expectoration and used up to 4 to 6 times per day (see **Table 4**). High-potency corticosteroid gels are effective for managing limited areas of involvement and can also be used as an adjunct to topical solutions in patients with extensive oral involvement. In this context, the application of tacrolimus ointment can be considered, although, because of its high viscosity and hydrophobic properties, it is less preferred for intraoral use and is usually the treatment of choice for lip involvement.[67] For intraoral use, tacrolimus can be compounded as a solution and used in combination with a corticosteroid solution in patients that do not have an adequate response to topical steroid therapy alone.[63,68] Finally, intralesional injections of triamcinolone acetonide (10–40 mg/mL) may be beneficial for resolution of refractory and symptomatic localized ulcerative lesions.

Oral moisturizing agents and saliva substitutes help to reduce salivary gland cGVHD-associated xerostomia.[11,69] Salivation can be stimulated by gustatory and masticatory means through the use of sugar-free chewing gums and candies.[69] More severe hyposalivation is managed by systemic therapy with the cholinergic agonists pilocarpine and cevimeline in the absence of contraindications, such as glaucoma, cardiac arrhythmias, or pulmonary disease.[11,33,67,69] Both agents have parasympathomimetic activity and similar safety profiles and are approved for symptomatic treatment of Sjögren syndrome. In salivary gland hypofunction associated with cGVHD, both agents have been reported to improve symptoms of dry mouth and increase salivary output.[70,71] The decision to use these agents should be balanced against the potential side effects, most commonly excessive sweating and flushing, and must be avoided in patients with pulmonary disease.[72]

Topical supportive care and antimicrobial prophylaxis are complementary to definitive treatment. Viscous lidocaine is the most frequently used palliative agent for relief of discomfort and pain and may be mixed with other soothing solutions, such as diphenhydramine and bismuth subsalicylate (Kaopectate) or aluminum hydroxide, magnesium hydroxide, and simethicone (Maalox).[31,37,67] Chronic GVHD is associated with a higher rate of oral infections that may exacerbate oral symptoms and dysfunction. Moreover, topical immunosuppressive treatment of oral cGVHD increases the risk of developing secondary oropharyngeal candidiasis. For these reasons, a prophylactic antifungal treatment, in the form of oral solution or troche, is generally recommended for patients receiving topical immunosuppressive therapy.[33,34,37]

Nonpharmacologic Strategies

Several types of intraoral phototherapy have been anecdotally reported to be beneficial in the management of oral mucosal cGVHD. These types include psoralen–UV-A (PUVA) using intraoral psoralen sensitizers, UV-B therapy, low-level laser therapy, and carbon dioxide laser therapy.[73–77] Although the results are encouraging, specifically in cases of refractory oral cGVHD, available data are limited, and further studies are required for determining safety, efficacy, and understanding the underlying mechanisms of action.[11,37]

Although not specific treatments for oral cGVHD, basic oral care is critical for eliminating local factors that might aggravate oral symptoms of GVHD and for preventing odontogenic infections. This care includes brushing, flossing, and application of remineralization agents on a regular basis (**Box 3**).[11,33,37] Patients should undergo a dental

---

Box 3
Basic oral care recommendations

Basic oral hygiene

- Brush at least twice daily, using a soft toothbrush
- Consider use of children's flavored toothpaste to minimize sensitivity associated with mint flavors
- Floss daily

Lip care

- Apply lip-coating agents with UV protection

Caries prevention

- Minimize intake of refined carbohydrates (sugars)
- Increase water intake
- Apply prescription fluoride 1.1% gel: brush on teeth or use in custom trays, daily
- Apply remineralizing agent in addition to fluoride
- Professional fluoride varnish applications

---

evaluation 6 to 12 months after HCT and subsequent routine follow-ups on an annual basis (once a year or more, as needed) including necessary bitewing radiographs to screen for interproximal caries.[38,78] Importantly, patients should be provided with appropriate literature on their condition as part of patient education and empowerment (www.aaom.com, see patient information sheets).

LATE COMPLICATIONS OF ORAL GVHD

A history of oral cGVHD is associated with an increased risk for the development of several late complications, in some cases many years after diagnosis and management. Perioral sclerodermatoid changes, resulting from fibrosis of the facial skin and mucosal cGVHD, may lead to restricted oral range of motion and reduced mouth opening. When severe, there can be significant limitation in oral intake of food and the ability to maintain oral hygiene. Additionally, fibrosis may lead to a loss of vestibular depth and attached gingiva, creating periodontal defects resulting in tooth loss. These changes may respond to systemic cGVHD treatment and physical therapy; however, severe cases may necessitate surgical intervention.[11,33,37,67]

It has long been known that allo-HCT is associated with an increased risk of developing secondary malignancies, including new solid cancers, such as squamous cell carcinoma (SCC) of the skin and oral cavity.[44,79–82] The increased risk of developing SCC of the skin and oral cavity has been associated with cGVHD and its therapy, and oral cGVHD specifically seems to be directly related with the occurrence of secondary oral cancer.[83,84] With a median time from transplantation to solid tumor diagnosis of 7 years and increasing risk with time since transplantation, annual comprehensive screening for oral malignancies is critical for all allo-HCT survivors.[37,80,83]

SUMMARY

Despite advances in the understanding of transplant immunology and clinical care, GVHD remains a significant cause of morbidity and mortality for allo-HCT recipients.

The oral cavity is one of the most frequent sites affected by cGVHD, with mucosal, salivary, and/or sclerotic manifestations that are associated with pain, impaired function and diminished quality of life. Accurate diagnosis and effective management of oral GVHD and its associated complications is a critical component of the overall care of patients with GVHD.

REFERENCES

1. Blazar BR, Murphy WJ, Abedi M. Advances in graft-versus-host disease biology and therapy. Nat Rev Immunol 2012;12(6):443–58.
2. Perez-Simon JA, Sanchez-Abarca I, Diez-Campelo M, et al. Chronic graft-versus-host disease: pathogenesis and clinical management. Drugs 2006; 66(8):1041–57.
3. Billingham RE. The biology of graft-versus-host reactions. Harvey Lect 1966;62: 21–78.
4. Vogelsang GB, Lee L, Bensen-Kennedy DM. Pathogenesis and treatment of graft-versus-host disease after bone marrow transplant. Annu Rev Med 2003; 54:29–52.
5. Ferrara JL, Reddy P. Pathophysiology of graft-versus-host disease. Semin Hematol 2006;43(1):3–10.
6. Pavletic SZ, Fowler DH. Are we making progress in GVHD prophylaxis and treatment? Hematology Am Soc Hematol Educ Program 2012;2012:251–64.
7. Lee SJ, Klein J, Haagenson M, et al. High-resolution donor-recipient HLA matching contributes to the success of unrelated donor marrow transplantation. Blood 2007;110(13):4576–83.
8. Spellman SR, Eapen M, Logan BR, et al. A perspective on the selection of unrelated donors and cord blood units for transplantation. Blood 2012;120(2): 259–65.
9. Warren EH, Zhang XC, Li S, et al. Effect of MHC and non-MHC donor/recipient genetic disparity on the outcome of allogeneic HCT. Blood 2012;120(14): 2796–806.
10. Weiden PL, Sullivan KM, Flournoy N, et al. Antileukemic effect of chronic graft-versus-host disease: contribution to improved survival after allogeneic marrow transplantation. N Engl J Med 1981;304(25):1529–33.
11. Schubert MM, Correa ME. Oral graft-versus-host disease. Dent Clin North Am 2008;52(1):79–109 viii-ix.
12. Filipovich AH, Weisdorf D, Pavletic S, et al. National Institutes of Health consensus development project on criteria for clinical trials in chronic graft-versus-host disease: I. Diagnosis and staging working group report. Biol Blood Marrow Transplant 2005;11(12):945–56.
13. Bolanos-Meade J, Vogelsang GB. Acute graft-versus-host disease. Clin Adv Hematol Oncol 2004;2(10):672–82.
14. Mielcarek M, Martin PJ, Leisenring W, et al. Graft-versus-host disease after non-myeloablative versus conventional hematopoietic stem cell transplantation. Blood 2003;102(2):756–62.
15. Goker H, Haznedaroglu IC, Chao NJ. Acute graft-vs-host disease: pathobiology and management. Exp Hematol 2001;29(3):259–77.
16. Deeg HJ, Antin JH. The clinical spectrum of acute graft-versus-host disease. Semin Hematol 2006;43(1):24–31.
17. Imanguli MM, Alevizos I, Brown R, et al. Oral graft-versus-host disease. Oral Dis 2008;14(5):396–412.

18. Przepiorka D, Weisdorf D, Martin P, et al. 1994 Consensus Conference on Acute GVHD Grading. Bone Marrow Transplant 1995;15(6):825–8.
19. Dignan FL, Clark A, Amrolia P, et al. Diagnosis and management of acute graft-versus-host disease. Br J Haematol 2012;158(1):30–45.
20. Gratwohl A, Hermans J, Apperley J, et al. Acute graft-versus-host disease: grade and outcome in patients with chronic myelogenous leukemia. Working Party Chronic Leukemia of the European Group for Blood and Marrow Transplantation. Blood 1995;86(2):813–8.
21. Kansu E. The pathophysiology of chronic graft-versus-host disease. Int J Hematol 2004;79(3):209–15.
22. Kataoka Y, Iwasaki T, Kuroiwa T, et al. The role of donor T cells for target organ injuries in acute and chronic graft-versus-host disease. Immunology 2001; 103(3):310–8.
23. Shimabukuro-Vornhagen A, Hallek MJ, Storb RF, et al. The role of B cells in the pathogenesis of graft-versus-host disease. Blood 2009;114(24):4919–27.
24. Allen JL, Fore MS, Wooten J, et al. B cells from patients with chronic GVHD are activated and primed for survival via BAFF-mediated pathways. Blood 2012; 120(12):2529–36.
25. Kharfan-Dabaja MA, Cutler CS. Rituximab for prevention and treatment of graft-versus-host disease. Int J Hematol 2011;93(5):578–85.
26. Shulman HM, Sale GE, Lerner KG, et al. Chronic cutaneous graft-versus-host disease in man. Am J Pathol 1978;91(3):545–70.
27. Lee SJ, Vogelsang G, Flowers ME. Chronic graft-versus-host disease. Biol Blood Marrow Transplant 2003;9(4):215–33.
28. Baird K, Pavletic SZ. Chronic graft versus host disease. Curr Opin Hematol 2006;13(6):426–35.
29. Kuzmina Z, Eder S, Bohm A, et al. Significantly worse survival of patients with NIH-defined chronic graft-versus-host disease and thrombocytopenia or progressive onset type: results of a prospective study. Leukemia 2012;26(4):746–56.
30. Subramaniam DS, Fowler DH, Pavletic SZ. Chronic graft-versus-host disease in the era of reduced-intensity conditioning. Leukemia 2007;21(5):853–9.
31. Woo SB, Lee SJ, Schubert MM. Graft-vs-host disease. Crit Rev Oral Biol Med 1997;8(2):201–16.
32. Treister NS, Cook EF Jr, Antin J, et al. Clinical evaluation of oral chronic graft-versus-host disease. Biol Blood Marrow Transplant 2008;14(1):110–5.
33. Treister N, Duncan C, Cutler C, et al. How we treat oral chronic graft-versus-host disease. Blood 2012;120(17):3407–18.
34. Mays J, Fassil H, Edwards D, et al. Oral chronic graft-versus-host disease: current pathogenesis, therapy, and research. Oral Dis 2012;19(4):327–46.
35. Nagler RM, Nagler A. Sialometrical and sialochemical analysis of patients with chronic graft-versus-host disease–a prolonged study. Cancer Invest 2003; 21(1):34–40.
36. Coracin FL, Pizzigatti Correa ME, Camargo EE, et al. Major salivary gland damage in allogeneic hematopoietic progenitor cell transplantation assessed by scintigraphic methods. Bone Marrow Transplant 2006;37(10):955–9.
37. Meier JK, Wolff D, Pavletic S, et al. Oral chronic graft-versus-host disease: report from the International Consensus Conference on Clinical Practice in cGVHD. Clin Oral Investig 2011;15(2):127–39.
38. Castellarin P, Stevenson K, Biasotto M, et al. Extensive dental caries in patients with oral chronic graft-versus-host disease. Biol Blood Marrow Transplant 2012; 18(10):1573–9.

39. Pavletic SZ, Lee SJ, Socie G, et al. Chronic graft-versus-host disease: implications of the National Institutes of Health consensus development project on criteria for clinical trials. Bone Marrow Transplant 2006;38(10):645–51.

40. Shulman HM, Kleiner D, Lee SJ, et al. Histopathologic diagnosis of chronic graft-versus-host disease: National Institutes of Health Consensus Development Project on Criteria for Clinical Trials in Chronic Graft-versus-Host Disease: II. Pathology working group report. Biol Blood Marrow Transplant 2006;12(1):31–47.

41. Schubert MM, Sullivan KM, Morton TH, et al. Oral manifestations of chronic graft-v-host disease. Arch Intern Med 1984;144(8):1591–5.

42. Soares AB, Faria PR, Magna LA, et al. Chronic GVHD in minor salivary glands and oral mucosa: histopathological and immunohistochemical evaluation of 25 patients. J Oral Pathol Med 2005;34(6):368–73.

43. Sato M, Tokuda N, Fukumoto T, et al. Immunohistopathological study of the oral lichenoid lesions of chronic GVHD. J Oral Pathol Med 2006;35(1):33–6.

44. Socie G, Stone JV, Wingard JR, et al. Long-term survival and late deaths after allogeneic bone marrow transplantation. Late Effects Working Committee of the International Bone Marrow Transplant Registry. N Engl J Med 1999;341(1): 14–21.

45. Pidala J. Graft-vs-host disease following allogeneic hematopoietic cell transplantation. Cancer Control 2011;18(4):268–76.

46. Fraser CJ, Bhatia S, Ness K, et al. Impact of chronic graft-versus-host disease on the health status of hematopoietic cell transplantation survivors: a report from the Bone Marrow Transplant Survivor Study. Blood 2006;108(8):2867–73.

47. Lee SJ, Klein JP, Barrett AJ, et al. Severity of chronic graft-versus-host disease: association with treatment-related mortality and relapse. Blood 2002;100(2): 406–14.

48. Lee SJ, Kim HT, Ho VT, et al. Quality of life associated with acute and chronic graft-versus-host disease. Bone Marrow Transplant 2006;38(4):305–10.

49. Fall-Dickson JM, Mitchell SA, Marden S, et al. Oral symptom intensity, health-related quality of life, and correlative salivary cytokines in adult survivors of hematopoietic stem cell transplantation with oral chronic graft-versus-host disease. Biol Blood Marrow Transplant 2010;16(7):948–56.

50. Hull KM, Kerridge I, Schifter M. Long-term oral complications of allogeneic haematopoietic SCT. Bone Marrow Transplant 2012;47(2):265–70.

51. Imanguli MM, Atkinson JC, Mitchell SA, et al. Salivary gland involvement in chronic graft-versus-host disease: prevalence, clinical significance, and recommendations for evaluation. Biol Blood Marrow Transplant 2010;16(10):1362–9.

52. Fassil H, Bassim CW, Mays J, et al. Oral chronic graft-vs-host disease characterization using the NIH scale. J Dent Res 2012;91(Suppl 7):45S–51S.

53. Treister N, Chai X, Kurland B, et al. Measurement of oral chronic GVHD: results from the Chronic GVHD Consortium. Bone Marrow Transplant 2013;48(8):1123–8.

54. Bacigalupo A. Management of acute graft-versus-host disease. Br J Haematol 2007;137(2):87–98.

55. Bolanos-Meade J. Update on the management of acute graft-versus-host disease. Curr Opin Oncol 2006;18(2):120–5.

56. Lee SJ, Flowers ME. Recognizing and managing chronic graft-versus-host disease. Hematology Am Soc Hematol Educ Program 2008;134–41.

57. Perkins J, Field T, Kim J, et al. A randomized phase II trial comparing tacrolimus and mycophenolate mofetil to tacrolimus and methotrexate for acute graft-versus-host disease prophylaxis. Biol Blood Marrow Transplant 2010;16(7): 937–47.

58. Cutler C, Kim HT, Hochberg E, et al. Sirolimus and tacrolimus without methotrexate as graft-versus-host disease prophylaxis after matched related donor peripheral blood stem cell transplantation. Biol Blood Marrow Transplant 2004;10(5):328–36.

59. Cutler C, Li S, Ho VT, et al. Extended follow-up of methotrexate-free immunosuppression using sirolimus and tacrolimus in related and unrelated donor peripheral blood stem cell transplantation. Blood 2007;109(7):3108–14.

60. Dignan FL, Amrolia P, Clark A, et al. Diagnosis and management of chronic graft-versus-host disease. Br J Haematol 2012;158(1):46–61.

61. Cutler C, Antin JH. Chronic graft-versus-host disease. Curr Opin Oncol 2006; 18(2):126–31.

62. Wolff D, Schleuning M, von Harsdorf S, et al. Consensus conference on clinical practice in chronic GVHD: second-line treatment of chronic graft-versus-host disease. Biol Blood Marrow Transplant 2011;17(1):1–17.

63. Wolff D, Gerbitz A, Ayuk F, et al. Consensus conference on clinical practice in chronic graft-versus-host disease (GVHD): first-line and topical treatment of chronic GVHD. Biol Blood Marrow Transplant 2010;16(12):1611–28.

64. Koc S, Leisenring W, Flowers ME, et al. Therapy for chronic graft-versus-host disease: a randomized trial comparing cyclosporine plus prednisone versus prednisone alone. Blood 2002;100(1):48–51.

65. Arora M, Burns LJ, Davies SM, et al. Chronic graft-versus-host disease: a prospective cohort study. Biol Blood Marrow Transplant 2003;9(1):38–45.

66. Stewart BL, Storer B, Storek J, et al. Duration of immunosuppressive treatment for chronic graft-versus-host disease. Blood 2004;104(12):3501–6.

67. Couriel D, Carpenter PA, Cutler C, et al. Ancillary therapy and supportive care of chronic graft-versus-host disease: national institutes of health consensus development project on criteria for clinical trials in chronic graft-versus-host disease: V. Ancillary Therapy and Supportive Care Working Group Report. Biol Blood Marrow Transplant 2006;12(4):375–96.

68. Mawardi H, Stevenson K, Gokani B, et al. Combined topical dexamethasone/tacrolimus therapy for management of oral chronic GVHD. Bone Marrow Transplant 2010;45(6):1062–7.

69. Fox PC. Salivary enhancement therapies. Caries Res 2004;38(3):241–6.

70. Nagler RM, Nagler A. The effect of pilocarpine on salivary constituents in patients with chronic graft-versus-host disease. Arch Oral Biol 2001;46(8): 689–95.

71. Carpenter PA, Schubert MM, Flowers ME. Cevimeline reduced mouth dryness and increased salivary flow in patients with xerostomia complicating chronic graft-versus-host disease. Biol Blood Marrow Transplant 2006;12(7):792–4.

72. Chainani-Wu N, Gorsky M, Mayer P, et al. Assessment of the use of sialogogues in the clinical management of patients with xerostomia. Spec Care Dentist 2006; 26(4):164–70.

73. Elad S, Garfunkel AA, Enk CD, et al. Ultraviolet B irradiation: a new therapeutic concept for the management of oral manifestations of graft-versus-host disease. Oral Surg Oral Med Oral Pathol Oral Radiol Endod 1999;88(4):444–50.

74. Menillo SA, Goldberg SL, McKiernan P, et al. Intraoral psoralen ultraviolet A irradiation (PUVA) treatment of refractory oral chronic graft-versus-host disease following allogeneic stem cell transplantation. Bone Marrow Transplant 2001; 28(8):807–8.

75. Elad S, Or R, Shapira MY, et al. CO2 laser in oral graft-versus-host disease: a pilot study. Bone Marrow Transplant 2003;32(10):1031–4.

76. Wolff D, Anders V, Corio R, et al. Oral PUVA and topical steroids for treatment of oral manifestations of chronic graft-vs.-host disease. Photodermatol Photoimmunol Photomed 2004;20(4):184–90.
77. Chor A, de Azevedo AM, Maiolino A, et al. Successful treatment of oral lesions of chronic lichenoid graft-vs-host disease by the addition of low-level laser therapy to systemic immunosuppression. Eur J Haematol 2004;72(3):222–4.
78. Rizzo JD, Wingard JR, Tichelli A, et al. Recommended screening and preventive practices for long-term survivors after hematopoietic cell transplantation: joint recommendations of the European Group for Blood and Marrow Transplantation, the Center for International Blood and Marrow Transplant Research, and the American Society of Blood and Marrow Transplantation. Biol Blood Marrow Transplant 2006;12(2):138–51.
79. Hasegawa W, Pond GR, Rifkind JT, et al. Long-term follow-up of secondary malignancies in adults after allogeneic bone marrow transplantation. Bone Marrow Transplant 2005;35(1):51–5.
80. Demarosi F, Lodi G, Carrassi A, et al. Oral malignancies following HSCT: graft versus host disease and other risk factors. Oral Oncol 2005;41(9):865–77.
81. Majhail NS. Secondary cancers following allogeneic haematopoietic cell transplantation in adults. Br J Haematol 2011;154(3):301–10.
82. Socie G, Rizzo JD. Second solid tumors: screening and management guidelines in long-term survivors after allogeneic stem cell transplantation. Semin Hematol 2012;49(1):4–9.
83. Curtis RE, Metayer C, Rizzo JD, et al. Impact of chronic GVHD therapy on the development of squamous-cell cancers after hematopoietic stem-cell transplantation: an international case-control study. Blood 2005;105(10):3802–11.
84. Mawardi H, Elad S, Correa ME, et al. Oral epithelial dysplasia and squamous cell carcinoma following allogeneic hematopoietic stem cell transplantation: clinical presentation and treatment outcomes. Bone Marrow Transplant 2011; 46(6):884–91.

Antiresorptive Drug–Related Osteonecrosis of the Jaw

Jettie Uyanne, DDS[a,b,]*, Colonya C. Calhoun, DDS, PhD[c,d],
Anh D. Le, DDS, PhD[a,e]

KEYWORDS

- Bisphosphonate • Denosumab • Osteonecrosis of the jaw • Zoledronate

KEY POINTS

- Nitrogen-containing and non–nitrogen-containing bisphosphonates have been implicated in the development of osteonecrosis of the jaw, a condition termed bisphosphonate-related osteonecrosis of the jaw.
- Other antiresorptive drugs have recently been implicated in the development of osteonecrosis of the jaw, hence the new term antiresorptive drug–related osteonecrosis of the jaw (ARONJ).
- Cofactors such as infection, diabetes, steroids, cancer, and chemotherapy may direct immune suppression and potentiate ARONJ development sooner.
- The risk of ARONJ is associated with the type of antiresorptive medication, route, and dosage.

INTRODUCTION

Osteonecrosis of the jaw (ONJ) is a debilitating bone disorder of the jaw and is defined by the advisory tasks forces from both the American Association of Oral and Maxillofacial Surgeon (AAOMS) and the American Society for Bone and Mineral Research (ASBMR) as the persistence of exposure of bone in the oral cavity for more than 8 weeks refractory to treatment, current or previous history of bisphosphonate (BP)

The authors have nothing to disclose.
[a] Division of Oral and Maxillofacial Surgery, Herman Ostrow School of Dentistry of USC, 925 West 34th Street, Los Angeles, CA 90089-0641, USA; [b] Division of Oral and Maxillofacial Surgery, Harbor UCLA, 1000 West Carson Street, Torrance, CA 90509, USA; [c] Division of Oral and Maxillofacial Surgery, Harbor UCLA, 1000 West Carson Street, Mailbox #19, Torrance, CA 90509, USA; [d] Charles R. Drew University, Los Angeles, CA, USA; [e] Department of Oral and Maxillofacial Surgery and Pharmacology, University of Pennsylvania School of Dental Medicine, Penn Medicine Hospital of the University of Pennsylvania, 240 South 40th Street, Philadelphia, PA 19104-6030, USA
* Corresponding author. Division of Oral and Maxillofacial Surgery, Herman Ostrow School of Dentistry of USC, Norris Dental Science Center, 925 West 34th Street, DEN 146, Los Angeles, CA 90089-0641.
E-mail addresses: uyanne@usc.edu; JUyanne@dhs.lacounty.gov

Dent Clin N Am 58 (2014) 369–384
http://dx.doi.org/10.1016/j.cden.2013.12.006
0011-8532/14/$ – see front matter Published by Elsevier Inc.

use, no evidence of malignancy, and no prior radiotherapy to the affected region.[1–5] Antiresorptive drug–related ONJ (ARONJ) is a recent concept adapted and recommended by the 2008 American Dental Association (ADA) Council on Scientific Affairs. The ADA council recommended that all cases related to the administration of antiresorptive agents be termed antiresorptive agent–induced ONJ.[6] This recommendation encompasses all antiresorptive drugs that could cause development of ONJ. Many patients are being treated with antiresorptive or antiremodeling agents such as hormonal replacement therapy, selective estrogen receptor modulators, calcitonin (direct inhibitor of osteoclasts), BPs, or the monoclonal antibody (eg, denosumab).

At present, ARONJ development has been associated with the use of BPs and anti–receptor activated nuclear factor KB ligand (anti-RANKL) monoclonal antibody such as denosumab. It has been postulated that ARONJ results from reduced bone turnover caused by the antiresorptive drugs, by which denosumab seems to have an equal or greater extent of bone turnover suppression than BP. Besides BP and anti-RANKL drugs, other antiresorptive agents have a low risk of ARONJ, which may in part be because they do not suppress bone turnover by more than 50%.[7,8]

Antiresorptive Drugs Associated with ONJ

BP

BPs have been widely used as antiresorptive agents for management of skeletal-related events in neoplasia, hypercalcemia of malignancy, osteoporosis, Paget disease, osteogenesis imperfecta, and fibrous dysplasia.[9] BP has been linked to the development of ARONJ. The currently accepted theory for the development ARONJ is through direct and indirect effects on bone turnover via apoptosis of osteoclasts.[10] BP is the synthetic analogue of inorganic pyrophosphate, containing a phosphorus-carbon-phosphorus (PCP) backbone and a variable side chain (nitrogen or non-nitrogen) that determines the potency for inhibition of bone resorption.

BPs that lack a nitrogen functional group (etidronate, clodronate, tiludronate) condense to form the nonhydrolyzable analogue of ATP, which inhibits ATP-dependent intracellular enzyme, resulting in osteoclast cell death.[11,12] In contrast, the nitrogen-containing BP (pamidronate, ibandronate, zoledronate, risedronate, alendronate) inhibit the activity of farnesyl diphosphate synthase, which is a key enzyme in the mevalonate pathway. Inhibition of this enzyme creates an intracellular deficiency of geranylgeranyl diphosphate and farnesyl diphosphate, which are both required for prenylation of small signaling proteins with GTPase activity. This process results in dysfunctional osteoclasts and eventually apoptosis.[11,13] The nitrogen-containing BP has a higher potency and thus is effective in therapeutic management of skeletal-related events in cancer but also results in a higher risk ONJ. Zoledronic acid is the most potent BP (500–1000 times more potent than pamidronate) and was the first drug approved for use in all solid tumors with bone metastasis such as breast cancer, prostate, multiple myeloma, and lung cancer.[14] Intravenous (IV) BP exposure in the setting of managing malignancy remains the major risk factor for ARONJ, whereas treatment with oral BP therapy is at a considerably lower risk for ARONJ, possibly because IV administration of BP results in a higher skeletal accumulation caused by the high mineral-binding affinity and is also associated with earlier onset of ARONJ than oral BP.[15]

Anti-RANK ligand: denosumab

Denosumab is an antiresorptive agent that also inhibits osteoclast-mediated bone resorption. Denosumab has US Food and Drug Administration approval for the treatment of osteoporosis and skeletal-related events (SREs) in patients with cancer. Prolia

(Amgen) was approved for treatment of osteoporosis and Xgeva (Amgen) for prevention of skeletal-related events in patients with bone metastases from solid tumors (Prolia/Xgeva [denosumab], prescribing information. Amgen, Thousand Oaks, CA; 2010). Denosumab works in a different pathway than BP in that it is a human monoclonal antibody (immunoglobulin G2) that inhibits receptor-activated nuclear factor KB ligand (RANKL) by mimicking the effect of osteoprotegerin on RANKL.[14,16] RANKL plays an important role in bone remodeling. It is a cytokine that is expressed on many cells including osteoblasts, bone marrow stomal cells, and immune cells. It plays a vital role in osteoclast cell function, activation, and differentiation and thus decreases bone turnover.[14,17] Because RANKL is expressed on the subset of T and B cells, there is a possibility that denosumab may be immunosuppressive.

In the FREEDOM (Fracture Reduction Evaluation of Denosumab in Osteoporosis every 6 Months) trial of 7000 patients with osteoporosis, there was a significant reduction of fractures in the treatment group; however, no cases of ARONJ were observed.[18] Denosumab significantly increases bone mass density by reducing osteoclast numbers and other parameters of bone turnover including levels of the bone resorption marker serum C-telopeptide. Reduced turnover significantly increases bone mass density.[19] Besides ARONJ, other adverse effects associated with denosumab include hypocalcemia, pancreatitis, and severe infection.[17]

Differences between BP and denosumab

Both BP and denosumab are associated with development of ARONJ and are approved for postmenopausal osteoporosis in women at increased risk of fracture and for the treatment of bone loss associated with cancer.[14] Denosumab has several advantages, including better tolerability, ease of subcutaneous injection, and decreased incidence of nephrotoxicity compared with BP. In terms of drug half-life, denosumab has an advantage compared with BP, with a shorter half-life of 25.4 days,[20] compared with 10 to 12 years for BP. In a phase II trial, denosumab suppressed bone resorption markers including urinary collagen type I cross-linked N-telopeptide (NTx) within 24 hours after initial dose and a greater reduction of these markers by 74% compared with 63% in BP-treated patients.[14] Denosumab has a shorter half-life and is therefore reversible. It is eliminated via the immunoglobin clearance pathway in the reticuloendothelial system, which makes it less nephrotoxic and possibly the drug of choice for renal patients or diseases with the propensity toward renal dysfunction, such as renal cell cancer and prostate cancer. In the phase III clinical trials of 5677 patients with bone metastasis, the risk of ARONJ was similar for both BP with 37 (1.3%) cases (zoledronic acid) and denosumab with 52 (1.8%) cases.[21]

EPIDEMIOLOGY

Since 2003, ARONJ has been reported as a serious side effect of BP treatment.[22–24] The reported rate of incidence for ARONJ from a population-based study is 0.8% to 1.5% for IV BP and 0.01% to 0.04% for oral BP.[3,23,25] However, dental extractions or trauma may significantly increase the BP risk of ARONJ from 1 in 10,000 and 1 in 100,000 to a risk of 1 in 300 (**Table 1**). It is recognized that 60% of cases occurred following a tooth extraction or other dentoalveolar surgery versus the remaining cases, which occur spontaneously. It is estimated that the incidence of ARONJ in patients with malignancy ranges from 1% to 10%.[3] A systematic review of 368 reported cases of ARONJ from 2003 to 2006 revealed that 94% of these patients were treated with IV BP (primarily pamidronate and zoledronate), and 85% of the patients had either multiple myeloma or metastatic breast cancer,[4,26] whereas the remaining patients were on oral BP for osteoporosis or Paget disease of bone. The oncologic doses for BP

Table 1
Risk factors associated with BP-related ONJ

Medical Comorbidities	Dental Comorbidities
Cancer	Periodontitis
Anemia	Infection
Smoking	Failed root canal therapy
Chemotherapy	Extraction
Radiation	Implants
Steroid	Trauma
Rheumatoid arthritis	Periodontal surgery
Antimetabolite medications	Apicoectomy
Diabetes	—
Obesity	—
Immunosuppression	—
Age	—
Alcohol	—
Malnutrition	—

are 10 to 12 times higher than osteoporosis doses and are usually given in combination with steroids. The cumulative effect was higher for zoledronate compared with pamidronate, with a 1% versus 0% risk, respectively, within the first year, and a 21% versus 4% risk, respectively, after 3 years of treatment. The estimated incidence of ARONJ in patients receiving IV BP for malignant disease ranges from 0.8% to 12%,[27] which is 900 times higher than that of the general patient with osteoporosis.[26,28] In a case-controlled study by Wessel and colleagues,[29] patients with cancer who had received zoledronate showed a significant 30-fold increase in their risk to develop ARONJ. Incidence of ARONJ is significantly higher in patients with cancer compared with patients with osteoporosis. In a study of risk of ARONJ among patients with different types of cancer (breast cancer, prostate cancer, multiple myeloma), the International Myeloma Association study showed that patients with cancer with multiple myeloma were more likely to have a higher risk of ARONJ than breast or prostate cancer. In a retrospective cohort study by Tennis and colleagues,[30] the incidence of ARONJ in the cancer cohort group was 5.3% among IV BP and 0.15% in the osteoporosis group using oral BP. Patients with multiple myeloma had an incidence 4.5 times that of patients with breast cancer. Among patients with cancer, the incidence of ARONJ was reported as 3.8%, 2.5%, and 2.9% for multiple myeloma, breast cancer, and prostate cancer, respectively.[31] In the patients with cancer treated with BP, the incidence rates for ARONJ were related to (1) length of exposure to the drug, (2) history of dental procedures, (3) number of treatment cycles, and (4) delivery method (IV or oral).[32,33]

WORLDWIDE INCIDENCE

The association between BP and ARONJ has been well established. With the increased rate of aging of the population, the World Health Organization predicts that people older than 65 years will comprise 20% of the world's population by 2030.[34,35] More than 24 million prescriptions for BP were issued in the United States and more than 190 million internationally.[34] A postal survey of oral surgeons and members of the Commonwealth of Australia Adverse Drug Reaction Committee indicates that the rate of ARONJ for inpatients receiving alendronate was between 1 per 2260 and 1 per 8470 patients (0.01%–0.04%).[36]

CLINICAL PARAMETERS
Diagnostic Guidelines and Staging of ARONJ

ARONJ can be a debilitating complication of BP therapy. The diagnostic criteria for ARONJ were formulated by the advisory task forces from AAOMS and the ASBMR in 2007, and revised in 2009. The diagnostic criteria for ARONJ include (1) an exposed, necrotic bone in the maxillofacial region that has persisted for more than 8 weeks; (2) current or previous history of BP use; and (3) no history of radiation therapy to the head and neck area. In addition to exposed nonhealing bone, other signs and symptoms may be present in suspected cases of ARONJ including pain, swelling, paresthesia, suppuration, nonhealing soft tissue ulcerations, sinus tracts, mobile or periodontally involved teeth, and radiographic variability including radiolucencies or radiopacities.[3] Lesions can occur spontaneously but most cases of ARONJ occur after dental extraction or traumatic insult.

The revised guideline in 2009 was established to include patients with stage 0 disease, characterized as having no evidence of exposed necrotic bone.[9] The current AAOMS guideline for ARONJ classifies the condition into 4 stages based on clinical findings to include stage 0 patients, who have no evidence of bone necrosis with nonspecific clinical findings and symptoms; stage 1 is characterized by the presence of exposed and necrotic bone, without evidence of infection; stage 2 patients have clinically exposed/necrotic bone with evidence of infection (pain, erythema, with or without purulent drainage); stage 3 patients have severely exposed and necrotic bone with severe infection extending beyond the alveolar bone region, osteolysis extending to the inferior border of the mandible or sinus floor, a predisposition to pathologic fracture, and oral-antral or oral-nasal communication.[4,37–39] Several reports of a clinical variant of ARONJ have recently been described, in which clinical features reported persistent bone pain, bone enlargement with gingival swelling, but no evidence of dental disease or exposure of bone.[39–43] Hutchinson and colleagues[43] reported that 30 patients out of 1005 presented no evidence of bone exposure and 10 of the 30 patients were stage 0 with radiographic changes of osteosclerosis in the symptomatic area. Such cases present a dilemma for the clinician both in diagnosis and management of ARONJ. Exposed necrotic bone is an important clinical characteristic of ARONJ. In these variant cases, the absence of the clinical signs of ARONJ can lead to late diagnosis, prolonged disease course, and a condition that is refractory to treatment.[39] Patel and colleagues[39] proposed a modification of the current staging system and treatment guidelines for the management of the variant form, nonexposed BP-related ONJ. Patel and colleagues[39] also proposed to add to the current AAOMS staging guideline the term nonexposed to each stage to accurately reflect the clinical presentation of the ARONJ.[39]

Imaging

ARONJ is a well-defined clinical disease with consistent radiographic findings to include osteosclerosis, osteolysis, dense woven bone, thickened lamina dura, subperiosteal bone deposition, and failure of postsurgical remodeling.[44] Panoramic radiography is routinely used because it is one of the least expensive modalities for viewing the jaw. On the panoramic radiograph, bony sequestra, osteonecrosis, and metastatic lesion(s) are readily identifiable. In ARONJ diagnosis, panoramic imaging can be used as an initial study for evaluating the jaw,[3,45] although it may not reveal any significant changes for early stage ARONJ, but late stages may resemble periapical inflammatory lesions or osteomyelitis.[46]

Computed tomography (CT) is another modality that can be used for differential diagnosis. CT may reveal a higher bone density with bony sequestration in advanced ARONJ cases. Cone beam CT gives details on thickness of cortex, integrity and bone marrow involvement, cancellous bone mineral density, and irregularities after tooth extraction.[47,48]

Magnetic resonance imaging (MRI) can be useful in assessing osteonecrosis or ischemia with the use of contrast; however, it may give false-positive results.[48] The histopathologic changes of necrotic bone are comparable and are depicted similarly by MRI. MRI can show bone marrow changes associated with edema or inflammation resulting from an increase in water content, which replaces the normal fatty bone marrow. On MRI, these changes in marrow are seen as low signal intensity on T1-weighted imaged and a high signal intensity on T2-weighted images.[49] There is speculation that marrow edema is not a part of the pathogenesis of ARONJ as seen in avascular bone necrosis and MRI may be of limited use in the diagnosis of ARONJ.[3]

Bone scintigraphy is mostly used in diagnosis and management of metastatic disease. It can provide information regarding local metabolic and vascular changes, is highly sensitive to detecting bony involvement, and facilitates earlier diagnosis than conventional radiographs.[50] In a retrospective study conducted at Kaiser by O'Ryan and colleagues,[50] 35 patients with previous plantar technetium (Tc) 99 methylene diphosphate or hydroxymethylene diphosphonate bone scintigraphy, 23 (65.7%) showed positive tracer uptake in the areas that later developed ARONJ. ^{18}F-fluorodeoxyglucose positron emission tomography (FDG-PET)/CT is another diagnostic tool used in the evaluation of patients with metastatic disease and can also be used to identify subclinical areas of hypermetabolic activity in the jaw of patients with ARONJ. However, definitive diagnosis can only be determined by biopsy because FDG-PET cannot differentiate between malignancy and ARONJ.[49,51]

PATHOGENICITY

Since the presentation of ARONJ in 2003, many hypotheses have been proposed as to the possible cause of ARONJ. To date, the exact pathogenesis of ARONJ remains unclear. The most popular hypothesis for ARONJ proposes that BP suppresses bone remodeling by inducing osteoclast death or apoptosis. The non-nitrogen BP and nitrogen-containing BP work in different pathways but both inhibit osteoclast function by interfering with important cellular enzymes or production of toxic metabolites that ultimately cause osteoclast cell death. Recent reports of denosumab's involvement in the development of ARONJ reveal that the pathogenicity of ARONJ might be multifactorial.[52-55]

Impaired Epithelial Repair

It has been suggested that the local toxic effects of BPs may have osteonecrotic effects on nonbone cells that might contribute to ARONJ. Several studies have implicated epithelial cells as one target for BP. Scheller and colleagues[52] examined human tissue from individuals with ARONJ who were taking BP and compared them with individuals who were not taking BP to identify changes in oral epithelium and connective tissue. The BP ARONJ sites had reduced numbers of basal progenitor cells, suggesting that BP treatment may delay oral epithelial healing via the mevalonate pathway. Another implicated target for BP is macrophages. Coxon and colleagues[53] showed uptake of BP into macrophages adjacent to active osteoclasts on a bone surface which also suggests that nonbone cells can be affected by BP in this special situation.

Bacterial Colonization and Biofilm

Several studies have shown the presence of microorganisms, especially oral *Actinomyces* species, and multispecies microbial biofilms in bone specimens collected from patients with ARONJ.[54,56–58] Some of the bacterial morphotypes identified in ARONJ lesions are capable of bone resorption and are thought to play an important role in the pathogenesis of ARONJ. Furthermore, approximately 85% of patients with ARONJ have a history of periodontitis concurrently with the diagnosis of ARONJ.[58] Most patients with ARONJ present clinically with obvious bone exposure and infection that is similar to osteomyelitis, osteoradionecrosis,[59] trauma, or genetic bone disorders. Further evidence supporting a key role for infection in ARONJ is the observed high incidence of ARONJ in patients with cancer who are on chemotherapy regimens that include immunosuppressants and corticosteroids, which also render them more susceptible to odontogenic infections. Other medical comorbidities such as diabetes are common in patients with ARONJ and may be associated with chronic periodontitis and impaired wound healing leading to bacteria-induced bone loss.[60] Bone resorption is seen in all ARONJ bone specimens, and this destruction is potentially caused by oral microbial biofilm organisms because there is no evidence of eukaryotic cells, such as osteoclasts, within or adjacent to the observed resorption pits.[56] Certain oral bacteria are capable of inducing pathologic bone loss through various mechanisms.[61] Given the large numbers of gram-negative bacteria observed in the specimens in our study, it is conceivable that the porins they carry may play a major role in causing bone destruction and exposure of nonvital jaw bone (sequestration).[62] Porins are beta barrel proteins located on the outer membrane of gram-negative bacteria that render the membrane permeable to metabolites and small molecules (<1500 Da); in addition, porins are involved in the synthesis of proinflammatory mediators. Once bacterial growth is established, further colonization, biofilm growth, and antimicrobial resistance may be conferred to the microbial community through conjugation, transformation, and coaggregation. Sedghizadeh and colleagues[62] reported that patients with ARONJ harbor different microbial assemblages than patients without ARONJ.

Three genetic groups or phyla of microbes were found in 99% of ARONJ samples, including (1) 70% that were in the Proteobacteria phylum (*Klebsiella* and *Serratia*), (2) 26.9% Firmicutes (*Streptococcus*, *Bacillus*), and (3) 1.95% Actinobacteria. Hence it may be evident that specific bacteria play a role in infection and infection can contribute to the pathogenicity of ARONJ by enhancing osteoclast-independent bone resorption.[7]

Immunosuppression

There is increasing evidence, both in vitro and in vivo, supporting the hypothesis that nitrogen-containing BPs are able to influence the immune system by modulating both innate and adaptive immune responses.[55,63] Immunomodulation by BP treatment can result in either immunosuppression or generalized enhanced immune responses[28] that may subsequently promote the development of ARONJ.

Several studies have shown that patients with cancer treated with IV BP have a greater risk of developing ARONJ. Most of the patients with cancer are on multiple immunosuppressant drugs, including dexamethasone and chemotherapeutic agents; therefore, they may experience some degree of impaired immunity. Hence, it is likely that immunosuppression contributes to an increased susceptibility to ARONJ. Our group[64] recently developed an experimental model of murine ARONJ disease that recapitulates the major and radiographic manifestations of the human disease. Administration of zoledronate, a potent nitrogen-containing BP, was capable of inducing ARONJ in part by suppressing the adaptive regulatory T cell, (T_{regs}), and activating the inflammatory T helper producing interleukin-17 cell, thereby suppressing the ratio of T_{reg}/Th17 ratio. In addition, systemic infusion of cells of the immune system (pan T cells or T_{regs}) alone significantly decreases the incidence of ARONJ-like lesions in immunocompromised mice, confirming the role of T_{regs} in preventing ARONJ. Also, pan T-cell treatment improves healing of the extraction socket both at the mucosal and bone level. Based on these findings, we hypothesize that altered immune homeostasis may contribute to the pathogenesis of ARONJ. We have also proposed to evaluate the immune profile (T_{reg}, T-cell profile, and cytokines) in high-risk patients with cancer and low-risk patients with osteoporosis who are being treated with BP. Preliminary data from our ARONJ case control study of 23 patients with cancer and osteoporosis show that there is a significant decrease in the T_{reg}/Th17 ratio in the ARONJ patient group compared with the patients without ARONJ receiving BP and healthy patients (Le A. unpublished data, 2012).

DIAGNOSTIC DILEMMAS

Since the initial presentation of ARONJ in 2003, many researchers have conducted studies to investigate diagnostic methods to predict the risk of ARONJ. The bone turnover marker C-terminal cross-linking telopeptide (CTX) was recently proposed as a predictor of risks of ARONJ.[65] Serum CTX (sCTX) can determine bone turnover and act as a biologic marker for osteoclast activity; it is used to assess the level of bone resorption in many bone diseases, including rheumatoid arthritis, multiple myeloma, breast cancer, and liver cirrhosis.[66–68] In the process of bone metastasis, the primary mechanism of bone destruction is cancer cell–mediated stimulation of osteoclastic bone resorption[69] and degradation of type I collagen, which comprises more than 90% of organic bone, resulting in the release of CTX. CTX is derived from alpha-1 chain C-telopeptide of type I collagen that has undergone aging-associated peptide chain arrangement (beta) isomerization.[67] Marx and colleagues[70] reported that an sCTX value of 100 pg/mL was considered a high risk, whereas a value of 100 to 150 pg/mL was a moderate risk and an sCTX greater than 150 pg/mL has minimal risk. In addition, Marx and colleagues[70] suggested that dental surgery should not be performed until an sCTX greater than 150 pg/mL is achieved and that BP therapy be suspended for 4 to 6 months, if necessary, to attain this level. Although sCTX is recommended in the management of patients on BP, its use in predicting ARONJ are being challenged by many studies. In the literature analysis by Baim and Miller,[67] they reported that the ability of sCTX to act as predictive marker of ARONJ risk had not been explored in a large clinical trial, and no current available clinical data supported the use of an sCTX threshold as a guide to minimizing the risk of ARONJ in patients receiving oral BP treatment. They also reported that sCTX shows a wide range of al variability in both healthy patients and patients with bone disease. The Kunchur and colleagues[71] study showed the variability of the CTX test. They evaluated CTX tests on a total 348 patients, of whom 215 were on oral BP for osteoporosis and 7 patients were taking IV BP for multiple myeloma or metastatic cancer. The mean average sCTX values were 238 ± 144 pg/mL and 329 ± 354 pg/mL, respectively, in the osteoporosis and cancer groups. The oral BP group had 1 case of ARONJ development. Because of controversy concerning the use of sCTX in predicting the risk of ARONJ, more research is needed to find an alternative in the diagnosis, prevention, and management of ARONJ.

MANAGEMENT STRATEGIES
Surgical Strategies

In the past, the goals of treatment have been to reduce or eliminate pain, prevent or manage infection, and to prevent development of any new necrotic foci. Recent additions of elimination of necrotic foci and mucosal closure have been advocated and studied.[72] Since the publication of the original AAOMS position paper, staging has been critical to determining treatment strategies. Despite changes in staging and management, there is no clear agreement on a standard ARONJ treatment with predictable clinical outcomes. In the past, stage-directed treatment has been based primarily on clinical signs of exposed necrotic bone pain and infection, but recent studies show that this can lead to a misinterpretation of disease severity and poor treatment in the patient with no apparent necrotic bone exposure. In our review article[39] we propose a staging/treatment algorithm (**Fig. 1**) that considers the patient with atypical clinical features of persistent jaw bone pain, bone enlargement, and gingival swelling in the absence of significant dental disease or necrotic bone exposure.[40,42,43,73] With these modifications, patients showing a nonexposed variant of ARONJ will be managed as if the lesions were stage 2 or 3, rather than stage 0 or 1,[40,74,75] which may improve clinical outcomes for these atypical cases.

In addition to changes in staging, some clinicians have recommended surgical management at stage 1 in an attempt to eradicate the necrotic foci and obtain complete mucosal coverage.[71,76,77] Stanton and Balasanian[76] described their experience in using sequestrectomy or debridement to treat patients with exposed bone as their main inclusion criteria. These patients were placed on a 2-month drug holiday before and after surgery in coordination with their other treating physicians

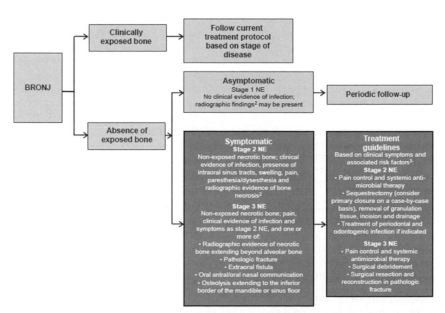

Fig. 1. Modified staging and treatment guidelines for nonexposed BP-related ONJ (BRONJ). (*From* Patel S, Choyee S, Uyanne J, et al. Non-exposed bisphosphonate-related osteonecrosis of the jaw: a critical assessment of current definition, staging, and treatment guidelines. Oral Dis 2012;18:629).

before surgery. Three of the 4 patients treated with sequestrectomy healed without incident. Of the 30 debridement cases, 25 healed completely, although 7 patients required additional sequestrectomy or debridements. Carlson and Basile[72] suggested that resection, whether marginal or segmental, is necessary to eradicate necrotic foci. Patients were treated based solely on the presence of exposed bone; they were not directed to take a drug holiday and the determination to perform a marginal resection versus segmental resection depended on absence or presence of basal bone involvement. Of the 92 resected sites, 91.6% healed with complete resolution with complete mucosal coverage. In a recent retrospective cohort, Graziani and colleagues[77] reviewed 347 subjects affected by ARONJ who underwent either local debridement (66%) or resection. Fifty-nine percent of subjects showed improvement after surgery, 30% showed no change, and 11% showed a worsening of their clinical condition. In the local debridement group, 49% of cases showed improvement, with no improvement in 35% and worsening in the remaining 16%, whereas, in the resective surgical patients, the results were statistically significant because improvement was seen in 68%, with no improvement in 27% and a worse clinical condition in 5%. These articles all suggest that early aggressive surgery may have better outcomes in patients with ARONJ.

Table 2
Current AAOMS guidelines on BP-related ONJ staging and treatment

Stages of ONJ	AAOMS 2009 Recommendations for Management of ONJ
At-risk category: no apparent necrotic bone in patients who have been treated with either oral or IV BPs	No treatment indicated: patient education
Stage 0: no clinical evidence of necrotic bone, but nonspecific clinical findings and symptoms	Symptomatic treatment: conservatively manage other local factors such as caries periodontal disease; systemic management including pain medication and antibiotics
Stage 1: exposed and necrotic bone in patients who are asymptomatic and have no evidence of infection	Antimicrobial mouth rinse, clinical follow-up on a quarterly basis, patient education and review of indications for continued BP therapy
Stage 2: exposed and necrotic bone associated with infection as shown by pain and erythema in the region of the exposed bone with or without purulent drainage	Symptomatic treatment: oral antibiotics, oral antibacterial mouth rinse Chronic pain medication, superficial debridement to relieve soft tissue irritation
Stage 3: exposed and necrotic bone in patients with pain, infection, and one or more of the following: exposed and necrotic bone extending beyond the region of alveolar bone resulting in pathologic fracture, extraoral, oral-antral/oral-nasal fistula, or osteolysis extending to the inferior border of the mandible or sinus floor	Antibacterial mouth rinse, antibiotic therapy, and pain control Surgical debridement/resection for longer term palliation of infection and pain

From Ruggiero SL, Dodson TB, Assael LA, et al. American Association of Oral and Maxillofacial Surgeons position paper on bisphosphonate-related osteonecrosis of the jaws-2009 update. J Oral Maxillofac Surg 2009;67(Suppl 5):7.

Table 3 Adjunctive and nonsurgical approaches to ARONJ management	
New Approaches	**Citation**
Hyperbaric oxygen	Freiberger et al. J Oral Maxillofac Surg 2012[80]
Platelet-rich plasma	Curi et al. J Oral Maxillofac Surg 2011[81]
Pentoxifylline and a-tocopherol	Epstein M. Oral Surg Oral Med Oral Pathol Oral Radiol Endod 2010[82]
Systemic low-dose parathyroid hormone	Harper R, Fung E. J Oral Maxillofac Surg 2007[83]
Low-dose systemic parathyroid hormone with vitamin D	Cheung A, Seeman E. N Engl J Med 2010[84]
Fluorescence-guided bone resection	Pautke et al. J Oral Maxillofac Surg 2011[85]
Laser ± Platelet-rich plasma	Martins et al. Oral Oncology 48:2012[86]; Vescovi et al. Photomed Laser Surg 2012[87]
Ozone	Agrillo Eur Rev Med Pharmacol Sci 2012[79]

Nonsurgical and Adjunctive Strategies

The AAOMS 2009 position paper recommends various nonsurgical managements in treating stages 0, 1, and 2 using antibiotics, pharmacologic pain management, and antimicrobial rinses, and these are listed in **Table 2**. In addition to the generally accepted nonsurgical treatments, Ruggiero[78] reviewed several articles using new adjunctive and nonsurgical approaches, as shown in **Table 3**. One new technology that was not mentioned was the use of ozone to treat ARONJ. Agrillo and colleagues[79] reviewed 94 patients diagnosed with ARONJ treated with a combination of antibiotic and antimycotic therapy as well as minimally invasive surgery and ozone therapy. Of the 94 patients treated, 57 (60%) experienced complete resolution with a decrease in symptoms; in 28 cases (30%) there was a marked reduction of the lesions and improvement of symptoms, whereas 9 patients (10%) only had a partial healing from symptoms without any resolution of the lesion. Further research is needed in diagnosis and management to further validate these results.

SUMMARY

Until recently, BP-related ONJ (BRONJ) was considered a rare bone disease that manifests in patients who are being treated with BP. Hence, BP was stated as the cause of BRONJ, although the exact linkage remained unknown. The recent development of ONJ in patients taking denosumab suggests that the pathogenicity of BRONJ, or the newly termed ARONJ, is multifactorial. In the literature, many hypotheses have been reported as to the mechanism by which BP causes ONJ and all may seem plausible, but the complexity of the pathophysiology of ARONJ still eludes researchers. The findings on denosumab may provide information on the potential role of immunosuppression in the development of ARONJ. Cofactors such as infection, diabetes, steroids, cancer, and chemotherapy may direct immune suppression and potentiate ARONJ development sooner in patients. The risk of ARONJ is associated with the type of antiresorptive medication, route, and dosage. ARONJ is not a problem that will vanish. As the aging population increases, more physicians will place patients on antiresorptive medications for the management of osteoporosis and cancer. More research and collaboration among researchers are needed on this debilitating disorder. Our group recently developed the first ARONJ experimental animal model that reproduces the major clinical and radiographic manifestations of this disease. Our findings suggest that host immune response in conjunction with oral microbial biofilm plays a significant role in the pathogenesis of ARONJ. A pilot case-controlled study is currently underway to further evaluate the findings from our animal study. Preliminary results show some promise. For better understanding of the pathophysiology of ARONJ in humans, more multicenter clinical trials are needed. Since the first report of ARONJ in 2003, the slow progress in both pathophysiology and clinical research underscore the need for translational research on this high-priority topic.

REFERENCES

1. Ruggiero SL, Fantasia J, Carlson E. Bisphosphonate-related osteonecrosis of the jaw: background and guidelines for diagnosis, staging and management. Oral Surg Oral Med Oral Pathol Oral Radiol Endod 2006;102(4):433–41.
2. AAOMS: Advisory Task Force on Bisohosphonate-related Osteonecrosis of the Jaws, American Association of Oral and Maxillofacial Surgeons. American Association of Oral and Maxillofacial Surgeons position paper on bisphosphonate-related osteonecrosis of the jaws. J Oral Maxillofac Surg 2007;65:369–76.
3. Khosla S, Burr D, Cauley J, et al. Bisphosphonate-associated osteonecrosis of the jaws: report of a task force of the American Society for Bone and Mineral Research. J Bone Miner Res 2007;22:1479–91.
4. Ruggiero SL. Bisphosphonate-related osteonecrosis of the jaw (BRONJ): initial discovery and subsequent development. J Oral Maxillofac Surg 2009; 67(Suppl 5):13–8.
5. Allen M. The effects of bisphosphonates on jaw bone remodeling, tissue properties, and extraction healing. Odontology 2011;99:8–17.
6. Hellstein JW, Adler RA, Edwards B, et al. Managing the care of patients receiving antiresorptive therapy for prevention and treatment of osteoporosis. J Am Dent Assoc 2011;142(11):1243–51.
7. Allen MR, Burr DB. The pathogenesis of bisphosphonate-related osteonecrosis of the jaw: so many hypotheses, so few data. J Oral Maxillofac Surg 2009; 67(Suppl 5):61–70.
8. Lipton A, Steger GG, Figueroa J, et al. Randomized active-controlled phase II study of denosumab efficacy and safety in patients with breast cancer-related bone metastases. J Clin Oncol 2007;25:4431–7.
9. Ruggiero SL, Drew SJ. Osteonecrosis of the jaws and bisphosphonate therapy. J Dent Res 2007;86:1013–21.
10. Freiberger JJ. Utility of hyperbaric oxygen in treatment of bisphosphonate-related osteonecrosis of the jaws. J Oral Maxillofac Surg 2009;67(Suppl 5): 96–106.
11. Reszka AA, Rodan GA. Bisphosphonate mechanism of action. Curr Rheumatol Rep 2003;5:65–74.
12. Rogers MJ, Gordon S, Benford HL, et al. Cellular and molecular mechanisms of action of bisphosphonates. Cancer 2000;88:2961–78.
13. Van den Wyngaert T, Huizing MT, Vermorken JB. Bisphosphonates and osteonecrosis of the jaw: cause and effect or a post hoc fallacy? Ann Oncol 2006; 17:1197–204.
14. Brown-Glaberman U, Stopeck AT. Role of denosumab in the management of skeletal complications in patients with bone metastases from solid tumors. Biologics 2012;6:89–99.

15. Fleisher KE, Jolly A, Venkata UDC, et al. Osteonecrosis of the jaw onset times are based on the route of bisphosphonate therapy. J Oral Maxillofac Surg 2013;71(3):513–9.
16. Silva-Fernandez L, Rosario MP, Martinez-Lopez JA, et al. Denosumab for the treatment of osteoporosis: a systematic literature review. Rheumatalo Clin 2013;9(1):42–52.
17. Bridgeman MB, Pathak R. Denosumab for the reduction of bone loss in post-menopausal osteoporosis: a review. Clin Ther 2011;22(11):1547–59.
18. Steger G, Bartsch R. Denosumab for the treatment of bone metastases in breast cancer: evidence and opinion. Ther Adv Med Oncol 2011;2(5):233–43.
19. Lacey DL, Boyle WJ, Simonet WS, et al. Bench to bedside: elucidation of the OPG-RANK-RANKL pathway and the development of denosumab. Nat Rev Drug Discov 2012;11(5):401–19.
20. Prolia (Denosumab) [prescribing information]. Thousand Oaks (CA): Amgen; 2010.
21. Cavilli L, Brandi ML. Targeted approaches in the treatment of osteoporosis: differential mechanism of action of denosumab and clinical utility. Ther Clin Risk Manag 2012;8:253–66.
22. Marx RE. Pamidronate (Aredia) and Zoledronate (Zometa) induced avascular necrosis of the jaws: a growing epidemic. J Oral Maxillofac Surg 2003;61: 1115–7.
23. Ruggiero SL, Mehrotra B, Rosenberg TJ, et al. Osteonecrosis of the jaws associated with the use of bisphosphonates: a review of 63 cases. J Oral Maxillofac Surg 2004;62(5):527–34.
24. Wang J, Goodger NM, Progel MA. Osteonecrosis of the jaws associated with cancer chemotherapy. J Oral Maxillofac Surg 2003;61:1104–7.
25. Dimopoulos M, Kastritis E, Moulopoulos LA, et al. The incidence of osteonecrosis of the jaw in patients with multiple myeloma who receive bisphosphonates depends on the type of bisphosphonate. Blood 2005;106:637 [American Society of Hematology Annual Meeting Abstracts].
26. Bamias A, Kastritis E, Bamia C, et al. Osteonecrosis of the jaw in cancer after treatment with bisphosphonates: incidence and risk factors. J Clin Oncol 2005;23:8580–7.
27. Drake MT, Clark BL, Khosla S. Bisphosphonates: mechanism of action and role in clinical practice. Mayo Clin Proc 2008;83:1032–45.
28. Wimalawansa SJ. Insight into bisphosphonate-associated osteomyelitis of the jaw: pathophysiology, mechanisms and clinical management. Expert Opin Drug Saf 2008;7:491–512.
29. Wessel JH, Dodson TB, Zavras AI, et al. Zoledronate, smoking and obesity are strong risk factors for osteonecrosis of the jaw: a case-control study. J Oral Maxillofac Surg 2008;66(4):625–31.
30. Tennis P, Rothman KJ, Bohn RL, et al. Incidence of osteonecrosis of the jaw among users of bisphosphonates with selected cancers or osteoporosis. Pharmacoepidemiol Drug Saf 2012;21:810–7.
31. Wang EP, Kaban LB, Strewler GJ, et al. Incidence of osteonecrosis of the jaw in patients with multiple myeloma and breast or prostate cancer on intravenous bisphosphonate therapy. J Oral Maxillofac Surg 2007;65(7):1328–31.
32. Gliklich R, Wilson J. Epidemiology of bisphosphonate-related osteonecrosis of the jaw: the utility of a national registry. J Oral Maxillofac Surg 2009;67(4):850–5.
33. Woo SB, Helllstein JW, Kalmar JR. Systemic review: bisphosphonates and osteonecrosis of the jaws. Ann Intern Med 2006;144:753–6.

34. Knight RJW, Reddy C, Rtshiladze MA, et al. Bisphosphonate-related osteonecrosis of the jaw: tip of the iceberg. J Craniofac Surg 2010;21:25–32.
35. Hellstein JW, Marek CL. Bis-phossy jaw, phossy jaw, and the 21st century: bisphosphonate-associated complications of the jaws. J Oral Maxillofac Surg 2004;62:1563–6.
36. Mavrokokki T, Cheng A, et al. Nature and frequency of bisphosphonate-associated osteonecrosis of the jaws in Australia. J Oral Maxillofac Surg 2007; 65:415–23.
37. Ruggiero SL. Bisphosphonate-related osteonecrosis of the jaw: an overview. Ann N Y Acad Sci 2011;1218:38–46.
38. Khan AA, Sándor GK, Dore E, et al. Canadian consensus practice guidelines for bisphosphonate associated osteonecrosis of the jaw. J Rheumatol 2008;35: 1391–7.
39. Patel S, Choyee S, Uyanne J, et al. Non-exposed bisphosphonate-related osteonecrosis of the jaw: a critical assessment of current definition, staging, and treatment guideline. Oral Dis 2012;18(7):625–32.
40. Junquera L, Gallego L. Nonexposed bisphosphonate-related osteonecrosis of the jaws: another clinical variant? J Oral Maxillofac Surg 2008;66(7):1516–7.
41. Fedele S, Porter SR, D'Aiuto F, et al. Nonexposed variant of bisphosphonate-associated osteonecrosis of the jaw: a case series. Am J Med 2010;123(11): 1060–4.
42. Vescovi P, Nammour S. Bisphosphonate-related osteonecrosis of the Jaw (BRONJ) therapy. A critical review. Minerva Stomatol 2010;59(4):181–203, 204–13.
43. Hutchinson M, O'Ryan F, Chavez V, et al. Radiographic findings in bisphosphonate-treated patients with stage 0 disease in the absence of bone exposure. J Oral Maxillofac Surg 2010;68(9):2232–40.
44. Bedogni A, Blandamura S, Lokmic Z, et al. Bisphosphonate-associated jawbone osteonecrosis: a correlation between imaging techniques and histopathology. Oral Surg Oral Med Oral Pathol Oral Radiol Endod 2008;105(3):358–64.
45. Store G, Larheim TA. Mandibular osteoradionecrosis: a comparison of computed tomography with panoramic radiography. Dentomaxillofac Radiol 1999;28(5):295–300.
46. Ficarra G, Beninati F. Bisphosphonate-related osteonecrosis of the jaws: an update on clinical, pathological and management aspects. Head Neck Pathol 2007;1(2):132–40.
47. Marx RE. Reconstruction of defects caused by bisphosphonate-induced osteonecrosis of the jaws. J Oral Maxillofac Surg 2009;67(Suppl 5):107–19.
48. Ganapathy N, Gokulnathan S, Bajan N, et al. Bisphosphonates: an update. J Pharm Bioallied Sci 2012;4(Suppl 2):S410–3.
49. Arce K, Assael LA, Weissman JL. Imaging findings in bisphosphonate-related osteonecrosis of jaws. J Oral Maxillofac Surg 2009;67(Suppl 1):75–84.
50. O'Ryan FS, Khoury S, Liao W, et al. Intravenous bisphosphonate-related osteonecrosis of the jaw: bone scintigraphy as an early indicator. J Oral Maxillofac Surg 2009;67(7):1363–72.
51. Unger E, Moldofsky P, Gatenby R, et al. Diagnosis of osteomyelitis by MR imaging. AJR Am J Roentgenol 1988;150(3):605–10.
52. Scheller EL, Baldwin CM, Kuo S, et al. Bisphosphonates inhibit expression of p63 by oral keratinocytes. J Dent Res 2011;90(7):894–9.
53. Coxon FP, Thompson K, Roelofs AJ, et al. Visualizing mineral binding and uptake of bisphosphonate by osteoclasts and non-resorbing cells. Bone 2008; 42:848–60.

54. Hansen T, Kunkel M, Springer E, et al. Actinomycosis of the jaws–histopathological study of 45 patients shows significant involvement in bisphosphonate-associated osteonecrosis and infected osteonecrosis. Virchows Arch 2007;451:1009–17.
55. Wolf AM, et al. The effect of zoledronic acid on the function and differentiation of myeloid cells. Haematologica 2006;91:1165–71.
56. Sedghizadeh PP, Kumar SKS, Gorur A, et al. Identification of microbial biofilms in osteonecrosis of the jaws secondary to bisphosphonate therapy. J Oral Maxillofac Surg 2008;66:767–75.
57. Sedghizadeh PP, Kumar SK, Gorur A, et al. Microbial biofilms in osteomyelitis of the jaw and osteonecrosis of the jaw secondary to bisphosphonate therapy. J Am Dent Assoc 2009;140:1259–66.
58. Marx RE, Sawatari Y, Fortin M, et al. Bisphosphonate-induced exposed bone (osteonecrosis/osteopetrosis) of the jaws: risk factors, recognition, prevention, and treatment. J Oral Maxillofac Surg 2005;63(11):1567–75.
59. Epstein J, Van Der Meij E, McKenzie M, et al. Postradiation osteonecrosis of the mandible: a long-term follow up study. Oral Surg Oral Med Oral Pathol Oral Radiol Endod 1997;83:657–62.
60. He H, Lui R, Desta T, et al. Diabetes causes osteoclastogenesis, reduced bone formation and enhanced apoptosis of osteoblastic cell in bacteria stimulated bone loss. Endocrinology 2004;145:447–52.
61. Henderson B, Nair SP. Hard labour: bacterial infection of the skeleton. Trends Microbiol 2003;11:570–7.
62. Sedghizadeh PP, Yooseph S, Fadrosh DW, et al. Metagenomic investigation of microbes and viruses in patient with jaw osteonecrosis associated with bisphosphonate therapy. Oral Surg Oral Med Oral Pathol Oral Radiol 2012;114(6):764–70.
63. Melani C, Sangaletti S, Barazzetta FM, et al. Amino-biphosphonate-mediated MMP-9 inhibition breaks the tumor-bone marrow axis responsible for myeloid-derived suppressor cell expansion and macrophage infiltration in tumor stroma. Cancer Res 2007;67:11438–46.
64. Kikuiri T, Kim I, Yamaza T, et al. Cell-based immunotherapy with mesenchymal stem cells cures bisphosphonate-related osteonecrosis of the jaw-like disease in mice. J Bone Miner Res 2010;25(7):1668–79.
65. Marx RE. Bisphosphonate-induce osteonecrosis of the jaws: a challenge, a responsibility and an opportunity. Int J Periodontics Restorative Dent 2008;28:5–6.
66. Lee CY, Suzuki JB. CTX biochemical marker of bone metabolism. Is it a reliable predictor of bisphosphonate-associated osteonecrosis of the jaws after surgery? Part II: a prospective clinical study. Implant Dent 2010;19(1):29–38.
67. Baim S, Miller P. Perspective assessing the clinical utility of serum CTX in post-menopausal osteoporosis and its use in predicting risk of osteonecrosis of the jaw. J Bone Miner Res 2009;24:561–74.
68. Bagan JV, Jimenez Y, Gómez D, et al. Collagen telopeptide (serum CTX) and its relationship with size and number of lesion in osteonecrosis of the jaw in cancer patient on IV bisphosphonate. Oral Oncol 2006;44:1088–9.
69. Salem AM, Zohny SF, Abd El-Wahab MM, et al. Predictive value of osteocalcin and β-CrossLaps in metastatic breast cancer. Clin Biochem 2007;40:1201–8.
70. Marx RE, Cillo JE, Ulloa JJ. Oral bisphosphonate-induced osteonecrosis: risk factors, prediction of risk using serum CTX testing, prevention, and treatment. J Oral Maxillofac Surg 2007;65(12):2397–410.
71. Kunchur R, Need A, Hughes T, et al. Clinical Investigation of C-terminal cross-linking telopeptide test in prevention and management of bisphosphonate-associated osteonecrosis of the jaws. J Oral Maxillofac Surg 2009;67(6):1167–73.

72. Carlson ER, Basile JD. The role of surgical resection in the management of bisphosphonate-related osteonecrosis of the jaws. J Oral Maxillofac Surg 2009;67(Suppl 5):85–95.

73. Yarom N, Fedele S, Lazarovici TS, et al. Is exposure of the jawbone mandatory for establishing the diagnosis of bisphosphonate-related osteonecrosis of the jaw? J Oral Maxillofac Surg 2010;68(3):705.

74. Ruggiero SL, Dodson TB, Assael LA, et al. American Association of Oral and Maxillofacial Surgeons position paper on bisphosphonate-related osteonecrosis of the jaws–2009 update. J Oral Maxillofac Surg 2009;67(Suppl 5):2–12.

75. Mawardi H, Treister N, Richardson P, et al. Sinus tracts–an early sign of bisphosphonate-associated osteonecrosis of the jaws? J Oral Maxillofac Surg 2009;67(3):593–601.

76. Stanton DC, Balasanian E. Outcome of surgical management of bisphosphonate-related osteonecrosis of the jaws: review of 33 surgical cases. J Oral Maxillofac Surg 2009;67(5):943–50.

77. Graziani F, Vescovi P, Campisi G, et al. Resective surgical approach shows a high performance in the management of advanced cases of bisphosphonate-related osteonecrosis of the jaws: a retrospective survey of 347 cases. J Oral Maxillofac Surg 2012;70(11):2501–7.

78. Ruggiero SL. Emerging concepts in the management and treatment of osteonecrosis of the jaw. Oral Maxillofac Surg Clin North Am 2013;25(1):11–20.

79. Agrillo F, Filiaci F, Ramieri V, et al. Bisphosphonate-related osteonecrosis of the jaw (BRONJ): 5 year experience in the treatment of 131 cases with ozone therapy. Eur Rev Med Pharmacol Sci 2012;16(12):1741–7.

80. Freiberger JJ, Padilla-Burgos R, McGraw T, et al. What is the role of hyperbaric oxygen in the management of bisphosphonate-related osteonecrosis of the jaw: a randomized controlled trial of hyperbaric oxygen as an adjunct to surgery and antibiotics. J Oral Maxillofac Surg 2012;70(7):1573–83.

81. Curi MM, Cossolin GSI, Koga DH, et al. Bisphosphonate-related osteonecrosis of the jaws–an initial case series report of treatment combining partial bone resection and autologous platelet-rich plasma. J Oral Maxillofac Surg 2011;69(9):2465–72.

82. Epstein MS, Wicknick FW, Epstein JB. Management of bisphosphonate-associated osteonecrosis: pentoxifylline and tocopherol in addition to antimicrobial therapy. An initial case series. Oral Surg Oral Med Oral Pathol Oral Radiol Endod 2010;110:593–6.

83. Harper R, Fung E. Resolution of bisphosphonate-associated osteonecrosis of the mandible: possible application for intermittent low-dose parathyroid hormone [rhPTH(1-34)]. J Oral Maxillofac Surg 2007;65(3):573–80.

84. Cheung A, Seeman E. Teriparatide therapy for alendronate-associated osteonecrosis of the jaw. N Engl J Med 2010;363(25):2473–4.

85. Pautke C, Bauer F, Otto S, et al. Fluorescence-guided bone resection in bisphosphonate-related osteonecrosis of the jaws: first clinical results of a prospective pilot study. J Oral Maxillofac Surg 2011;69(1):84–91.

86. Martins MA, Martins MD, Lascala CA. Association of laser phototherapy with PRP improves healing of bisphosphonate-related osteonecrosis of the jaws in cancer patients: a preliminary study. Oral Oncology 2012;48:79–84.

87. Vescovi P, Merigo E, Manfredi M. Nd:YAG Laser Biostimulation in the Treatment of Bisphosphonate-Associated Osteonecrosis of the Jaw: Clinical Experience in 28 Cases. Photomedicine and Laser Surgery 2008;26(1):37–46.

The Role of Human Papillomavirus in Oral Disease

Gordon A. Pringle, DDS, PhD

KEYWORDS

- Human papillomavirus • Squamous papilloma • Condyloma acuminatum
- Oral squamous cell carcinoma • Multifocal epithelial hyperplasia • Verruca vulgaris

KEY POINTS

- A wide range of low-risk and high-risk human papillomavirus (HPV) genotypes have been detected in oral mucosa after infection. Clinical infections with low-risk genotypes manifest as squamous papilloma, condyloma acuminatum, verruca vulgaris, or multifocal epithelial hyperplasia.
- Clinical infections with high-risk genotypes have been associated with malignant lesions. The most common genotype isolated from subclinical infection is HPV-16.
- Unlike oropharyngeal carcinoma, a causal role for HPV in carcinogenesis of oral squamous carcinoma is minimal, with greater influence in a small subset of nonsmokers.
- Ongoing vaccination against HPV types 6, 11, 16, and 18 is expected to decrease spread of infection and decrease the carcinogenic potential of HPV-16 in the oropharynx and oral cavity.

INTRODUCTION

Human papillomavirus (HPV) is the cause of benign cutaneous and anogenital warts (condyloma acuminatum). HPV is also firmly established as an etiologic agent in cervical, vulvar, penile, and anal intraepithelial neoplasia (dysplasia) and carcinoma.[1,2] Low-risk and high-risk anogenital HPV genotypes are spread by sexual contact. The same viral genotypes have been identified in oral condylomata, squamous papillomas, and head and neck squamous cell carcinomas.[3,4] The same viral genotypes have also been detected in exfoliated cells of the oral cavity[5,6] or brushings of normal oral mucosa[7-9] in 6% to 30% of study populations; HPV-16, the high-risk genotype most commonly associated with cervical and genital carcinomas, is also the most common oral genotype[5,8,9] identified. Although the incidence of oral squamous carcinoma in the United States, largely as a result of environmental carcinogens derived from tobacco, alcohol, and areca nut use has remained relatively

Oral Pathology Laboratory, Department of Pathology and Laboratory Medicine, Temple University School of Medicine, Temple University Hospital, 3401 North Broad Street, Philadelphia, PA 19040, USA
E-mail address: gpringle@temple.edu

Dent Clin N Am 58 (2014) 385–399
http://dx.doi.org/10.1016/j.cden.2013.12.008
0011-8532/14/$ – see front matter © 2014 Elsevier Inc. All rights reserved.

dental.theclinics.com

stable, the incidence of oropharyngeal squamous carcinoma, strongly associated with HPV-16, has been increasing rapidly.[10–12]

THE VIRUS

HPVs constitute several species within 5 genera of the Papillomaviridae family. All HPVs share the same basic structure: a nonenveloped virus, 55 nm in diameter, with an icosahedral protein capsid consisting of 72 capsomeres. The viral genome is circular double-stranded DNA, approximately 7900 bp in length. All putative coding sequences are located on only 1 DNA strand.[1,2]

The HPV genome consists of 3 functional regions.[13–15] Soon after infection, early genes (E1-E7) are transcribed, and their protein products control viral replication and gene transcription and modulate epithelial cell growth and proliferation. The E2 gene product is a transcriptional repressor that inhibits transcription of oncogenic E6 and E7 proteins. Genes expressed later (L1 and L2) code for the capsid proteins and are transcribed before the final assembly of virions. An upstream regulatory region of the viral genome is noncoding and controls viral DNA replication and transcription of the early and late genes. Sequence analysis of the L1 major capsid protein gene derived from DNA isolated from various benign and malignant lesions has shown that considerable genomic variation exists in this gene. Less than 90% homology between L1 genes defines different HPV genotypes, and there are more than 120 well-characterized genotypes, with many more recognized (**Table 1**).

Much of the recent literature relating HPV genotypes with disease has focused on HPV in the cause of anogenital warts and dysplasia and cancer of the uterine cervix. At least 40 HPV genotypes can infect genital skin and mucosae.[1,2] HPV genotypes associated with high-grade dysplasia and carcinoma of cervical, vaginal, vulvar, penile, and anal epithelium are subclassified as high risk, whereas those genotypes associated with low-grade dysplasia, condylomata, and other warts are described

Table 1
HPV genotypes and associated epithelial lesions

Genotypes	Lesion
1, 2, 4, 26, 27, 57	Verruca vulgaris
3, 10, 26, 27, 75	Verruca plana
1, 2, 4, 63	Plantar warts
13, 32	Multifocal epithelial hyperplasia
6, 11, can also harbor high-risk genotypes	Condyloma acuminatum
6, 11, can also harbor high-risk genotypes	Oral squamous papilloma
6, 11, can also harbor high-risk genotypes	Recurrent respiratory papillomatosis
6, 11, can also harbor high-risk genotypes	Anogenital low-grade intraepithelial neoplasia
16, 18, 31, 33, 51, 52, 66 and other high-risk genotypes	Anogenital high-grade intraepithelial neoplasia
16, 18, 31, 33, 35, 51, 66, 73, 82 and other high-risk genotypes	Anogenital and cervical carcinoma
16, 33, 31, 18, 52 and other high-risk genotypes	Head and neck squamous cell carcinoma

The table lists the more common genotypes associated with the disease, as well as a small representative number of other genotypes. This list is not exhaustive; many other genotypes are also potentially involved in the various lesions listed.

as low risk. High-risk types 16 and 18 account for approximately 70% of high-grade anogenital disease,[1] whereas low-risk types 6 and 11 are the most common genotypes associated with condylomata and low-grade anogenital disease.[1,2] In low-risk infections, the viral genome remains as an episome in the nucleus, independent of the host DNA.[16] In this type of infection, E2 function is not disrupted, which allows E2 protein to potentially suppress transcription of E6/E7 gene(s). Replication of the viral genome occurs in parallel with host genome replication, resulting in a stable viral copy number distributed among daughter epithelial cells. In high-grade dysplasia and carcinomas, the high-risk HPV genome is present in high copy number, is typically integrated into the host DNA, and when integration involves disruption of the E2 gene and its regulatory function, there is increased transcription of E6 and E7 genes.[13,15] Whether simply a quantitative increase or a significant structural difference in the E6 and E7 proteins produced by high-risk genotypes, or both, it is the increased production of these 2 oncoproteins in high-risk HPV infections that account for the carcinogenic potential of HPV.

E7 protein interacts with pRb, the tumor suppressor protein that controls entry into the S phase of the cell cycle. The E7:pRb complex effectively inhibits pRb control of these critical restriction points, allowing the rate of cell cycling to increase.[16] Concomitantly, E6 protein interacts with several molecules in critical pathways that control cell replication, inhibiting mechanisms of suppression and enhancing the function of cellular oncoproteins. A major target of E6 is p53, the tumor suppressor protein that monitors critical cellular pathways and the integrity of the genome during DNA replication. DNA breakage, chromosomal loss, and mutations that potentially disrupt genome replication cause an increase in p53, which in turn halts the cell cycle to initiate DNA repair or, if irreparable, it initiates apoptosis. E6 protein inactivates p53 by targeting it for ubiquitination and degradation. With the resultant decrease in p53, defective host cell DNA can continue through the cell cycle. This process causes daughter cells to continually accumulate mutations and chromosomal loss caused by increased genetic instability, a hallmark of carcinogenesis. Inhibiting pRb function, as described earlier, accelerates the neoplastic transformation process.

HPV INFECTION

HPV infection is limited to epithelium, with most infections occurring in squamous epithelium of skin and mucosae.[14] After infection of basal epithelial cells and a variable incubation period, viral replication and assembly of virions occurs as squamous cells differentiate, with mature virus shed with sloughing superficial cells.[1,2,14] Latent HPV infections are considered noninfectious, because the viral copy number per cell is too low to transmit disease. In subclinical HPV infections, viral DNA replication and transcription are active, present in infectious epithelium not yet observable as a clinical lesion.[13] Clinical HPV infections contain active virus present in an infectious, clinically apparent lesion. Latent and subclinical infections are probably most common.[2,17] The clinical and microscopic features of HPV-induced epithelial lesions vary with the anatomic site infected and the genotype of the virus.[18] Thus, clinical lesions can be exophytic and flat, papillomatous or verruciform, or endophytic and less obvious. Histopathologically, subclinical and clinical lesions can be benign, dysplastic with varying degrees of intraepithelial neoplasia, or malignant. In clinical infections, virally affected epithelial cells can be visible microscopically in the upper spinous layer as koilocytes (cells with a small condensed nucleus and perinuclear clear space). Individual epithelial lesions can harbor more than 1 HPV genotype.

Persistent infection with high-risk HPV genotypes is necessary for HPV-induced carcinogenesis, but is not sufficient, because cervical cancer does not develop in most infected women. There are several factors that potentially govern the risk and rate of HPV-induced carcinogenesis. For example, a high-risk HPV infection that lacks effective translation of E6/E7 messenger RNA (mRNA) does not contribute significantly to carcinogenesis.[19] Transcription of E6/E7 genes may be influenced by the degree to which E2 is disrupted after viral integration. Hypermethylation of genes in other important pathways governing host cell growth and replication may also decrease the effectiveness of E6 and E7 proteins, as might structural polymorphisms in p53 and pRb, which could decrease binding affinity of the viral oncoproteins. Furthermore, although high-risk infections that actively transcribe E6/E7 mRNA foster genetic instability, they themselves are not directly mutagenic. Other promoting agents, such as cigarette smoking, or coinfections, seem to be required.

HPV IMMUNOLOGY

Because the growth cycle of HPV is limited to epithelium, HPV antigens are minimally exposed to the immune system. Nevertheless, cell-mediated immunity is believed to be the most effective means of controlling viral infection.[13] All aspects of infection are increased in immunosuppressed individuals.[13,17,20,21] Cell-mediated immunity is also believed to be the reason that most lesions and subclinical lesions undergo spontaneous regression.[22] It has been reported[1] that certain human leukocyte antigen (HLA) class II alleles that help govern the immune response are associated with persistence of viral infection and increased susceptibility for HPV-induced carcinogenesis.

Humoral immunity is limited, because the principal viral antigen, the L1 major capsid protein, is expressed only in the superficial epithelial layers.[1] Seroconversion has been estimated to occur in only 60% of infected patients and can take 6 months or more to develop.[2] Antibodies reactive to E6 and E7 proteins have also been detected and signify that the viral infection is transcriptionally active. Seropositivity for HPV16 E6 and E7 proteins has been used as a biomarker for increased survival of patients with oropharyngeal carcinoma.[23]

HPV TRANSMISSION

Transmission of HPV is caused by direct contact of skin or mucosa with an infected lesion. Minor trauma at the site is believed to facilitate infection of the basal epithelial cells. Cutaneous low-risk HPV infections include common warts (verruca vulgaris), juvenile flat warts (verruca plana), and plantar warts. They are widespread in the general population, with a prevalence of 3% to 20%.[1] Verrucae are more common in children, whereas plantar warts are more common in adolescents and young adults. Anogenital warts (condyloma acuminatum) are transmitted via sexual intercourse, orogenital and manual-genital contact, and autoinoculation.[24,25] Open mouth-to-mouth kissing is also a means of nonsexual transmission.[26] Nosocomial transmission of HPV present in fumes caused by laser ablation of lesions is believed to be possible.[2] HPV can be transmitted to the mouth and upper airway of a newborn from an infected mother during birth, which can result in recurrent respiratory papillomatosis and severe breathing difficulties in infants.[1]

EPIDEMIOLOGY

It has been estimated that 6 million new genital HPV infections occur annually in sexually active young people.[1] Genital HPV infection is one of the most common sexually transmitted diseases. Number of sexual partners, frequency of sex, and absence of condoms, immunization, and circumcision are important risk factors.[1,2] The prevalence of anogenital warts in the general population is estimated at 1%, with 5% to 6% of a study group ranging in age from 18 to 59 years reported having had them.[27]

The prevalence of oral HPV infection has also been studied using polymerase chain reaction (PCR) technique and subsequent genotyping of oral rinse samples or mucosal scrapings. The genotypes identified are typically the low-risk and high-risk types found genitally. Evaluation of rinse samples from a large study group in the United States ranging in age from 14 to 69 years showed that HPV DNA was detectable in 6.9% of the sample population.[5] A separate study estimated that 7.3% of the adult US population had 1 or more HPV types detected in oral rinse.[6] Low-risk, high-risk, and multiple type infections were found, and infection was more prevalent in men than women.[5,6] High-risk infections were slightly more common than low-risk infections. High-risk HPV-16 infection was most common (1.0%).[5] Oral infection was higher in those with a history of sexual contact and increased with number of sexual partners. Similar findings were reported in a smaller Finnish family study using scrapings from buccal mucosa analyzed by PCR and genotyping at various time points over 7 years.[7–9] Infection of males (15%–31%) and females (15%–24%) varied during the 7-year period. Females showed a greater prevalence of low-risk infections than males, and like previous studies, the most frequent infection was HPV-16, and it was most likely to persist.[22] Low-risk HPV infections cleared from the mouth faster than high-risk infections.[22] Although the oral mucosa may play a significant role in HPV transmission, these methods provide no measure of viral load or whether the high-risk types present are transcriptionally active.

A recent endodontic publication reported HPV in a small percentage (13%) of periapical abscesses using PCR and a non–type-specific L1 sequence.[28] Determination of the specific role of the virus in this location awaits further study.

HPV-16 has been detected in cyclosporine-induced gingival fibrous hyperplasia in renal allograft patients[29] and in acute gingivitis in patients with AIDS.[30] HPV-16 has also been detected in gingival tissues from patients with chronic periodontitis, and it has been postulated that oral, as well as sulcular and junctional epithelium, may serve as a source for infection or persistent infection of HPV. A recent study using real-time PCR with 104 gingival samples found no HPV-16 and concluded no association of HPV-16 with chronic periodontitis.[31]

Subclinical HPV infections are not readily identified in the oral cavity by clinical means. Detection of high-risk genotypes in oral rinse samples by PCR and subsequent genotype-specific hybridization indicates only that HPV DNA (infection) is present. This information may provide impetus for patients to alter their social behavior, with subsequent tests evaluating persistence or absence of infection. This method does not provide information as to the location of oral infection, the surface area of oral epithelium infected, or the risk of transmission of infection to others by way of oral or sexual contact.

ORAL CLINICAL LESIONS ASSOCIATED WITH HPV
Verruca Vulgaris (Common Wart)

Caused principally by HPV-2 and HPV-4, this cutaneous lesion is most commonly observed in children on the hands and fingers. Verruca vulgaris is uncommon in the mouth (**Fig. 1**A). This wart is a well-circumscribed growth of squamous epithelium with prominent hyperkeratosis, giving it a white pebbly or papillary surface (see **Fig. 1**B). A heavy granular layer and koilocytes are typically observed histologically

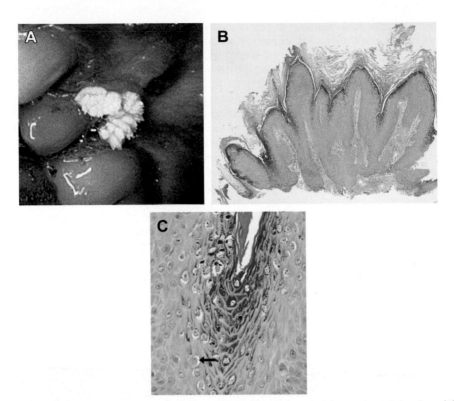

Fig. 1. (*A*) Verruca vulgaris on palatal gingival showing typical heavy keratinization. (*B*) Low-power photomicrograph depicting overall architecture of verruca vulgaris. (*C*) High-power photomicrograph depicting hyperorthokeratosis, prominent granular layer and koilocytes (*arrow*). ([A] *Courtesy of* Thomas Daley, DDS, MSc, London, Ontario, Canada.)

(see **Fig. 1**C). Oral lesions resemble skin lesions both clinically and microscopically and occur via autoinoculation of fingers to mouth.

Multifocal Epithelial Hyperplasia (Heck Disease)

Multifocal epithelial hyperplasia presents most commonly in children as multiple, small, slightly elevated and minimally keratinized papules located mainly on labial and buccal mucosa and tongue. Caused by HPV-13 and HPV-32, lesions occur in a tight cluster, giving a cobblestone appearance to the mucosa (**Fig. 2**). Risk factors for infection include crowded, unhygienic living conditions and the HLA-DR4 allele. Multifocal epithelial hyperplasia has also been reported in immunosuppressed patients.[32] Like verrucae, spontaneous regression of lesions is common after months to years.

Condyloma Accuminatum (Venereal Wart)

Condylomata are most common in the anogenital region and are regarded as a sexually transmitted disease. Most are caused by low-risk genotypes 6 and 11,[33] and can harbor high-risk HPV genotypes, such as 16 and 18. Oral condylomata are more common in adolescents and young adults but are not limited to that age group. Oral lesions are sessile or pedunculated, with papillary projections (**Fig. 3**A, B). Koilocytes may be observed in histopathologic sections (see **Fig. 3**C).

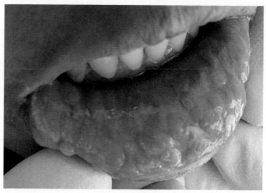

Fig. 2. Multifocal epithelial hyperplasia (Heck disease) with cluster of adjacent minimally keratinized lesions on lower labial mucosa extending on to upper lip mucosa. (*Courtesy of* Roman Carlos, DDS, Guatemala City, Guatemala).

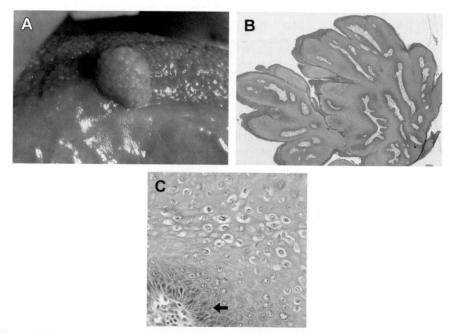

Fig. 3. (*A*) Condyloma acuminatum on the lateral border of tongue. (*B*) Low-power photomicrograph of overall architecture of condyloma acuminatum showing pedunculated growth of squamous epithelium with papillary projections and hyperkeratosis. (*C*) High-power photomicrograph of condyloma acuminatum showing virally affected cells (koilocytes) developing in the upper, maturing spinous layer. Note the relatively thin zone of virally induced hyperplasia of basal and parabasal cells (*arrow*) and rapid progression to epithelial maturation in the spinous layer in this benign lesion. ([A] *Courtesy of* Thomas Daley, DDS, MSc, London, Ontario, Canada.)

ORAL SQUAMOUS PAPILLOMA

The squamous papilloma occurs over a wide age range and with an estimated prevalence of 1 per 250 adults.[32] It is an exophytic, sessile, or pedunculated growth of squamous epithelium, with papillary projections (**Fig. 4**A). The lesion can appear pink or white, depending on the degree of keratinization. With its broad range of features, the squamous papilloma is often difficult to distinguish from condyloma acuminatum or verruca vulgaris clinically and pathologically (see **Fig. 4**B). The squamous papilloma is presumed to be caused by low-risk types of HPV, and genotypes 6 and 11 have been detected in approximately 50% of lesions.[34]

POTENTIALLY MALIGNANT PAPILLOMATOUS LESIONS

The presence of intraepithelial neoplasia (dysplasia) in anogenital condylomata has long been associated with high-grade dysplasia and squamous cell carcinoma in the anogenital region. Condylomata showing low-grade dysplasia may progress to high-grade dysplasia or carcinoma, particularly if infected or coinfected with a high-risk genotype. Oral papillomatous lesions (condylomata and squamous papillomas) can also show low-grade and high-grade dysplasia (**Fig. 5**). Compared with the number of benign squamous papillomas and condylomata diagnosed in an oral pathology laboratory, dysplastic papillomatous lesions are distinctly uncommon (<1%) with many occurring in immunosuppressed individuals.

ORAL LEUKOPLAKIA AND HEAD AND NECK SQUAMOUS CELL CARCINOMA

Oral leukoplakia has a strong association with tobacco (especially cigarette, pipe, and cigar smoking) and areca nut use. Leukoplakia is the most common premalignant oral lesion with dysplasia, present in 5% to 25% of biopsies.[32] Studies using PCR and genotyping have detected low-risk, high-risk, and multiple type HPV infections in oral leukoplakia.[34,35] Dysplastic leukoplakias (26.2%)[36] are more likely than normal mucosa (10%–13%)[7,36] to be infected with HPV. However, studies showing that oral precancerous lesions have a low viral load and that viral integration seldom occurs[37] strongly suggest that the virus is often passenger HPV,[38] having little role in neoplastic transformation of these lesions.

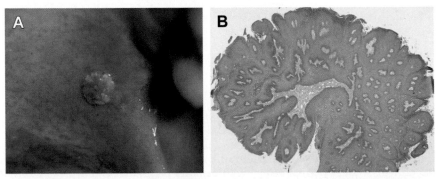

Fig. 4. (*A*) Oral squamous papilloma. (*B*) Low-power photomicrograph of overall architecture of oral squamous papilloma. Many clinical and histopathologic features are similar to condyloma acuminatum, including relatively thin zone of basal cell hyperplasia and broad zone of maturing spinous cells. ([A] *Courtesy of* Thomas Daley, DDS, MSc, London, Ontario, Canada.)

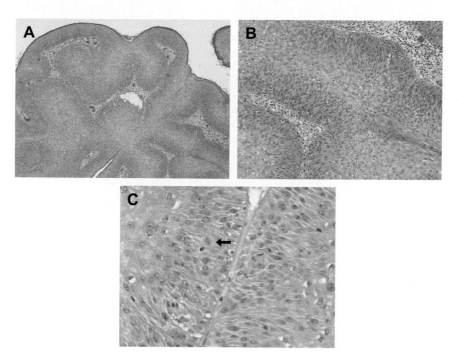

Fig. 5. (*A*) Low-power photomicrograph of a papillomatous lesion showing the same basic overall architecture as condyloma or squamous papilloma, but with moderate to focally severe epithelial dysplasia. (*B*) Note the expanded zone of proliferative basal and parabasal cells of the dysplastic epithelium. (*C*) High-power photomicrograph of dysplastic epithelium showing maturational disorganization of cells, cellular and nuclear pleomorphism, and increased numbers of mitotic figures (*arrow*). After surgical excision, periodic follow-up is recommended to rule out recurrent dysplasia.

Evidence of an etiologic role for HPV in head and neck squamous cell carcinoma has been accumulating, with high-risk HPV-16 detected in many carcinomas in this region. However, when cases are stratified according to location, HPV-16 DNA prevalence is lower (13%–47.5%) in squamous cell carcinoma (SCCa) of the oral cavity (lateral border of tongue, floor of mouth, soft palate, gingiva) compared with SCCa of the oropharyngeal tissues (60%–100%), which include the palatine tonsils and the tonsillar tissue at the base of the tongue.[39,40]

It has been proposed that there are 2 separate pathways of carcinogenesis for head and neck squamous cell carcinoma[41]: the first pathway promoted by environmental carcinogens, such as heavy tobacco and alcohol use, and the second pathway promoted by high-risk HPV infection. Support for this theory is based on the high percentage of oropharyngeal SCCa infected with high-risk HPV and that these HPV-cytopositive cancers occur predominantly in white men 40 to 55 years of age who in general report high-risk sexual behavior and a low level of alcohol and tobacco use. These cancers have a high viral load, a high degree of viral integration, a high degree of E6/E7 mRNA transcription,[19,42] and a large percentage overexpress p16INK4a (a cyclin-dependent kinase/cyclin inhibitor involved in controlling cell cycle progression).[42] Genomic mutation and chromosomal loss are also less pronounced, particularly with regard to 3p, 9p, and 17p (p53) gene regions.[19] The p53 gene is typically not mutated. Histopathologically, oropharyngeal SCCa is typically high grade, consisting of basaloid cells in a lobular growth pattern with comedo-type necrosis. The tumors are usually endophytic and can be difficult to detect clinically. At diagnosis, the tumor usually shows a low T stage, but an advanced N stage with cystic degeneration of lymph nodes according to the TNM (tumor size, nodal involvement, metastasis) staging criteria.[43]

In contrast, oral SCCa occurs in an older age group, typically does not consist of basaloid cells, and presents as an endophytic or exophytic mass, which is often ulcerated. Like precancerous leukoplakia and erythroplakia, oral SCCa is strongly associated with environmental carcinogens and shows a higher degree of genomic mutation, loss of heterozygosity, and chromosomal loss, particularly in the 3p, 9p, and 17p regions. Oral SCCa has been shown to harbor high-risk HPV genotypes,[4,7,44,45] but unlike the strong causal relationship apparent in studies of oropharyngeal SCCa, the causal relationship between HPV and oral SCCa is minimal[46,47] or limited to a subset of HPV-positive oral SCCa occurring in patients with a lifestyle more likely to be lacking environmental carcinogens.[4] Most HPV-16-cytopositive oral SCCa have a low viral load, a low level of viral integration, and only a small percentage are E6/E7 transcriptionally active.[19,44,48–50] Expression of p16INK4a is also typically low, with low specificity.[48]

Despite the high grade and advanced presentation of high-risk HPV-induced oropharyngeal SCCa, nonsmoking patients with this tumor have a definite survival advantage compared with SCCa present in other head and neck sites.[3] A large meta-analysis study[51] found that HPV-positive oropharyngeal SCCa had a 28% reduced risk of death and a 49% reduced risk of treatment failure compared with HPV-negative oropharyngeal SCCa. Survival of patients with HPV-positive oropharyngeal SCCa is lower if they were also smokers,[3,52,53] suggesting that when both carcinogenic pathways are active in the same tumor, they have a synergistic effect with regard to tumor growth and behavior. The same holds true for the small percentage of HPV-infected oral SCCa in which the virus is transcriptionally active. The risk of oral cavity SCCa was reportedly greater in HPV E6/E7 seropositive heavy tobacco or heavy alcohol users than in seronegative heavy tobacco or heavy alcohol users.[44] A separate study reported an increased risk of metastasis and lower survival in patients with advanced oral SCCa infected with HPV-16.[54]

TREATMENT OF ORAL HPV-RELATED CLINICAL LESIONS

The benign cutaneous warts have been treated by a variety of modalities. Spontaneous remission of many verrucae and plantar warts occurs within 1 to 2 years, and many warts are untreated. Over-the-counter topical medications containing agents such as salicylic acid have been used to treat cutaneous warts. Surgical excision, cryotherapy, laser ablation, and electrosurgery have also been used for persistent or recurrent cutaneous and mucosal lesions. Anogenital warts can be treated medically with imiquimod and podophyllotoxin as well as the various ablative techniques.[1,2] Treatment of these lesions is intended to decrease spread of infection and remove lesions that are potentially dysplastic.

Oral verruca vulgaris, multifocal epithelial hyperplasia, squamous papilloma, and condyloma acuminatum are also infectious and because only a few oral squamous papillomas and condylomata can be dysplastic, surgical excision is the recommended treatment.

Recurrence of these types of warts is unusual and is believed to be caused by incomplete removal of infected epithelium at the base of the lesion. Continued reinfection or the transition of an ongoing subclinical lesion to a clinical lesion cause new lesions to appear. Malignant transformation has not been reported in verrucae or multifocal epithelial hyperplasia. Oral condylomata and squamous papillomas that harbor high-risk HPV genotypes are associated with increased risk for dysplasia and development of squamous cell carcinoma.[32] Excisional biopsies of squamous papillomas and condylomata are not routinely evaluated for the presence of high-risk HPV genotypes; histopathologic examination determines the presence of dysplasia and adequacy of clear surgical margins. Similar to dysplastic leukoplakia, dysplastic papillomatous lesions require continued periodic follow-up to rule out recurrence of dysplasia.

There is no method to treat subclinical oral infection other than prevention.

Oropharyngeal SCCa is treated with surgery and concomitant chemoradiotherapy. Nonsmokers with HPV-positive oropharyngeal SCCa have a better prognosis than smokers with HPV-negative oropharyngeal SCCa, and it has been hypothesized that a major factor for the improved prognosis is increased sensitivity to radiotherapy caused by the presence of a functional, nonmutated p53 protein.[3] The mechanism for increased survival may be more complex, because improved prognosis of HPV-associated oropharyngeal carcinoma is also observed in patients not treated by radiotherapy, suggesting that increased survival may be independent of primary treatment modality. As a result of better survival, excessive toxicity caused by over-treatment using standard treatment regimens has led to several clinical trials evaluating the efficacy of less toxic protocols.[55]

Oral SCCa is treated with surgery or radiotherapy for smaller lesions, or combined therapy for larger lesions involving lymph nodes. Further studies are required to assess whether changes in treatment protocols would increase survival in (advanced) oral SCCa infected with high-risk HPV.

PREVENTION

Prevention of HPV infection depends on avoidance of contact with infected lesions and reducing the susceptibility of infection by immunization. Avoidance of sexual contact, use of condoms, and male circumcision have been reported to reduce the risk of HPV infection.[1,2] The recent introduction of a quadrivalent vaccine (Gardasil) directed against low-risk HPV types 6 and 11, and high-risk genotypes 16 and 18, and a bivalent vaccine (Cervarix) directed against HPV genotypes 16 and 18 only, provides the best means of prevention. Both vaccines contain viruslike particles composed of the L1 major capsid protein of each type. The vaccine is administered over 6 months in 3 equal doses (at 0, 2, and 6 months). Initially recommended for females 11 to 12 years of age, it is currently recommended for females as young as 9 years and females from 13 to 26 years as catchup vaccination for those not receiving the full vaccination earlier.[2] It is also recommended for males 9 to 26 years of age to help reduce the likelihood of genital warts and decrease risk of anal intraepithelial neoplasia. Vaccination is intended to prevent HPV infection in unexposed patients. It provides no therapeutic protection against existing infections and lesions. Several studies have shown that the vaccine has efficacy.[56,57] The effectiveness of the vaccine to prevent oral infection with HPV types 6, 11, 16, and 18 has yet to be evaluated, although from a theoretic standpoint, the benefits of the vaccine should be systemic.

SUMMARY

- HPV infection of the oral cavity is common and is increasing.
- Low-risk HPV genotypes are responsible for the oral clinical infections of squamous papilloma, condyloma acuminatum, verruca vulgaris, and multifocal epithelial hyperplasia. These lesions can be coinfected with high-risk genotypes.
- Subclinical HPV infection is believed to be more common than clinical infection. A wide range of low-risk and high-risk genotypes have been detected in the oral

cavity in those with subclinical infection. High-risk HPV-16 is the most common genotype detected.
- A causal role for high-risk, transcriptionally active HPV genotypes (particularly HPV-16) has been established for oropharyngeal carcinoma. Environmental carcinogens such as smoking can modify the neoplastic transformation process and survival.
- Oral leukoplakia and oral squamous cell carcinoma are strongly associated with environmental carcinogens such as smoking and areca nut use. The percentage of these lesions with transcriptionally active high-risk HPV infections seems to be low, but evidence suggests that viral oncoproteins can modify the neoplastic transformation process of oral squamous carcinoma and survival.
- High-risk HPV infection may have more of a causal role in a smaller subset of oral squamous cell carcinoma occurring in nonsmokers as opposed to oropharyngeal squamous cell carcinoma.
- Vaccination of teenage males and females will potentially decrease spread of infection and subsequent development of oral disease caused by certain low-risk and high-risk genotypes.

ACKNOWLEDGMENTS

The author wishes to thank Dr Tom Daley and Dr Roman Carlos for figures depicting the clinical manifestations of oral HPV infection.

REFERENCES

1. Douglas JM Jr. Papillomavirus. In: Goldman L, Schafer AI, editors. Goldman's Cecil medicine. 24th edition. Philadelphia: Elsevier Saunders; 2012. p. 2121–5.
2. Bonnez W, Reichman RC. Papillomaviruses. In: Mandell GL, Bennett JE, Dolin R, editors. Mandell, Douglas and Bennett's principles and practice of infectious diseases. 7th edition. Philadelphia: Churchill Livingstone; 2010. p. 2035–49.
3. Adelstein DJ, Rodriguez CP. Human papillomavirus: changing paradigms in oropharyngeal cancer. Curr Oncol Rep 2010;12:115–20.
4. Chen SF, Yu FS, Chang YC, et al. Role of human papillomavirus infection in carcinogenesis of oral squamous cell carcinoma with evidence of prognostic association. J Oral Pathol Med 2012;41:9–15.
5. Gillison ML, Broutian T, Pickard RK, et al. Prevalence of oral HPV infection in the United States, 2009-2010. JAMA 2012;307:693–703.
6. Sanders AE, Slade GD, Patton LL. National prevalence of oral HPV infection and related risk factors in the US adult population. Oral Dis 2012;18:430–41.
7. Luo CW, Roan CH, Liu CJ. Human papillomaviruses in oral squamous cell carcinoma and precancerous lesions detected by PCR-based gene-chip array. Int J Oral Maxillofac Surg 2007;36:153–8.
8. Kero K, Rautava J, Syrjanen K, et al. Oral mucosa as a reservoir of human papillomavirus: point prevalence, genotype distribution, and incident infections among males in a 7-year prospective study. Eur Urol 2012;62:1063–70.
9. Rautava J, Willberg J, Louvanto K, et al. Prevalence, genotype distribution and persistence of human papillomavirus in oral mucosa of women: a six-year follow-up study. PLoS One 2012;7:e42171. http://dx.doi.org/10.1371/journal.pone.0042171.
10. Chaturvedi AK, Engels EA, Anderson WF, et al. Incidence and trends for human papillomavirus-related and -unrelated oral squamous cell carcinomas in the United States. J Clin Oncol 2008;26:612–9.

11. Shiboski CH, Schmidt BL, Jordan RC. Tongue and tonsil carcinoma: increasing trends in the US population ages 20-44 years. Cancer 2005;103:1843–9.
12. Marur S, D'Souza G, Westra WH, et al. HPV-associated head and neck cancer: a virus-related cancer epidemic. Lancet Oncol 2010;11:781–9.
13. Bonnez W. Papillomavirus. In: Richman RD, Whitley RJ, Hayden FG, editors. Clinical virology. 3rd edition. Washington, DC: American Society for Microbiology; 2009. p. 603–44.
14. Doorbar J, Quint W, Banks L, et al. The biology and life cycle of human papillomaviruses. Vaccine 2012;30S:F55–70.
15. Feller L, Khammissa RA, Wood NH, et al. Epithelial maturation and molecular biology of HPV. Infect Agent Cancer 2009;4:16–24.
16. Wiest T, Schwarz E, Enders C, et al. Involvement of intact HPV16 E6/E7 gene expression in head and neck cancers with unaltered p53 status and perturbed pRb cell cycle control. Oncogene 2002;21:1510–7.
17. Trottier H, Franco EL. The epidemiology of genital human papillomavirus infection. Vaccine 2006;24:S1–15.
18. Reichman RC. Human papillomavirus infections. In: Kasper DL, Braunwald E, Fauci AS, Hauser SL, Lango DL, Jameson JL, editors. Harrison's principles of internal medicine. 16th edition. New York: McGraw-Hill; 2005. p. 1056–8.
19. Braakhuis BJ, Snijders PJ, Keune WJ, et al. Genetic patterns in head and neck cancers that contain or lack transcriptionally active human papillomavirus. J Natl Cancer Inst 2004;96:998–1006.
20. Kojic EM, Cu-Uvin S. Update: human papillomavirus infection remains highly prevalent and persistent among HIV-infected individuals. Curr Opin Oncol 2007;19:464–9.
21. Frisch M, Biggar RJ, Goedert JJ. Human papillomavirus-associated cancers in patients with human immunodeficiency virus infection and acquired immunodeficiency syndrome. J Natl Cancer Inst 2000;92:1500–10.
22. Louvanto K, Rautava J, Willberg J, et al. Genotype-specific incidence and clearance of human papillomavirus in oral mucosa of women: a six-year follow-up study. PLoS One 2013;8:e53413. http://dx.doi.org/10.1371/journal.pone.0053413.
23. Liang C, Marsit CJ, McClean MD, et al. Biomarkers of HPV in head and neck squamous cell carcinoma. Cancer Res 2012;72:5004–13.
24. D'Souza G, Agrawal Y, Halpern J, et al. Oral sexual behaviors associated with prevalent oral human papillomavirus infection. J Infect Dis 2009;199:1263–9.
25. Kreimer AR, Alberg AJ, Daniel R, et al. Oral human papillomavirus infection in adults is associated with sexual behavior and HIV serostatus. J Infect Dis 2004;189:686–98.
26. Fakhry C, D'Souza G, Sugar E, et al. Relationship between prevalent oral and cervical human papillomavirus infections in human immunodeficiency virus-positive and negative women. J Clin Microbiol 2006;44:4470–85.
27. Dinh TH, Ternberg M, Dunne EF, et al. Genital warts among 18-59 year-olds in the United States; National Health and Nutrition Examination Survey 1999-2004. Sex Transm Dis 2008;35:357–60.
28. Ferreira DC, Paiva SS, Carmo FL, et al. Identification of herpesviruses types 1 to 8 and human papillomavirus in acute apical abscesses. J Endod 2011;37:10–6.
29. Bustos DA, Grenon MS, Benitez M, et al. Human papillomavirus infection in cyclosporine-induced gingival overgrowth in renal allograft recipients. J Periodontol 2001;72:741–4.
30. Hormia M, Willberg J, Ruokonen H, et al. Marginal periodontium as a potential reservoir of human papillomavirus in oral mucosa. J Periodontol 2005;76:358–63.

31. Horewicz VV, Feres M, Rapp GE, et al. Human papillomavirus-16 prevalence in gingival tissue and its association with periodontal destruction: a case-control study. J Periodontol 2010;81:562–8.

32. Neville BW, Damm DD, Allen CM, et al. Oral pathology. 3rd edition. St Louis: Saunders Elsevier; 2009. p. 362.

33. Syrjanen S. Human papillomavirus infections and oral tumors. Med Microbiol Immunol 2003;192:123–8.

34. Ostwald C, Rutsatz K, Schweder J, et al. Human papillomavirus 6, 11, 16, and 18 in oral carcinomas and benign oral lesions. Med Microbiol Immunol 2003; 192:145–8.

35. Nielsen H, Norrild B, Vedtofte P, et al. Human papillomavirus in human premalignant lesions. Eur J Cancer B Oral Oncol 1996;32:264–70.

36. Miller CS, Johnstone BM. Human papillomavirus as a risk factor for oral squamous cell carcinoma: a meta-analysis, 1982-1997. Oral Surg Oral Med Oral Pathol Oral Radiol Endod 2001;91:622–35.

37. Feller L, Lemmer J. Oral leukoplakia as it relates to HPV infection: a review. Int J Dent 2012;2012:540561. http://dx.doi.org/10.1155/2012/540561.

38. Evans MF, Matthews A, Kandil D, et al. Discrimination of 'driver' and 'passenger' HPV in tonsillar carcinomas by the polymerase chain reaction, chromogenic in situ hybridization, and p16INK4a immunohistochemistry. Head Neck Pathol 2011;5:344–8.

39. Allen CT, Lewis JS Jr, El-Mofty SK, et al. Human papillomavirus and oropharynx cancer: biology, detection and clinical implications. Laryngoscope 2010;120: 1756–72.

40. Laco J, Vosmikova H, Novakova V, et al. The role of high-risk human papillomavirus infection in oral and oropharyngeal squamous cell carcinoma in non-smoking and non-drinking patients: a clinicopathological and molecular study of 46 cases. Virchows Arch 2011;458:179–87.

41. Gillison ML, Koch WM, Capone RB, et al. Evidence for a causal association between human papillomavirus and a subset of head and neck cancers. J Natl Cancer Inst 2000;92:2875–84.

42. Jung AC, Briolat J, Millon R, et al. Biological and clinical relevance of transcriptionally active human papillomavirus (HPV) infection in oropharynx squamous cell carcinoma. Int J Cancer 2010;126:1882–94.

43. Fakhry C, Westra WH, Li S, et al. Improved survival of patients with human papillomavirus-positive head and neck squamous cell carcinoma in a prospective clinical trial. J Natl Cancer Inst 2008;100:261–9.

44. Smith EM, Rubenstein LM, Haugen TH, et al. Complex etiology underlies risk and survival in head and neck cancer human papillomavirus, tobacco, and alcohol: a case for multifactor disease. J Oncol 2012;2012:571862. http://dx.doi.org/10.1155/2012/571862.

45. Furrer VE, Benitez MB, Furnes M, et al. Biopsy vs superficial scraping: detection of human papillomavirus 6, 11, 16, and 18 in potentially malignant and malignant oral lesions. J Oral Pathol Med 2006;35:338–44.

46. Hobbs CG, Sterne JA, Bailey M, et al. Human papillomavirus and head and neck cancer: a systemic review and meta-analysis. Clin Otolaryngol 2006;31:259–66.

47. Liang XH, Lewis J, Foote R, et al. Prevalence and significance of human papillomavirus in oral tongue cancer: the Mayo Clinic experience. J Oral Maxillofac Surg 2008;66:1875–80.

48. Lewis JS Jr, Ukpo OC, Ma XJ, et al. Transcriptionally-active high-risk human papillomavirus is rare in oral cavity and laryngeal/hypopharyngeal squamous

cell carcinomas–a tissue microarray study utilizing E6/E7 mRNA in situ hybridization. Histopathology 2012;60:982–91.

49. Schlecht NF, Brandwein-Gensler M, Nuovo GJ, et al. A comparison of clinically utilized human papillomavirus detection methods in head and neck cancer. Mod Pathol 2011;24:1295–305.

50. Ha PK, Pai SI, Westra WH, et al. Real-time quantitative PCR demonstrates low prevalence of human papillomavirus type 16 in premalignant and malignant lesions of the oral cavity. Clin Cancer Res 2002;8:1203–9.

51. Ragin CC, Tailoi E. Survival of squamous cell carcinoma of the head and neck in relation to human papillomavirus infection: review and meta-analysis. Int J Cancer 2007;121:1813–20.

52. Gillison ML, Harris J, Westra W, et al. Survival outcomes by tumor human papillomavirus status in stage III/IV oropharyngeal cancer in RTOG 0129 [abstract 6003]. J Clin Oncol 2009;27:27s.

53. Hafkamp HC, Manni JJ, Haesevoets A, et al. Marked differences in survival rate between smokers and nonsmokers with HPV-16-associated tonsillar carcinomas. Int J Cancer 2008;122:2656–64.

54. Lee LA, Huang CG, Liao CT, et al. Human papillomavirus-16 infection in advanced oral cavity cancer patients is related to an increased risk of distant metastases and poor survival. PLoS One 2012;7:e40767. http://dx.doi.org/10.1371/journal.pone.0040767.

55. Ang KK, Sturgis EM. Human papillomavirus as a marker of the natural history and response to therapy of head and neck squamous cell carcinoma. Semin Radiat Oncol 2012;22:128–42.

56. Barr E, Gause CK, Bautista OM, et al. Impact of a prophylactic quadrivalent human papillomavirus (types 6, 11, 16, 18) L1 virus-like particle vaccine in a sexually active population of North American women. Am J Obstet Gynecol 2008; 198:261.e1–11.

57. Munoz N, Manalastas R Jr, Pitisuttithum P, et al. Safety, immunogenicity, and efficacy of quadrivalent human papillomavirus (types 6, 11, 16, 18) recombinant vaccine in women aged 24-45 years: a randomized, double-blind trial. Lancet 2009;373:1949–57.

Perioral Lesions and Dermatoses

Geoffrey F.S. Lim, BS[a],*, Carrie Ann R. Cusack, MD[a],
Joseph M. Kist, MD[b]

KEYWORDS

- Perioral • Seborrheic keratosis • Warts • Actinic keratoses • Actinic cheilitis
- Squamous cell carcinoma • Basal cell carcinoma • Perioral dermatitis

KEY POINTS

- Neoplasms, infections, and inflammatory dermatoses may present around or near the mouth.
- Dental professionals are well positioned to evaluate perioral skin conditions.
- Early recognition and treatment of perioral lesions and dermatoses provide best clinical outcomes.

INTRODUCTION

The purpose of this article is to review the common neoplasms, infections, and inflammatory dermatoses that may present around or near the mouth. Dental professionals are well positioned to evaluate perioral skin conditions, further contributing to patients' general health. This article includes a review of seborrheic keratosis, warts, actinic keratoses, actinic cheilitis, and squamous cell carcinoma, among several other perioral cutaneous lesions.

SEBORRHEIC KERATOSIS

Introduction

Seborrheic keratoses are very common and usually multiple, presenting as oval, slightly raised, tan or light brown to black, sharply demarcated papules or plaques that usually measure less than 3 cm in diameter.[1]

Cause

The pathogenesis of seborrheic keratosis is unknown. In about one-third or more of cases, mutations in FGFR3 and PI3K have been implicated.[2] Advanced age is a

Conflicts of Interest: None.
[a] Department of Dermatology, Drexel University College of Medicine, The Arnold T. Berman, M.D. Building, 219 North Broad Street, Philadelphia, PA 19107, USA; [b] Department of Dermatology, Perelman School of Medicine, University of Pennsylvania, South Pavilion, 1st Floor, 3400 Civic Center Boulevard, Philadelphia, PA 19104, USA
* Corresponding author.
E-mail address: gfl25@drexel.edu

well-established risk factor, although the relationship between seborrheic keratosis and sun exposure has been debated.[3–6]

Epidemiology

The age of onset usually falls within the fourth to fifth decade,[3] and males and females are equally affected.[7]

Prognosis

These lesions are benign with no risk of malignant transformation.

Clinical Features

Seborrheic keratoses have a characteristic stuck-on appearance and are often described as waxy and smooth. When removed, the underside of the warty lesions reveals a raw, moist base. Although most are asymptomatic, some lesions cause itching, bleeding, or pain. The chest and back tend to be the primary sites affected; but seborrheic keratosis commonly involves the scalp, face, neck, and extremities.[3,7] Some patients, particularly Caucasians, may have hundreds of these lesions on the trunk.[7] A variant of the central face, known as *dermatosis papulosa nigra*, is common in African Americans and Asians.[7,8]

Because of its classic appearance, the diagnosis of seborrheic keratosis is primarily clinically based. Although the histology does vary, seborrheic keratoses universally show a proliferative process, with hyperkeratosis and acanthosis without dysplasia.[4] Biopsy is rarely indicated unless lesions are difficult to distinguish from melanoma.[4,7] Clinicians should also be aware that the sudden onset of multiple seborrheic keratoses has been thought to represent a paraneoplastic syndrome from an occult malignancy, such as stomach or colon cancer.[9–11] However, this phenomenon, known as the *sign of Leser-Trélat*, has recently been questioned.[12]

Management

As a benign lesion, seborrheic keratosis may be treated electively. The primary indication for surgical removal is cosmetic, though chronic bleeding, irritation, and blistering may warrant treatment. Removal is also considered when the diagnosis is unclear. Shave excision, electrodessication and curettage, and cryotherapy are common surgical options but may be associated with recurrence, scarring, and changes in pigmentation.[4] Consequently, the use of lasers (erbium YAG, carbon dioxide [CO_2], and 532 diode) has become more popular.[13] Medical therapies, such as topical and systemic vitamin D, have shown limited efficacy.[4]

WARTS
Introduction

Warts (verrucae) are caused by human papillomaviruses (HPVs), small DNA viruses of the papovavirus family, with more than 100 different HPV types being described.[14] Cutaneous lesions often present as small papules, single or multiple, throughout all age groups.

Cause

HPVs are classified according to mucosal and cutaneous types caused by HPV 1, 2, and 4.[14,15] Planar or flat warts on the face are caused by HPV-3 and 10.[14,15] Mucosal types are divided into low risk and high risk. Low risk (HPV-6, 11) is defined by never being found in invasive squamous cell carcinomas (SCC), whereas high-risk types, such as HPV-16, 18, and others, are prevalent in this instance.[14–16]

Epidemiology

Estimates suggest a prevalence of common warts in 3.5% of adults and up to 33% of children.[14,15,17] There is an increased incidence in immunosuppressed patients, including those with human immunodeficiency virus (HIV) disease and organ transplantation recipients.[15,18]

Prognosis

Warts may cause pain or cosmetic distortions; however, treatment may cause similar issues. Regression is often spontaneous, with immune mechanisms playing an important role; however, this is often slow.[17–19] Although rare, malignant transformation may occur.[16] It is mostly noted in the setting of immunosuppression.

Clinical Features

HPVs demonstrate a variety of mucocutaneous manifestations: common warts, plantar warts, verruca plana, anogenital warts, epidermodysplasia verriculoformis, oral warts, condyloma, focal epithelial hyperplasia (Heck disease), nasal and conjunctival papillomas, laryngeal papillomatosis, and cervical lesions.[14,15]

Common warts typically present as small papules with a verrucous and hyperkeratotic surface, ranging in size from 1 to 10 mm.[15] Although lesions typically occur on the hands and fingers, they may occur in other locations. Periorally, lesions may also appear flat, as verruca plana, or filiform with fingerlike projections (**Fig. 1**).[14,15] Histologically, verrucae are characterized by hyperkeratosis, acanthosis, and papillomatosis. Often the edges of the lesions project inward, known as arborization. Tiers of parakeratosis are often noted, with an increased granular cell layer and coarse keratohyalin granules. Koilocytes, cells with a pyknotic nucleus and clear halo, are often but not always noted.

Flat warts are usually multiple, flat-topped, smooth papules, often skin colored. They may regress. Before regression, they may be preceded by an eruption of multiple lesions.[14,15,18] Histologically, the features are similar to common warts; however, papillomatosis is mild and parakeratosis is often absent.

Management

The treatment of warts is difficult and failures are common. Multiple treatment options are available, and it is important to note that none are completely effective. Treatments range from observation, because warts may regress spontaneously,

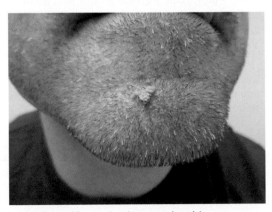

Fig. 1. Filiform wart with fingerlike projections on the chin.

to topical therapy, surgical therapy, and even systemic therapies. Topical therapy includes salicyclic acid; cantharidin (an extract from a blister beetle); contact sensitizers, such as squaric acid and diphencyclopropenone, tricholoacetic acid, podophyllin, imiquimod, tretinoin; and the application of duct tape.[23] Liquid nitrogen cryotherapy is a frequently used technique, which may induce blistering.

For more recalcitrant lesions, topical cidofovir, photodynamic therapy with amino-levulinic acid and blue light exposure, 5-fluorouracil, intralesional bleomycin, and intra-lesional candida antigen can be used.[17,19,20] CO_2, pulsed dye, and Nd:YAG lasers have been used for more resistant lesions.[21] Electrodessication and curettage may be used; however, it has a high risk of scarring.

Systemic oral therapies for multiple and recalcitrant warts have been tried, including cimetidine and oral retinoids. It has been shown that cimetidine activates Th1 cells to produce interleukin 2 (IL-2) and interferon (IFN)-γ, which correlates with wart remission.[22] High-dose cimetidine (30–40 mg/kg/d) has been helpful for recalcitrant warts, although the treatment time is often lengthy, requiring weeks to months of therapy.[18,22] Vaccines are available currently for low and high-risk types. The vaccines are effective against diseases caused by HPV types 16 and 18. One vaccine additionally protects again HPV types 6 and 11.[23] Vaccination is recommended for females and males aged 9 through 26 years in a series of 3 doses. Of note, the vaccine produces higher antibody titers when given at 11 to 12 years of age compared with older ages.[23]

FACIAL ACTINIC KERATOSIS
Introduction

Actinic keratoses are scaly, erythematous skin lesions that are induced by UV solar radiation. They are considered a premalignant lesion.[24–26]

Cause

Besides sun exposure, other risk factors include fair skin, advanced age, male sex, and immunosuppression.[26] The inciting event in the process of photodamage that leads to actinic keratosis is a mutation in the tumor suppressor factor p53 initiated from solar radiation.[27]

Epidemiology

In the United States and Europe, the incidence of actinic keratosis is approximately 10% to 15%.[24] Actinic keratosis is important to recognize because it may progress to SCC in nearly 15% of cases.[24–26] Actinic keratoses are most common in fair-skinned Caucasian individuals.

Prognosis

The progression of actinic keratosis to squamous cell is variable but may occur within carcinoma and takes approximately 2 years.[28]

Clinical Features

Actinic keratosis is usually diagnosed clinically. Characteristically, the affected areas present as slightly erythematous, rough, scaly macules, distributed on sun-exposed areas of the skin. However, because it is on a continuum with SCC, there are instances when actinic keratosis cannot reliably be distinguished from its malignant counterpart without a biopsy.[1]

Management

The management of actinic keratosis includes medical and surgical therapies. Local-directed approaches include cryotherapy and electrodessication with curettage; field-directed treatment encompasses photodynamic therapy; topical chemotherapeutic agents, including 5-fluorouracil and imiquimod; dermabrasion; and CO_2 laser resurfacing.[28,29] The most common technique for managing actinic keratosis is liquid nitrogen cryotherapy, although topical chemotherapy using 5-fluorouracil has been shown to be one of the most effective methods.[29–31] The therapy of choice depends on a variety of factors, such as the number and extent of lesions, patient compliance with medical therapies, surgical experience of the clinician, and previously failed therapies.[29]

ACTINIC CHEILITIS
Introduction

Actinic cheilitis is a premalignant lesion of the lips that has the potential to develop into invasive SCC. Caused by solar damage, it occurs more commonly in fair-skinned (primarily Caucasian) individuals.[32–37]

Cause

Sun exposure, especially among fair-skinned middle-aged to older patients, is the primary risk factor for actinic cheilitis.[32]

Epidemiology

Women are less often affected, possibly because of the protective barrier effects of lipstick.

Prognosis

Actinic cheilitis has similar malignant potential to actinic keratosis, with advanced disease leading to the development of SCC.[34–37] The presence of actinic cheilitis may more than double the risk of SCC. Of note, the risk of invasion and involvement of the cervical lymph nodes is higher in SCC of the lip than that of the skin.[35]

Clinical Features

The lower lip is the most common site of involvement likely because of its direct exposure to sunlight.[32] Clinically, these lesions are multifocal and are most often characterized as dry, atrophic, and scaly. Some patients may present with a blurred demarcation between the lip vermilion border and the skin or marked folds along the lip vermilion.[33] These presentations require careful evaluation including biopsy.

Management

The ultimate goal in the management of actinic cheilitis is preventing UV light–induced skin damage by applying sunscreen when outdoors and reducing sun exposure.[33]

The multifocal nature of the disease makes it difficult to correlate clinical findings with histologic findings. Therapies include those used for actinic keratosis, such as CO_2 laser, cryotherapy, and 5-fluoracil,[38–40] in addition to vermilionectomy in cases of severe dysplasia.[41,42]

SCC OF THE LIP
Introduction

SCC of the lip is a common head and neck malignancy.[43] Most lesions occur on the lower lip from the vermillion border.[44–46]

Cause

SCC of the lip is related to chronic sun exposure.[44–46] It may be seen in younger individuals who are immunosuppressed.[44,47,48] Solar/UV radiation is the most important risk factor, with UVB (290–320 nm) being more carcinogenic than UVA (320–400 nm).[44] Other factors also play a role, including smoking, excessive alcohol use, HPV, race, family and genetic predisposition, immunosuppressive state, poor diet, and socioeconomic situation.[45–52]

Epidemiology

SCC of the lip has a higher incidence in Caucasian men and primarily affects people greater than 60 years of age.[44–46]

Prognosis

SCC of the lip is typically considered a disease of low aggressiveness and favorable prognosis because it tends to progress slowly.[48,52] When diagnosed early, it has a cure rate of 80% to 90% and a mortality rate between 10% and 15%.[53,54] Metastases tend to occur at a later stage; in these cases, the mean survival in 5 years decreases to 25%.[53,55,56]

Clinical Features

Initially, it may be difficult to distinguish from actinic cheilitis because it is often asymptomatic.[48,52–54] Lesions present as white or pink atrophic plaques, which may have persistent fissuring, scaling, or crusting. Over time, the lesion may ulcerate, cause pain, and demonstrate infiltration at the base. In more advanced stage, ulcerations with indurated borders persist without healing. Exophytic, verrucous nodules may also be appreciated.[44,48,52,53] It is helpful to palpate both the internal mucosa and external surface to help identify the true extent of the lesion.[48,52]

Histopathologically, SCC of the lip is characterized by invasive islands of malignant squamous epithelial cells.[48,52] The cells are enlarged with hyperchromatic nuclei, an increased nuclear-to-cytoplasmic ratio, and an eosinophilic glassy cytoplasm. Keratin pearl formation occurs, and individual cells may prematurely keratinize. SCC of the lip is characterized as well, moderately, and poorly differentiated.[48,52,57] Well-differentiated tumors tend to grow slowly. Poorly differentiated tumors are characterized by atypical mitoses, nuclear pleomorphism, little or no keratinization, and rapid growth. Tumors with characteristics between these are classified as moderately differentiated.[48,52,57,58] Tumor thickness greater than 4 to 5 mm has been shown to be a predictor for developing nodal disease.[59–61] Perineural invasion has been shown to increase the risk for both local recurrence and metastasis.[58,59]

Management

Treatment of SCC of the lip without nodal involvement is either by Mohs micrographic surgery, surgical excision, or radiation therapy, depending on the functionality and cosmetic outcomes.[58,59] Adjuvant radiation therapy should be considered in the setting of close or positive margins to reduce the risk of local recurrence, in the range of 40 to 70 Gy, fractionated.[61,62] Currently, there is no consensus defining an acceptable surgical margin in cutaneous SCC, ranging from 2 to 4 mm.[58,59] It is important to note that margin status, including the lip, is a well-documented risk for developing local relapse, thus local adjuvant radiation therapy may benefit in reducing local recurrence.[59] SCC of the lip is considered a higher-risk lesion and has a greater risk of metastasis compared with other cutaneous sites. There is growing evidence showing the prognostic benefits of sentinel node biopsy in high-risk patients with SCC with clinically negative regional nodal disease.[63–65] Although this has been adopted for cutaneous malignant melanoma, further studies are needed to address its utility in SCC of the lip.[66]

BASAL CELL CARCINOMA
Introduction

Basal cell carcinoma is the most common malignancy in man, with more than 2 million cases diagnosed in the United States annually.[67] In most cases, it is very treatable, with a very low risk of metastasis.

Cause

Exposure to sunlight, particularly to UVB radiation, is the primary risk factor for basal cell carcinoma, with regions of higher altitude and closer proximity to the equator exhibiting a greater prevalence.[68] Fair-skinned individuals, such as those of Scandinavian or Irish descent, tend to sunburn easily and are more prone to basal cell carcinoma compared with those with more darkly pigmented skin.[69,70]

Epidemiology

Basal cell carcinoma composes 75% of all nonmelanoma skin cancers and is responsible for 25% of all cancers diagnosed in the United States.[71,72] Incidence estimates range from 124 to 849 per 100,000 people per year and has been increasing over the past 2 decades.[69,73] Most basal cell carcinomas are identified between the ages of 40 and 60 years, with a male-to-female ratio of 2:1. Risk increases substantially with advancing age, although an increasing number of younger people are presenting with basal cell carcinoma, presumably caused by sunbathing.[74]

Prognosis

Basal cell carcinomas are slow growing, ranging from a few millimeters to several centimeters in diameter. They rarely metastasize and, thus, are associated with low mortality. However, they have the potential to cause significant morbidity through local invasion and subsequent loss of function and disfigurement. Therefore, appropriate and timely diagnosis and management is essential. Lesions suspicious for basal cell carcinoma should be biopsied. The type of biopsy—shave, punch, or complete excision—depends on the size and architecture of the lesion. Any pigmented tumor suspicious for melanoma always warrants a full-thickness biopsy.

Clinical Features

Basal cell carcinoma arises from the keratinocytes of the epidermis, hair follicles, and eccrine sweat ducts. Basophilic cells with large nuclei are observed histologically, and 5 major patterns are recognized: nodular (21%), superficial (17%), micronodular (15%), infitrative (7%), and morpheaform (1%).[75] Nearly 40% of all cases exhibit a mixed pattern of 2 or more subtypes.[75] Clinically, the nodular subtype most commonly presents as a pearly pink or white, dome-shaped papule that develops sizable telangiectasias with growth.[76] There is a predilection for the head and neck areas, most commonly the nasal tip and ala followed by the cheeks and forehead. Other nodular forms can present as blue, brown, or black on account of melanin accumulation, mimicking melanoma.[77] If left alone, these lesions can reach a large size and be locally destructive to areas like the nose, eyelid, ear, or lip, leaving a significant ulcer (rodent ulcer).[78] Micronodular and infiltrative basal cell carcinomas are are more aggressive and have a higher risk of recurrence.[79–82] Superficial basal cell carcinoma occurs most commonly on the trunk and extremities, although they have been reported on the head and neck.[79,83] It features a scaly plaque similar to eczema or psoriasis, but it also has pearly raised borders similar to the nodular type. Morpheaform basal cell carcinoma may resemble a scar or localized scleroderma in that it is an indurated, ill-defined, ivory lesion sometimes with overlying telangiectasia. It is known for its subclinical spread and high recurrence rate following treatment.[84]

Management

When diagnosed early, basal cell carcinoma can be removed by one of several methods. Surgical excision is the most common treatment, although electrodessication and curettage or cryosurgery may also be used.[85–87] Radiation therapy and topical agents like imiquimod and fluorouracil are used in some cases.[88,89] Mohs micrographic surgery is the most effective therapy and has a recurrence rate of less than 1% after 5 years, compared with 5% for surgical excision.[87] However, Mohs is usually reserved for more invasive subtypes (micronodular, infiltrative, and morpheaform); high-risk locations, such as the nose, eyelids, and ear; as well as for recurrences given its cost. Regardless of the treatment used, all patients with basal cell carcinomas require follow-up to monitor for the development of new tumors and for recurrence at the treated site.

LABIAL MELANOTIC MACULE
Introduction

A labial melanotic macule is a benign pigmented lesion on the lip that arises secondary to increased melanin within basal layer keratinocytes and melanocytes.[90,91]

Cause

Labial melanotic macules may result from racial pigmentation or they may be idiopathic.

Epidemiology

Females present more commonly than males, and the highest incidence is reported during the fifth decade.[92,93]

Prognosis

Unlike ephelides (freckles), melanotic macules do not darken with exposure to solar radiation.[94] Multiple lesions are rare unless associated with systemic syndromes, such as Peutz-Jeghers and Laugier-Hunziker syndromes, or endocrine disorders such as Addison disease, McCune-Albright syndrome, hyperthyroidism, and Nelson syndrome.[95]

Clinical Features

A labial melanotic macule is characterized as a tan-brown, irregular macule with well-defined borders on the cutaneous or mucosal lip that usually measures less than 1 cm (**Fig. 2**).[96,97] Labial lesions almost exclusively affect the lower lip.[93] The central lip is the

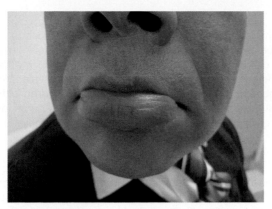

Fig. 2. Labial melanotic macule on the central lower lip.

most common site, and some cases may involve the vermilion border. Although often darkly pigmented, labial melanotic macules are evenly pigmented with a uniform pigment network. Furthermore, they tend to remain stable over time. Although a labial melanotic macule may occasionally be difficult to differentiate from melanoma clinically, the former does not show any significant increase in melanocytes histologically.[91]

Management

Treatment is unnecessary because this lesion is without malignant potential. For elective removal, cryotherapy, laser therapy, and surgical excision may be used.

NEVI
Introduction

A nevus is a benign proliferation of melanocytes. Nevi are divided according to their histology—junctional, compound or intradermal proliferation of melanocytes—or by their appearance—halo or blue.

Cause

Nevi may be congenital (present at birth or acquired in the first year of life) or acquired. Nevi arise from the neural crest and migrate during embryonic development to their final location in the brain, eyes, and skin.

Epidemiology

Common acquired melanocytic nevi are the most frequent neoplasms in Caucasians.[98] They develop in children even in the first years of life, and their number increases continually into adulthood.[99–102] Melanocytic nevi develop predominantly in childhood and adolescence. Studies demonstrate that sun exposure at a young age promotes the development of melanocytic nevi.[99,103,104] When children grow up in sunny climates, the number of nevi on sun-exposed skin is increased.[105] High, intermittent UV exposure also promotes the development of a greater number of melanocytic nevi, along with sunburn. Genetic factors also play a role, including somatic mutations of the RAS and RAF genes.[106]

Prognosis

The number of common melanocytic nevi represents an independent risk factor for the development of melanoma. With greater than 50 nevi, the melanoma risk is increased by about a factor of 4 to 5.[107,108] Because the number of nevi impacts the risk of melanoma, this indicates the importance of UV light for the development of melanoma. Freckles are associated with a greater number of nevi. Children with fair skin (Fitzpatrick types I and II, which are defined as skin that "always burns, does not tan" and "burns easily, tans with difficulty," respectively) have significantly more nevi than those with darker skin.[98]

Clinical Features

Junctional melanocytic nevi are round or oval macules with brown pigmentation, regular in color and contour. Compound nevi are round to oval, flat papules with light to dark brown pigmentation (**Fig. 3**). Dermal melanocytic nevi usually present as flesh-colored nodules with a smooth surface, usually dome shaped, but papillomatous and pedunculated forms also exist.

Histologically, nests of melanocytic cells are found at the dermoepidermal junction for junctional nevi. Compound nevi have additional nests and cordlike nevus cell formations in the dermis, whereas intradermal nevi no longer have melanocytes along the dermoepidermal junction.

A congenital melanocytic nevus is a melanocytic nevus that is present at birth or within the newborn period. It is a hamartoma of melanocytes derived from the neural crest.[109,110] It is categorized as either small (<1.5 cm), medium (1.5 to <20 cm), or giant (>20 cm).[108] Giant congenital melanocytic nevi affect a substantial portion of an anatomic region and do have an increased risk of developing melanoma.[111,112] Congenital melanocytic nevi present as homogeneous light to dark brown pigmented macules or plaques with sharp borders, a smooth surface, and increased hair. They increase in size proportionally as the skin grows.[113] As lesions age, they may have an irregular surface or have their pigment lighten.[114] Some larger lesions may display color variations with darker areas.

Atypical or dysplastic nevi are those that are larger, have irregular borders, and variable pigmentation. Originally described in association with familial melanomas, it was later recognized that these nevi appear in individuals from nonmelanoma families. The clinical criteria for atypia in melanocytic nevi overlap with the ABCD rule for early melanoma (A, asymmetry; B, border; C, color; D, diameter). Dermoscopy, a noninvasive

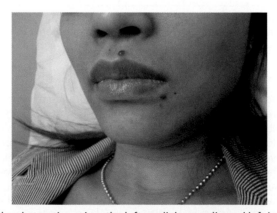

Fig. 3. Compound melanocytic nevi on the left medial upper lip and left lateral lower lip.

examination of the skin with a magnifier and a nonpolarized light source, can play an important role in identifying atypical melanocytic lesions and assist in differentiating benign versus malignant lesions.[115] Additionally, the ugly duckling sign has gained importance in the differentiation from melanoma. In this instance, a pigmented lesion is suspicious for melanoma if that lesion is distinctive and dissimilar relative to the patient's other nevi.[116–118]

Management

The most important goal of surgical treatment of melanocytic nevi is the histologic differentiation from melanoma.[98] Whether or not to excise melanocytic lesions depends on the risk of developing into melanoma. Because this may be difficult clinically at times, an excision is indicated for diagnostic purposes.

MELANOMA
Introduction

Melanoma, a malignancy that develops from melanocytes either de novo or from within a nevus, is an important public health issue throughout the world, including the United States. A melanoma may present as a changing mole or a new dark brown or black macule, papule, or nodule. Diagnosing melanoma early is of utmost importance because the primary treatment modality is surgical excision.

Cause

The causes of malignant melanoma have not been fully elucidated; however, multiple risk factors have been identified, including brief, intense exposure to UV light (UVA 315–400 nm), environmental exposures, skin type, the presence of nevi, and genetic mutations.

Exposure to the sun is the most important environmental cause of melanoma, with the UV radiation being most associated with development of the disease.[119] There is a documented role for UVA radiation inducing carcinogenesis.[119–123] In light-skinned populations, tanning beds have become the main nonsolar source of exposure to UV light. Multiple studies over the past 30 years show that the risk of melanoma is increased by 20% for those who ever used indoor tanning.[119]

Acquired melanocytic nevi are important markers for the risk of melanoma development, with the total number of melanocytic nevi on the whole body being the most important independent risk factor.[124,125] Additionally, the presence of dysplastic nevi is an additional independent risk factor for the development of melanoma.[126] The development of potential precursors to melanoma, such as dysplastic nevi, is inhibited by the regular use of sunscreen.[127–129] Sun protection at an early age may lower the subsequent risk of melanoma.[130]

Approximately 10% of melanomas occur in familial clusters. There is a relationship between a prior personal or family history and melanoma risk.[131–133] Mutations have been identified in 2 high-penetrance susceptibility genes, the cyclin-dependent kinase inhibitor 2A (CDKN2A) on chromosome 19p21 and cyclindependent kinase 4 (CDK4) on chromosome 12q14.[134] Mutations in CDKN2A account for approximately 20% to 40% of hereditary melanoma and 0.2% to 1.0% of all melanomas.[135] In a more recent study, the melanocortin 1 receptor gene, which encodes the melanocyte-stimulating hormone receptor and determines pigment development, has been identified as a low penetrance melanoma susceptibility gene.[136,137] Thus, the inability to tan is also associated with an increased risk of melanoma.[137]

Epidemiology

The incidence of melanoma has been increasing faster than that of any other cancer in the United States.[124,138] Each year, melanoma is diagnosed in more than 70,000 Americans.[138] At current rates, the lifetime risk of developing invasive melanoma is 1 in 52 overall, 1 in 38 for Caucasian men, and 1 in 56 in Caucasian women.[124] In the United States, melanoma is more common in men than in women overall; however, more recently, incidence seems to be increasing in younger women possibly because of increased tanning bed use.[139] The incidence of melanoma also differs between races, with a lower incidence in nonwhite populations.[140]

Prognosis

The prognosis is usually good for thin melanomas; however, greater thickness and advanced-staged melanomas have a much lower 5-year survival. Metastatic melanoma has a well-known predilection for distant spread, with a median survival time of 6 to 9 months.[141] In advanced regional disease, it commonly metastasizes hematogenously to other skin regions, soft tissues, the lung, the liver, and the brain.[142,143] Lungs are the second most common sites of metastatic disease, after lymph node involvement.[142,143]

Clinical Features

Cutaneous melanoma can have a variety of clinical appearances, either occurring de novo or within preexisting melanocytic nevi, often with a change in clinical appearance. Early lesions are often characterized by a macule or plaque with different hues (brown, black, blue, red, or white) or occasionally as an ulceration that does not heal. Pigmented cutaneous lesions can be initially evaluated using the ABCDE acronym (asymmetry, border irregularity, color variegation, diameter, and evolving lesions).[144,145] Not all melanomas present with all 5 features, and it is the combination of the different ABCDE parameters that makes a cutaneous lesion suspect for melanoma.[146]

The anatomic distribution differs by sex and age. In men, they are commonly located on the trunk (55%), especially the back (39%).[147] In women, 42% of melanoma lesions were localized to the lower extremities, with 24% on the lower leg. Lentigo maligna melanoma, a variant more common in the elderly, has a predilection for the head and neck.[148]

Melanoma is diagnosed by skin biopsy. Excisional biopsy with a 1- to 2-mm margin of adjacent normal-appearing skin is the preferred technique for cutaneous lesions suspicious for melanoma.[149] This technique allows the entire lesion to be removed while providing important prognostic information for staging.[150,151]

Four major clinical subtypes of melanoma have been described: superficial spreading melanoma, nodular melanoma, lentigo maligna melanoma, and acral lentiginous melanoma. Superficial spreading melanoma is the most common subtype, accounting for 50% to 80% of all melanoma diagnoses.[150,152] Although they can arise from a precursor nevus, most occur de novo. Clinically, a superficial spreading melanoma appears variegated with a sharply marginated, irregular border. Multiple hues and shades are often noted.[153] Histopathologically, there are pagetoid and nested epithelioid melanocytes cells in the intraepidermal portion with poor circumscription.[153]

Nodular melanoma composes 20% to 30% of cases and is more common in men.[150] Typically, they are found on the trunk and are thickened dark brown or black papules.[148,153]

Lentigo maligna melanoma commonly occurs in older individuals with sun-damaged skin. It has a predilection for sun-exposed areas, such as the nose, malar region, temple, forehead, neck, and forearms.[148] It presents as a slowly enlarging patch that is flat and variably pigmented with tan, brown, and black colors. It is typically asymmetrical with irregular borders.[148] Transformation is slow, often taking 10 to 50 years before invasive growth becomes apparent.[154]

Acral lentiginous melanoma, the least common subtype, accounts for less than 5% of all melanomas.[148,155] This subtype accounts for 70% of melanomas seen in African Americans and occurs on hairless areas like the subungual, palmar, and plantar regions.[150,152,156] Clinically, a variably colored macule develops irregular borders and variegated pigment, usually brown or black, and increases in size over time.[150]

Staging of melanoma is based on the tumor, node, metastasis (TNM) staging criteria. The TNM categories described by the American Joint Committee on Cancer consider histopathologic factors, such as primary tumor thickness, ulceration status, and rate of mitosis.[152]

Because the current research suggests that UV light exposure contributes to the development of nonmelanoma skin cancers and possibly melanoma, limiting exposure may prevent the development of skin cancers.[157,158] The United States Preventive Services Task Force currently recommends that primary care physicians counsel patients on sunprotective strategies, including regular application of sunscreen and avoidance of indoor tanning.[159]

Management

Surgical excision is the primary treatment modality. Wide excision is recommended; but the recommended surgical margin varies, depending on the depth of the tumor.[160] Mohs micrographic surgery has emerged as a surgical option in cases in which tissue preservation is important, such as on the head and neck, particularly in cases of lentigo maligna.[161]

Sentinel lymph node biopsy is important in melanoma staging. The results from sentinel lymph node biopsy may provide important prognostic information.[143] It is often recommended for melanomas that are more than 1 mm in depth. Adjuvant systemic therapies have limited success in the treatment of advanced-stage melanoma.[143] IFN-a is an adjuvant treatment approved by the US Food and Drug Administration (FDA) for stage III melanoma; however, there is very limited efficacy.[162–164]

High-dose IL-2, another immunotherapeutic recently been approved by the FDA for the treatment of metastatic melanoma, has been found to induce remission in 6% of cases of metastatic melanoma.[164] In 2011, ipilimumab, a monoclonal antibody against cytotoxic T-lymphocyte antigen 4 that induces a T-cell–mediated response against the tumor, was approved for metastatic disease.[165] Bevacizumab, an endothelial growth factor antibody, and vemurafenib, a BRAF cellular pathway inhibitor, have also shown some efficacy in advanced melanoma.[143] Radiotherapy plays a limited role since melanoma is radioresistant compared with other cancers.[143]

TRICHOEPITHELIOMA
Introduction

Trichoepitheliomas are benign follicular neoplasms, 2- to 3-mm dome-shaped papules on the nasolabial folds and upper lip.[166]

Cause

Multiple familial trichoepithelioma is a disseminated autosomal dominant form of this disease characterized by numerous papules on the central face.[167,168] Another heritable condition, known as Brooke-Spiegler syndrome, consists of trichoepitheliomas accompanied by other neoplasms, cylindromas and spiradenomas, as a result of mutations in the *CYLD* tumor suppressor gene.[169,170]

Epidemiology

They are increasingly probable with advancing age, though inherited forms can be seen in children.[166]

Prognosis

Trichoepitheliomas are characterized by slow growth.[166] Recurrence may occur with partial removal of lesions. The familial variant may have an aggressive, recurrent course with numerous tumors.

Clinical Features

A solitary lesion presents as a small 2- to 3-mm, smooth, firm, dome-shaped, skin-colored papule that is commonly seen on the nasolabial folds, nose, upper cutaneous lip, and scalp.[166] Trichoepitheliomas can be clinically suspicious for a malignancy.[171] A certain phenotype, known as desmoplastic trichoepithelioma, may resemble basal cell carcinoma and presents as firm papules with raised annular borders and a slightly indented center.[172] Such lesions are found most commonly among young women, and familial solitary and multiple lesions have been described. Shave or small punch biopsies allow a histologic diagnosis of trichoepithelioma, which shows nodules of basaloid cells in a fibrous stroma with prominent follicular germs and papillae and small horn cysts.[173]

Management

Treatment is primarily surgical excision. Multiple lesions can be resurfaced with laser surgery, dermabrasion, or electrosurgery[174,175]; but the results of these procedures vary and tend to be repeated because of the gradual regrowth of elevated papules or nodules.

SEBACEOUS HYPERPLASIA

Introduction

Sebaceous hyperplasia is characterized by yellowish or skin-colored papules with a predilection for the face.[176]

Cause

The risk of development of sebaceous hyperplasia is dramatically increased by chronic immunosuppression with cyclosporin A or infection with HIV.[177–180] Although the cause is unclear, murine experiments have suggested that topical irritants and carcinogens may be implicated in the pathogenesis of sebaceous hyperplasia.[181,182] Growth factors or other cytokines produced by young fibrocytes may explain why some sebaceous hyperplasias overly other lesions, including neurofibromas, melanocytic nevi, verruca vulgaris, and acrochordons.[183–187]

Epidemiology

Lesions may be seen at any age, although prevalence is highest in the fifth decade and increases over time.[188–190] Sebaceous hyperplasia is more common in men.

Prognosis

Although sebaceous hyperplasia does not have malignant potential, it is associated with an increased risk of nonmelanoma skin cancer in patients undergoing a renal transplant.[178] Additionally, an association with Muir-Torre syndrome, an autosomal dominant genodermatosis characterized by at least a single sebaceous gland tumor and one or more internal malignancies, has been postulated, although this is controversial because the high prevalence of sebaceous hyperplasia renders it essentially nonspecific for the syndrome.[191–193]

Clinical Features

Several rare forms of sebaceous hyperplasia exist, which are classified as giant, linear, diffuse, functional familial, and juxtaclavicular beaded lines.[176] The most common variant, however, is senile sebaceous hyperplasia, which is recognized by its yellow color, dome-shaped morphology, and ductal opening.[194] The diagnosis of sebaceous hyperplasia can be made clinically, but biopsy is confirmatory when there is uncertainty.[195,196] Lesions may clinically resemble basal cell carcinoma, making histologic examination necessary.

Management

Treatment is usually for cosmetic purposes and may elicit the use of photodynamic therapy, chemical peeling, isotretinoin, bichloracetic acid, cryosurgery, electrodessication, and laser therapy.[176]

MILIA
Introduction

Milia are small, white, benign, superficial cysts that generally measure less than 4 mm.[197]

Cause

Milia are classified as either primary or secondary. Primary milia arise spontaneously and include the following subtypes: congenital milia, benign primary milia of children and adults, milia en plaque, nodular grouped milia, multiple eruptive milia, nevus depigmentosus with milia, and genodermatosis-associated milia. Secondary milia are associated with blistering disease, medication, or trauma.[197]

Epidemiology

Milia are noted to occur in those of all ages. Primary milia are seen in newborns. Multiple eruptive milia, although rare, are more common in women.

Prognosis

Milia in infancy tend to spontaneously disappear within the first few weeks of life. When they occur in adults or older children, they often persist.

Clinical Features

Milia have walls of stratified squamous epithelium that resemble the epidermis or the follicular infundiblulum, and they have a granular cell layer adjacent to the keratinous cyst lumen.[197] They are white to yellow cystic-appearing papules, dome shaped, and asymptomatic. Overwhelmingly, the most common type encountered in clinical practice is benign primary milia of children and adults, with lesions of the head commonly seen on the cheeks, eyelids, forehead, and, rarely, the nasal crease.[197,198]

Management

Milia can be safely left alone; but if treatment is desired, the contents of the cyst may be extruded by making a small incision with a needle, scalpel blade, or even a paper clip and applying tangential pressure with a comedone extractor or curette.[197,199] Topical retinoids and mild electrocautery or electrodesiccation are other therapeutic options for multiple milia.[200–202]

ACNE VULGARIS
Introduction

Acne vulgaris is a common, inflammatory disease of the pilosebaceous units affecting adolescents and young adults, characterized by the development of comedones (keratin and sebum-plugged pilosebaceous units), inflammatory papules, and pustules.[203]

Cause

The formation of acne depends on 4 primary factors: increased sebum production from the sebaceous glands, hyperkeratinization of the follicle that leads to an enlarged comedo, colonization of the follicle by the anaerobe *Propionibacterium acnes*, and an inflammatory reaction.[204]

Epidemiology

Acne is the most common skin disorder in the United States, affecting 40 to 50 million people of all ages and races.[203] Acne usually begins in adolescence and often resolves by the mid 20s, with girls peaking in prevalence at a younger age than boys.[205] Males are usually more frequently and more severely affected than females on account of greater androgen levels, which correlate with greater sebaceous gland activity.[206]

Prognosis

Acne is generally self-limited, lasting from months to a few years. Adult woman with chronic acne can be an exception to this rule and may be affected by acne for several years. Cystic acne variants, seen most commonly in young men, may persist from adolescence to the fifth decade of life and can be complicated by profound scarring despite treatment.[207]

Clinical Features

The main features of acne range from noninflammatory open (blackheads) or closed (whiteheads) comedones to inflammatory papules, pustules, nodules, and cysts.[208] Lesions occur in areas with the highest concentration of sebaceous glands, such as the face, neck, chest, and back. Inflammatory lesions may be superficial or deep, and deeper lesions may be complicated by scarring.[209] In patients with darker skin types, postinflammatory hyperpigmentation is commonly observed.

The presence of comedones can help distinguish acne from the following conditions: folliculitis, rosacea, or perioral dermatitis.[210]

Management

The goals of treating acne include acute control of flare-ups; long-term maintenance therapy; scar prevention; and reduction of accompanying psychologic sequelae, such as embarrassment and anxiety. Accordingly, the severity of the condition and patients' motivation dictate aggressiveness and risk of the therapy to be undertaken. Current therapies are aimed at the aforementioned 4 major factors of acne development. Topical retinoids are effective in the reduction and prevention of comedones, making them suitable for the treatment of inflammatory and noninflammatory lesions.[211] Benzoyl peroxide is an over-the-counter bactericidal agent that does not lead to bacterial resistance.[212] Topical and oral antibiotics are especially effective in combination with topical retinoids and benzoyl peroxide but may be used as monotherapy. Systemic hormonal therapy may be useful in adult women with chronic acne. Severe, recalcitrant acne, especially if associated with scarring, may warrant the use of oral isotretinoin.[213] Finally, patients should be counseled to avoid picking or squeezing acne lesions, which may prolong healing.

GRAM-NEGATIVE FOLLICULITIS
Introduction

Gram-negative folliculitis is an uncommon superficial or deep bacterial infection of the hair follicle.

Cause

The normal gram-positive flora of the facial skin and mucous membranes of the nose are replaced and invaded by gram-negative bacteria, which include *Escherischia coli*, *Pseudomonas aeruginosa*, *Serratia marescens*, *Klebsiella*, and *Proteus mirabilis*.[214] The infection is considered to be a complication of long-term antibacterial treatment in patients with acne and rosacea.[215,216]

Epidemiology

Anyone using antibiotics for a prolonged period of time may be affected, with a greater likelihood among older men with severe seborrhea.[215,216]

Prognosis

The prognosis for cure is excellent once the diagnosis is accurately established and appropriate therapy is rendered.

Clinical Features

Typical features include perioral and perinasal erythematous papules and pustules or, less commonly, a deep, nodular, and cystic lesion.[215,216] Gram-negative folliculitis should be suspected in patients with acne with flare of these characteristic lesions, who are being treated with chronic, oral tetracycline antibiotics.[214] The differential diagnosis includes acne, rosacea, and pseudofolliculitis barbae. Diagnosis is confirmed by swabbing a lesion for gram stain, culture, and sensitivities.

Management

Gram-negative folliculitis may be treated with oral antibiotics selected based on the sensitivity and resistance pattern of the culture. Isotretinoin, a systemic retinoid, is also effective.[214]

PSEUDOFOLLICULITIS BARBAE
Introduction

Pseudofolliculitis barbae is a common, chronic, irritating, and potentially scarring and disfiguring dermatologic disorder of the hair follicles that usually develops as a complication of shaving.[217]

Cause

Following a shave of tightly curled hair, sharp, tapered, and pointed tips of hair are created and may produce either extrafollicular or transfollicular penetration of the skin.[217,218] Extrafollicular penetration involves the shaved tip of hair exiting the follicle and curving back to pierce the skin with subsequent inflammation of the epidermis.

Transfollicular penetration usually occurs when the skin is shaved under tension and against the grain. With the release of tension, hairs retract underneath the surface of the skin and grow, penetrating the follicular wall, resulting in an inflammatory reaction.

Epidemiology

This condition commonly affects African Americans.[217]

Prognosis

Pseudofolliculitis barbae often improves with discontinuation of shaving within a few months.

Clinical Features

The bearded areas of the anterior neck, submandibular area, chin, and lower jaw are the most commonly affected sites.[217,219] The severity ranges from fewer than a dozen lesions in mild cases to more than 100 in severe presentations. Primary lesions included erythematous follicular papules, pustules, and nodules. Hyperpigmentation, scarring, and keloid formation may complicate this condition.[217,220]

Management

Treatment involves the temporary avoidance of shaving and the use of topical and/or oral acne medications.[218,221–223] Combing and gentle massaging the skin can help in dislodging ingrown hairs. Definitive treatment is the discontinuation of shaving but is impractical for many patients. Another mode of permanent cure is depilation, or hair removal, via electrical or laser methods.[217] Education about proper shaving techniques is essential for prevention and consists of advising patients to shave in the direction of hair growth, not to attempt to achieve a very close shave (particularly on the neck), to use moisturizing products that soften the hair before shaving, and to maintain the best-tolerated shaving system.[224]

IMPETIGO
Introduction

Impetigo is a contagious superficial skin infection most frequently caused by *Streptococcus pyogenes* and secondarily infected with *Staphylococcus aureus*.[225,226]

Cause

Risk of infection is associated with colonization in the nasal, axillary, pharyngeal, or perineal areas.[227,228] The spread of causative bacteria between patients can occur via fingers, towels, or clothing[229]; it is enhanced by atopic diathesis, injured skin, high humidity, and poor hygiene. Areas on the body adjacent to or in close contact with the primary lesion may form satellite lesions.

Epidemiology

It is the most common infection among children worldwide, primarily seen between 2 and 5 years of age.[225,230]

Prognosis

With the use of appropriate antibiotics, the prognosis is excellent. Spontaneous resolution may occur with nonbullous impetigo.

Clinical Features

Impetigo classically presents in 2 forms: nonbullous and bullous. Lesions of both types are frequently seen on the face and extremities.[229] Approximately 70% of cases are nonbullous, which are characterized by erythematous papules and thin-walled vesicles that heal with a honey-colored crusted plaque usually less than 2 cm in diameter.[231,232] These lesions may be preceded by insect bites, abrasions, lacerations, chickenpox, scabies pediculosis, and burns.[232] Regional lymphadenopathy and fever are occasionally present. In contrast, bullous impetigo infects intact skin on account of exfoliative toxins produced by *S aureus*, resulting in thin-roofed bullae and shallow erosions.[230] Rare complications of either type include sepsis, osteomyelitis, septic arthritis, pneumonia, and poststreptococcal glomerulonephritis.[233]

The differential diagnosis includes atopic dermatitis, pemphigus foliaceous, and herpes simplex virus infection.

The diagnosis of impetigo can be made clinically. Gram stain and culture is confirmatory and provide information about bacterial sensitivity and resistance patterns.

Management

Nonbullous impetigo lesions generally resolve spontaneously in 2 to 3 weeks.[225] In cases requiring treatment, the number of lesions and their locations must be considered, and antibiotics should be targeted to the causative pathogen. However, the increase in antibacterial resistance has complicated the therapeutic paradigm.[234] Impetigo and other limited skin and soft tissue infections should be treated with topical agents, such as mupirocin, fusidic acid, and retapamulin, to reduce resistance and minimize the incidence of adverse events. Systemic antibiotics may be prescribed for patients with widespread involvement.[235]

ROSACEA
Introduction

Rosacea is a chronic disorder affecting the facial skin of adults characterized by one or a combination of features, including centrofacial erythema, telangiectasia, a tendency to flush, inflammatory papules and pustules, and phymatous changes.[236,237]

Cause

The cause of rosacea is not completely understood. Individuals affected by rosacea may have a genetic susceptibility toward vasomotor instability of the facial skin, in addition to an inflammatory response.[238] Rosacea flushing may be precipitated by several factors, including sun, wind, cold, alcohol, and other triggers.[237,238]

Epidemiology

Rosacea is a common condition affecting approximately 14 million Americans.[239] Rosacea affects men and women, and it usually begins after 30 years of age.[236]

Prognosis

Rosacea is a chronic condition of adults, which can be effectively managed but not cured. The condition may be, but is not necessarily, progressive.[238]

Clinical Features

The clinical features of rosacea mainly affect the skin the central face.[236,237] Patients may exhibit one or a combination of symptoms and signs, including persistent facial erythema; a tendency to flush; acnelike papules and pustules; and telangiectasia

(**Fig. 4**). An uncommon and late-stage finding is the development of rhynophyma, characterized by a bulbous appearance of the nose with thickened skin and patulous follicles. Patients may also have associated features of ocular rosacea, including burning, stinging, and conjunctival injection.

The differential diagnosis includes acne, seborrheic dermatitis, contact dermatitis, and photosensitivity disorders.[237]

Management

The management of rosacea is best planned and executed according to patients' clinical features or subtype because different features respond to different interventions.[239,240] For example, inflammatory papules and pustules are usually very responsive to oral tetracycline therapy. Remission can then be maintained by topical metronidazole therapy.[241] Topical metronidazole has also been shown to reduce erythema of rosacea. Telangiectases can be successfully treated with vascular lasers. Ablative lasers and electrocautery can be used to sculpt the nose and enhance the appearance of rhynophyma. Patients with rosacea often have sensitive skin. Irritating products, such as benzoyl peroxide and tretinoin, may cause significant stinging and erythema and should be used cautiously in carefully selected patients.[238]

PERIORAL DERMATITIS
Introduction

Perioral dermatitis is a common condition predominately affecting the skin of women characterized by fine erythematous papules and/or pustules on a background of erythema on the perioral and peranasal skin.[242,243]

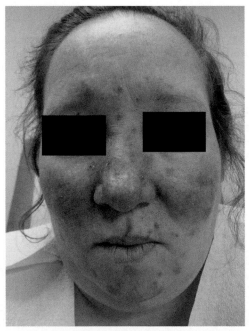

Fig. 4. Rosacea exhibiting centrofacial erythema, acneiform papules and pustules, telangiectasias, and early rhinophymatous changes.

Cause

The cause of perioral dermatitis is uncertain; however, the use of topical steroids on affected regions has often been associated with this condition.[242–244] More recently, intranasal steroids have also been associated with this condition.[245] Other agents, such as cosmetics and fluoride-containing toothpaste, have also been implicated.

Epidemiology

Perioral dermatitis mostly affects women in the second through fifth decades.[242,243] Children and men may be less commonly affected.

Prognosis

The condition may persist until appropriately treated.

Clinical Features

Patients typically present with fine erythematous papules and/or pustules on a background of erythema on the perioral and paranasal skin.[242,243] Perioral lesions most often appear on the side of the chin and the cutaneous lip, sparing a small zone of skin around the vermilion lip. Less frequently, lesions may occur on the periocular skin, and the term *periorificial dermatitis* has been applied. Patients may report that the affected skin feels irritated with mild, burning, stinging, or itching.

The differential diagnosis may include acne, rosacea, seborrheic dermatitis, and contact dermatitis.

Management

Despite the lack of precise knowledge regarding the cause of perioral dermatitis, the condition is often highly responsive to certain therapy. Oral antibiotic therapy with the antibiotics tetracycline or doxycycline in doses of 250 mg or 50 mg, respectively, twice daily can either induce cure or provide durable remission in most cases with 4 to 6 weeks of treatment.[242,243,246] Patients who are using topical steroids or other exacerbating products on the skin should be advised to discontinue these agents. It should be noted that abrupt cessation of a high-potency topical steroid may induce a rebound flare of perioral dermatitis, and patients may benefit from a gradual tapering off of topical steroids. Topical therapy with antimicrobial agents, such as erythromycin or metronidazole, may provide some benefit and are especially useful for patients in whom systemic tetracycline therapy is contraindicated. Potentially irritating products, such as topical retinoids and benzoyl peroxide, can inflame the affected skin and should be avoided.

CONTACT CHEILITIS
Introduction

As the names implies, contact cheilitis is an inflammatory condition of the lips caused by exposure to a contactant, an allergenic, or irritating substance.[247] The reaction pattern is typically eczematous and is responsive to topical steroids. Identification and avoidance of the offending contactant is essential for optimal management.

Cause

Contact cheilitis may be subdivided into 2 main categories, irritant and allergic, based on whether the contactant elicits inflammatory reaction by way of a nonspecific irritant process or by way of a specific immunologic reaction.[247]

Irritants are substances that have a direct toxic effect on the skin, which can be strong or weak. Thus, irritant contact cheilitis is not a specific reaction to a particular antigen. In addition to the intrinsic strength of the irritant, the extent of the reaction often depends on the duration and frequency of the exposure, the concentration of the irritant, and patients' susceptibility to the irritant.[248] Irritant contact cheilitis may result from lip licking, harsh or extreme environmental conditions, and alkaline tartar-control compounds.[249]

In contrast, allergic contact cheilitis is a cell-mediated immune response mediated by epidermal antigen-presenting cells (Langerhans cells) and memory T cells in response to exposure to a specific antigen.[248] Common allergens include fragrance and flavorings present in oral hygiene products, such as toothpastes and mouthwash; cosmetics; and foods.[250–255] The metal nickel and topical medications, including neomycin and bacitracin, may also cause allergic contact cheilitis.

Epidemiology

Allergic contact cheilitis tends to increase with age and exhibits an overwhelming female predominance; as high as 90% of patients are female.[251,253,254] The theoretical explanation for this is the assumption that females are more frequently exposed to potential contact allergens via the use of cosmetics and lip products as compared with men.

Prognosis

If the offending irritant and/or allergen can be identified and eliminated, the cheilitis should resolve.

Clinical Features

Contact cheilitis is an inflammatory condition that typically affects the vermilion zone with variable extension onto the adjacent skin. It is caused by exposure to a contactant, an allergenic, or irritating substance. The condition generally manifests with eczematous changes, which may include the sensation of itching, burning, or stinging, and physical characteristics, including erythema, edema, scaling, vesiculation, crusting, and fissuring.[247,249,250]

The differential diagnosis includes atopic dermatitis, nutritional deficiency, or perioral dermatitis.

Management

Patch testing is a diagnostic test that is highly useful in the identification and confirmation of allergens that may cause allergic contact dermatitis and cheilitis.[250–255] Avoidance of relevant contactants is a mainstay of therapy and may be curative. It is important to bear in mind that contact cheilitis may be multifactorial, and removing all exacerbating factors is necessary. Some factors, such as lip licking, may be habitual and challenging to correct. Signs and symptoms of contact cheilitis usually respond to therapy with topical corticosteroids.[249] Ointments are generally preferred to creams. As the inflammation subsides, patients are transitioned off of topical cortisosteroids onto bland ointment emollients, such as petrolatum.[249]

SEBORRHEIC DERMATITIS
Introduction

Seborrheic dermatitis is a common, chronic inflammatory skin condition characterized by scaling, erythematous patches that may affect the scalp, face, ears, and occasionally the sternum and intertriginous sites.[256]

Cause

The cause of seborrheic dermatitis is incompletely understood. However, active sebum production, as in the neonatal period and during puberty, may be permissive.[256] Fungi of the genus *Malassezia* have been thought to play a role in the pathogenesis because they are lipid-dependent, ubiquitous inhabitants of the skin and antifungal agents are useful in treatment.[257–259]

Epidemiology

Newborns are frequently affected with seborrheic dermatitis, also known as cradle cap.[260] Seborrheic dermatitis also commonly affects adolescents and adults. Individuals with HIV are susceptible to more frequent and more severe cases.[261,262]

Prognosis

Seborrheic dermatitis is a chronic condition that can be controlled but not cured.

Clinical Features

Signs and symptoms include scaling (dandruff), erythema, and mild itch (**Fig. 5**). The scalp is almost invariably affected, followed by the nasolabial folds, eyebrows, bearded areas, conchal bowls and auditory canals of the external ears, retroauricular skin, presternal chest, and intertriginous regions.[263]

The differential diagnosis includes psoriasis, contact dermatitis, and atopic dermatitis.[254]

Management

Seborrheic dermatitis is usually highly responsive to therapy. Patients should be advised to cleanse their hair and scalp with a dandruff shampoo (containing zinc pyrithione, selenium sulfide, or ketoconazole, for example) at least 2 to 3 times weekly. If the response to proper shampooing is inadequate, topical agents are used. Ketoconazole and, if necessary, hydrocortisone cream will generally control dermatitis affecting the glabrous skin. Low- and midpotency topical corticosteroids are available in solution, lotion, and foam formulations for hair-bearing skin. Topical calcineurin inhibitors are used in selected cases that are refractory to other forms of treatment.

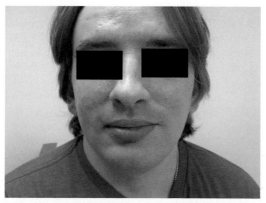

Fig. 5. Seborrheic dermatitis featuring scaling and erythema of eyebrows, glabella, malar regions, nasolabial folds, and upper lip.

REFERENCES

1. Brodsky J. Management of benign skin lesions commonly affecting the face: actinic keratosis, seborrheic keratosis, and rosacea. Curr Opin Otolaryngol Head Neck Surg 2009;17:315–20.
2. Hafner C, Stoehr R, Van Oers JM, et al. FGFR3 and PIK3CA mutations are involved in the molecular pathogenesis of solar lentigo. Br J Dermatol 2009; 160:546–51.
3. Gill D, Dorevitch A, Marks R. The prevalence of seborrheic keratoses in people aged 15 to 30 years: is the term senile keratosis redundant? Arch Dermatol 2000;136:759–62.
4. Hafner C, Vogt T. Seborrheic keratosis. J Dtsch Dermatol Ges 2008;6:664–77.
5. Kavak A, Parlak AH, Yesildal N, et al. Preliminary study among truck drivers in Turkey: effects of ultraviolet light on some skin entities. J Dermatol 2008;35: 146–50.
6. Kwon OS, Hwang EJ, Bae JH, et al. Seborrheic keratosis in the Korean males: causative role of sunlight. Photodermatol Photoimmunol Photomed 2003;19: 73–80.
7. James WD, Berger TG, Elston DM. Seborrheic keratosis. In: James WD, Berger TG, Elston DM, editors. Andrews' diseases of the skin: clinical dermatology. 11th edition. Philadelphia: Saunders; 2011.
8. Dunwell P, Rose A. Study of the skin disease spectrum occurring in an Afro-Caribbean population. Int J Dermatol 2003;42:287–9.
9. Wieland CN, Kumar N. Sign of Leser–Trélat. Int J Dermatol 2008;47:643–4.
10. Dasanu CA, Alexandrescu DT. Bilateral Leser–Trélat sign mirroring lung adenocarcinoma with early metastases to the contralateral lung. Southampt Med J 2009;102:216–8.
11. Li M, Yang LJ, Zhu XH. The Leser–Trélat sign is associated with nasopharyngeal carcinoma: case report and review of cases reported in China. Clin Exp Dermatol 2009;34:52–4.
12. Fink AM, Filz D, Krajnik G, et al. Seborrhoeic keratoses in patients with internal malignancies: a case-control study with prospective accrual of patients. J Eur Acad Dermatol Venereol 2009;23:1316–9.
13. Kilmer SL. Laser eradication of pigmented lesions and tattoos. Dermatol Clin 2002;20:37–53.
14. Cobb MW. Human papillomavirus infection. J Am Acad Dermatol 1990;22: 547–66.
15. Cardoso JC, Calonje E. Cutaneous manifestations of human papillomaviruses: a review. Acta Dermatovenerol Alp Panonica Adriat 2011;20(3):145–54.
16. Riddel C, Rashid R, Thomas V. Ungual and periungual human papillomavirus-associated squamous cell carcinoma: a review. J Am Acad Dermatol 2011; 64(6):1147–53.
17. Kwok CS, Gibbs S, Bennett C, et al. Topical treatments for cutaneous warts. Cochrane Database Syst Rev 2012;(9):CD001781.
18. Yilmaz E, Alpsoy E, Basaran E. Cimetidine therapy for warts: a placebo-controlled, double-blind study. J Am Acad Dermatol 1996;34:1005–7.
19. Horn TD, Johnson S, Helm RM, et al. Intralesional immunotherapy of warts with mumps, Candida, and Trichophyton skin test antigens. Arch Dermatol 2005;141: 589–94.
20. Lee Y, Baron ED. Photodynamic therapy: current evidence and applications in dermatology. Semin Cutan Med Surg 2011;30(4):199–209.

21. Street ML, Roenigk RK. Recalcitrant periungual verrucae: the role of carbon dioxide laser vaporization. J Am Acad Dermatol 1990;23:115–20.
22. Mitsuishi T, Iida K, Kawana S. Cimetidine treatment for viral warts enhances IL-2 and IFN-gamma expression but not IL-18 expression in lesional skin. Eur J Dermatol 2003;13(5):445–8.
23. Erickson BK, Alvarez RD, Huh WK. Human papillomavirus: what every provider should know. Am J Obstet Gynecol 2013;208(3):169–75.
24. Oppel T, Korting HC. Actinic keratosis: the key event in the evolution from photoaged skin to squamous cell carcinoma. Therapy based on pathogenetic and clinical aspects. Skin Pharmacol Physiol 2004;17:67–76.
25. Schwartz RA, Bridges TM, Butani AK, et al. Actinic keratosis: an occupational and environmental disorder. J Eur Acad Dermatol Venereol 2008;22:606–15.
26. Rossi R, Mori M, Lotti T. Actinic keratosis. Int J Dermatol 2007;46:895–904.
27. Kanellou P, Zaravinos A, Zioga M, et al. Genomic instability, mutations and expression analysis of the tumour suppressor genes p14(ARF), p15(INK4b), p16(INK4a) and p53 in actinic keratosis. Cancer Lett 2008;264:145–61.
28. Fuchs M, Marmur E. The kinetics of skin cancer: progression of actinic keratosis to squamous cell carcinoma. Dermatol Surg 2007;33:1099–101.
29. Ceilley RI, Jorizzo JL. Current issues in the management of actinic keratosis. J Am Acad Dermatol 2013;68:S28–38.
30. Kuflik EG. Cryosurgery updated. J Am Acad Dermatol 1994;31:925–34.
31. Jorizzo J, Weiss J, Furst K, et al. Effect of a 1-week treatment with 0.5% topical fluorouracil on occurrence of actinic keratosis after cryosurgery: a randomized, vehicle-controlled clinical trial. Arch Dermatol 2004;140:813–6.
32. Girard KR, Hoffman BL. Actinic cheilitis: report of a case. Oral Surg Oral Med Oral Pathol 1980;50:21–4.
33. Cavalcante AS, Anbinder AL, Carvalho YR. Actinic cheilitis: clinical and histological features. J Oral Maxillofac Surg 2008;66:498–503.
34. Main JH, Pavone M. Actinic cheilitis and carcinoma of the lip. J Can Dent Assoc 1994;60:113–6.
35. Robinson JK. Actinic cheilitis. A prospective study comparing four treatment methods. Arch Otolaryngol Head Neck Surg 1989;115:848–52.
36. Kaugars GE, Pillion T, Svirsky JA, et al. Actinic cheilitis: a review of 152 cases. Oral Surg Oral Med Oral Pathol Oral Radiol Endod 1999;88:181–6.
37. Markopoulos A, Albanidou-Farmaki E, Kayavis I. Actinic cheilitis: clinical and pathologic characteristics in 65 cases. Oral Dis 2004;10:212–6.
38. Dufresne RG Jr, Garrett AB, Bailin PL, et al. Carbon dioxide laser treatment of chronic actinic cheilitis. J Am Acad Dermatol 1988;19:876–8.
39. Sexton J. Carbon dioxide laser treatment for actinic cheilitis [letter]. J Oral Maxillofac Surg 1993;51:953.
40. Kutcher MJ, Rubenstein D. Fifteen inches from cancer: early recognition of facial lesions by the dentist. Compend Contin Educ Dent 2004;25:939–42.
41. La Riviere W, Pickett AB. Clinical criteria in diagnosis of early squamous cell carcinoma of the lower lip. J Am Dent Assoc 1979;99:972–7.
42. Zitsch RP 3rd. Carcinoma of the lip. Otolaryngol Clin North Am 1993;26:265–77.
43. Moore SR, Allister J, Roder D, et al. Lip cancer in South Australia, 1977–1996. Pathology 2001;33:167–71.
44. Kwa RE, Campana K, Moy RL, et al. Biology of cutaneous squamous cell carcinoma. J Am Acad Dermatol 1992;26:1–26.
45. Winn DM. Diet and nutrition in the etiology of oral cancer. Am J Clin Nutr 1995; 61:437S–45S.

46. Lindqvist C, Teppo L, Pukkala E. Occupations with low risk of lip cancer show high risk of skin cancer of the head. Community Dent Oral Epidemiol 1981;9:247–50.

47. Birkeland SA, Storm HH, Lamm LU, et al. Cancer risk after renal transplantation in the Nordic countries, 1964–1986. Int J Cancer 1995;60:183–9.

48. Vieira RA, Minicucci EM, Marques ME, et al. Actinic cheilitis and squamous cell carcinoma of the lip: clinical, histopathological and immunogenetic aspects. An Bras Dermatol 2012;87(1):105–14.

49. Frisch M, Biggar RJ, Engels EA, et al, AIDS-Cancer Match Registry Study Group. Association of cancer with AIDS-related immunosuppression in adults. JAMA 2001;285:1736–45.

50. Bilkay U, Kerem H, Ozek C, et al. Management of lower lip cancer: a retrospective analysis of 118 patients and review of the literature. Ann Plast Surg 2003;50: 43–50.

51. Broughman N, Dennett E, Cameron R, et al. The incidence of metastasis from cutaneous squamous cell carcinoma and the impact of its risk factors. J Surg Oncol 2012;106:811–5.

52. McGregor GI, Davis NL, Hay JH. Impact of cervical lymph node metastases from squamous cell cancer of the lip. Am J Surg 1992;163:469–71.

53. Ochsenius G, Ormeño A, Godoy L, et al. A retrospective study of 232 cases of lip cancer and pre cancer in Chilean patients. Clinical-histological correlation. Rev Med Chil 2003;131:60–6.

54. dos Santos LR, Cernea CR, Kowalski LP, et al. Squamous-cell carcinoma of the lower lip: a retrospective study of 58 patients. Sao Paulo Med J 1996;114: 1117–26.

55. Zitsch RP 3rd, Park CW, Renner GJ, et al. Outcome analysis for lip carcinoma. Otolaryngol Head Neck Surg 1995;113:589–96.

56. Scully C. Oral manifestations associated with human immunodeficiency virus (HIV) infection in developing countries–are there differences from developed countries? Oral Dis 2000;6:395.

57. Patel SG, Shah JP. TNM staging of cancers of the head and neck: striving for uniformity among diversity. CA Cancer J Clin 2005;55:242–58.

58. Bentley JM, Barankin B, Lauzon GJ. Paying more than lip service to lip lesions. Can Fam Physician 2003;49:1111–6.

59. Najim M, Cross S, Gebski V, et al. Early-stage squamous cell carcinoma of the lip: the Australian experience and the benefits of radiotherapy in improving outcome in high-risk patients after resection. Head Neck 2012;35(10):1426–30.

60. Kyrgidis A, Tzellos TG, Kechagias N, et al. Cutaneous squamous cell carcinoma (SCC) of the head and neck: risk factors of overall and recurrence free survival. Eur J Cancer 2010;46:1563–72.

61. Onercl M, Yilmaz T, Gedikoğlu G. Tumor thickness as a predictor of cervical lymph node metastasis in squamous cell carcinoma of the lower lip. Otolaryngol Head Neck Surg 2000;122:139–42.

62. Babington S, Veness MJ, Cakir B, et al. Squamous cell carcinoma of the lip: is there a role for adjuvantuvant radiotherapy in improving local control following incomplete or inadequate excision? ANZ J Surg 2003;73:621–5.

63. Renzi C, Caggiati A, Mannooranparampil TJ, et al. Sentinel lymph node biopsy for high risk cutaneous squamous cell carcinoma: case series and review of the literature. Eur J Surg Oncol 2007;33:364–9.

64. Ross AS, Schmults CD. Sentinel lymph node biopsy in cutaneous squamous cell carcinoma: a systematic review of the English literature. Dermatol Surg 2006;32: 1309–21.

65. Rastrelli M, Soteldo J, Zonta M, et al. Sentinel node biopsy for high-risk cutaneous nonanogenital squamous cell carcinoma: a preliminary result. Eur Surg Res 2010;44:204–8.
66. Murali R, Haydu LE, Quinn MJ, et al. Sentinel lymph node biopsy in patients with thin primary cutaneous melanoma. Ann Surg 2012;255:128–33.
67. Rogers HW, Weinstock MA, Harris AR, et al. Incidence estimate of nonmelanoma skin cancer in the United States, 2006. Arch Dermatol 2010;146: 283–7.
68. Johnson TM, Rowe DE, Nelson BR, et al. Squamous cell carcinoma of the skin (excluding lip and oral mucosa). J Am Acad Dermatol 1992;26:467–84.
69. Leman JA, McHenry PM. Basal cell carcinoma: still an enigma. Arch Dermatol 2001;137:1239–40.
70. Marcil I, Stern RS. Risk of developing a subsequent nonmelanoma skin cancer in patients with a history of nonmelanoma skin cancer: a critical review of the literature and meta-analysis. Arch Dermatol 2000;136:1524–30.
71. Crowson AN. Basal cell carcinoma: biology, morphology and clinical implications. Mod Pathol 2006;19(Suppl 2):S127–47.
72. Willey A, Swanson NA, Lee KK. Recognition and treatment of skin lesions. In: Flint PW, Haughey BH, Lund VJ, et al, editors. Cummings otolaryngology head and neck surgery. 5th edition. Philadelphia: Mosby; 2010. p. 281–94.
73. Alam M, Ratner D. Cutaneous squamous-cell carcinoma. N Engl J Med 2001; 344:975–83.
74. Christenson LJ, Borrowman TA, Vachon CM, et al. Incidence of basal cell and squamous cell carcinomas in a population younger than 40 years. JAMA 2005;294:681–90.
75. Sexton M, Jones DB, Maloney ME. Histologic pattern analysis of basal cell carcinoma. Study of a series of 1039 consecutive neoplasms. J Am Acad Dermatol 1990;23:1118–26.
76. Firnhaber JM. Diagnosis and treatment of basal cell and squamous cell carcinoma. Am Fam Physician 2012;86:161–8.
77. Maloney ME, Jones DB, Sexton FM. Pigmented basal cell carcinoma: investigation of 70 cases. J Am Acad Dermatol 1992;27:74–8.
78. Cockerell CJ, Tran KT, Carucci J, et al. Basal cell carcinoma. In: Rigel DS, Robinson JK, Ross MI, et al, editors. Cancer of the skin. 2nd edition. Philadelphia: Saunders; 2011. p. 99–123.
79. Raasch BA, Buettner PG, Garbe C. Basal cell carcinoma: histological classification and body-site distribution. Br J Dermatol 2006;155:401–7.
80. Rippey JJ. Why classify basal cell carcinomas? Histopathology 1998;32:393–8.
81. Milroy CJ, Horlock N, Wilson GD, et al. Aggressive basal cell carcinoma in young patients: fact or fiction? Br J Plast Surg 2000;53:393–6.
82. Saldanha G, Fletcher A, Slater DN. Basal cell carcinoma: a dermatopathological and biological update. Br J Dermatol 2003;148:195–202.
83. Bastiaens MT, Hoefnagel JJ, Bruijn JA, et al. Differences in age, site distribution, and sex between nodular and superficial basal cell carcinoma indicate different types of tumors. J Invest Dermatol 1998;110:880–4.
84. Salasche SJ, Amonette RA. Morpheaform basal-cell epitheliomas. A study of subclinical extensions in a series of 51 cases. J Dermatol Surg Oncol 1981;7: 387–94.
85. Silverman MK, Kopf AW, Grin CM, et al. Recurrence rates of treated basal cell carcinoma. Part 2: curettage-electrodesiccation. J Dermatol Surg Oncol 1991; 17:720–6.

86. Torre D. Cryosurgery of basal cell carcinoma. J Am Acad Dermatol 1986;15: 917–29.

87. Thissen MR, Neumann MH, Schouten LJ. A systematic review of treatment modalities for primary basal cell carcinoma. Arch Dermatol 1999;135:1177–83.

88. Hunter RD. Skin. In: Easson EC, Pointon RC, editors. The radiotherapy of malignant disease. New York: Springer-Verlag; 1985. p. 135.

89. Love WE, Bernhard JD, Bordeaux JS. Topical imiquimod or fluorouracil therapy for basal and squamous cell carcinoma: a systematic review. Arch Dermatol 2009;145:1431–8.

90. Lin J, Koga H, Takata M, et al. Dermoscopy of pigmented lesions on mucocutaneous junction and mucous membrane. Br J Dermatol 2009;161:1255–61.

91. Ho KK, Dervan P, O'Laughlin S, et al. Labial melanotic macule: a clinical histopathologic and ultrastructural study. J Am Acad Dermatol 1993;28:33–9.

92. Buchner A, Merrel PW, Carpenter WM. Relative frequency of solitary melanocytic lesions of the oral mucosa. J Oral Pathol Med 2004;33:550–7.

93. Kaugars GE, Heise AP, Riley WT, et al. Oral melanotic macules. A review of 353 cases. Oral Surg Oral Med Oral Pathol 1993;76:59–61.

94. Weathers DR, Corio RL, Crawford BE, et al. The labial melanotic macule. Oral Surg Oral Med Oral Pathol Oral Radiol Endod 1976;42:196–205.

95. Meleti M, Vescovi P, Mooi W, et al. Pigmented lesions of the oral mucoa and perioral tissues: a flow-chart for the diagnosis and some recommendations for the management. Oral Surg Oral Med Oral Pathol Oral Radiol Endod 2008; 105:606–16.

96. Eisen D. Disorders of pigmentation in the oral cavity. Clin Dermatol 2000;18: 579–87.

97. Kauzman A, Pavone M, Blanas N, et al. Pigmented lesions of the oral cavity: review, differential diagnosis, and case presentation. J Can Dent Assoc 2004;70: 682–3.

98. Hauschild A, Egberts F, Garbe C, et al. Melanocytic nevi. J Dtsch Dermatol Ges 2011;9(9):723–34.

99. English DR, Armstrong BK. Melanocytic nevi in children. I. Anatomic sites and demographic and host factors. Am J Epidemiol 1994;139:390–401.

100. Green A, Siskind V, Hansen ME, et al. Melanocytic nevi in schoolchildren in Queensland. J Am Acad Dermatol 1989;20:1054–60.

101. Luther H, Altmeyer P, Garbe C, et al. Increase of melanocytic nevus counts in children during 5 years of follow-up and analysis of associated factors. Arch Dermatol 1996;132:1473–8.

102. Wiecker TS, Luther H, Buettner P, et al. Moderate sun exposure and nevus counts in parents are associated with development of melanocytic nevi in childhood. Cancer 2003;97:628–38.

103. Gallagher RP, McLean DI, Yang CP, et al. Suntan, sunburn, and pigmentation factors and the frequency of acquired melanocytic nevi in children. Similarities to melanoma: the Vancouver Mole Study. Arch Dermatol 1990;126:770–6.

104. Harrison SL, Buettner PG, MacLennan R. Body-site distribution of melanocytic nevi in young Australian children. Arch Dermatol 1999;135:47–52.

105. Harrison SL, MacKie RM, MacLennan R. Development of melanocytic nevi in the first three years of life. J Natl Cancer Inst 2000;92:1436–8.

106. Dahl C, Guldberg P. The genome and epigenome of malignant melanoma. APMIS 2007;115:1161–76.

107. Garbe C, Buttner P, Weiss J, et al. Risk factors for developing cutaneous melanoma and criteria for identifying persons at risk: multicenter case-control study

of the Central Malignant Melanoma Registry of the German Dermatological Society. J Invest Dermatol 1994;102:695–9.

108. Bauer J, Garbe C. Risk estimation for malignant transformation of melanocytic nevi. Arch Dermatol 2004;140:127.

109. Barnhill RL, Fleischli M. Histologic features of congenital melanocytic nevi in infants 1 year of age or younger. J Am Acad Dermatol 1995;33:780–5.

110. Kopf AW, Levine LJ, Rigel DS, et al. Prevalence of congenital-nevus-like nevi, nevi spili, and cafe au lait spots. Arch Dermatol 1985;121:766–9.

111. Krengel S, Hauschild A, Schäfer T. Melanoma risk in congenital melanocytic nevi – a systematic review. Br J Dermatol 2006;155:1–8.

112. Hendrickson MR, Ross JC. Neoplasms arising in congenital giant nevi: morphologic study of seven cases and a review of the literature. Am J Surg Pathol 1981; 5:109–35.

113. Rhodes AR, Albert LS, Weinstock MA. Congenital nevomelanocytic nevi: proportionate area expansion during infancy and early childhood. J Am Acad Dermatol 1996;34:51–62.

114. Kinsler VA, Birley J, Atherton DJ. Great ormond street hospital for children registry for congenital melanocytic naevi: prospective study 1988–2007. Part 2 – evaluation of treatments. Br J Dermatol 2009;160:387–92.

115. Kittler H, Pehamberger H, Wolff K, et al. Diagnostic accuracy of dermoscopy. Lancet Oncol 2002;3:159–65.

116. Grob JJ, Bonerandi JJ. The "ugly duckling" sign: identification of the common characteristics of nevi in an individual as a basis for melanoma screening. Arch Dermatol 1998;134:103–4.

117. Gachon J, Beaulieu P, Sei JF, et al. First prospective study of the recognition process of melanoma in dermatological practice. Arch Dermatol 2005;141: 434–8.

118. Scope A, Dusza SW, Halpern AC, et al. The "ugly duckling" sign: agreement between observers. Arch Dermatol 2008;144:58–64.

119. Boniol M, Autier P, Peter Boyle P, et al. Cutaneous melanoma attributable to sunbed use: systematic review and meta-analysis. BMJ 2012;345:e4757.

120. Ridley AJ, Whiteside JR, McMillan TJ, et al. Cellular and sub-cellular responses to UVA in relation to carcinogenesis. Int J Radiat Biol 2009;85:177–95.

121. Rünger TM, Kappes UP. Mechanisms of mutation formation with long-wave ultraviolet light (UVA). Photodermatol Photoimmunol Photomed 2008;24:2–10.

122. Mouret S, Forestier A, Douki T. The specificity of UVA-induced DNA damage in human melanocytes. Photochem Photobiol Sci 2011;11:155–62.

123. Mouret S, Baudouin C, Charveron M, et al. Cyclobutane pyrimidine dimers are predominant DNA lesions in whole human skin exposed to UVA radiation. Proc Natl Acad Sci U S A 2006;103:13765–70.

124. Russak JE, Rigel DS. Risk factors for the development of primary cutaneous melanoma. Dermatol Clin 2012;30(3):363–8.

125. Snels DG, Hille ET, Gruis NA, et al. Risk of cutaneous malignant melanoma in patients with nonfamilial atypical nevi from a pigmented lesions clinic. J Am Acad Dermatol 1999;40(5 Pt 1):686–93.

126. Tucker MA. Melanoma epidemiology. Hematol Oncol Clin North Am 2009;23(3): 383–95, vii.

127. Marks R. Epidemiology of melanoma. Clin Exp Dermatol 2000;25(6):459–63.

128. Green A, Williams G, Neale R, et al. Daily sunscreen application and betacarotene supplementation in prevention of basal-cell and squamous-cell carcinomas of the skin: a randomised controlled trial. Lancet 1999;354:723–9.

129. Naylor MF, Boyd A, Smith DW, et al. High sun protection factor sunscreens in the suppression of actinic neoplasia. Arch Dermatol 1995;131:170–5.
130. MacLennan R, Kelly JW, Rivers JK, et al. The Eastern Australian Childhood Nevus Study: site differences in density and size of melanocytic nevi in relation to latitude and phenotype. J Am Acad Dermatol 2003;48(3):367–75.
131. Florell SR, Boucher KM, Garibotti G, et al. Population- based analysis of prognostic factors and survival in familial melanoma. J Clin Oncol 2005;23:7168–77.
132. Kang S, Barnhill RL, Mihm MC, et al. Multiple primary cutaneous melanomas. Cancer 1992;70:1911–6.
133. DiFronzo LA, Wanek LA, Elashoff R, et al. Increased incidence of second primary melanoma in patients with a previous cutaneous melanoma. Ann Surg Oncol 1999;6:705–11.
134. Meyer K, Guldberg P. Genetic risk factors for melanoma. Hum Genet 2009;120: 499–510.
135. Begg CB, Orlow I, Hummer AJ, et al. Lifetime risk of melanoma in CDKN2A mutation carriers in a population-based sample. J Natl Cancer Inst 2005;97: 1507–15.
136. Suzuki I, Cone RD, Im S, et al. Binding of melanotropic hormones to the melanocortin receptor MC1R on human melanocytes stimulates proliferation and melanogenesis. Endocrinology 1996;137:1627–33.
137. Lin JY, Fisher DE. Melanocyte biology and skin pigmentation. Nature 2007;445: 843–50.
138. Linos E, Swetter SM, Cockburn MG, et al. Increasing burden of melanoma in the United States. J Invest Dermatol 2009;129:1666–74.
139. Eide MJ, Weinstock MA. Epidemiology of skin cancer. In: Rigel DS, editor. Cancer of the skin. Philadelphia: Elevier; 2011.
140. Rigel DS. Epidemiology of melanoma. Semin Cutan Med Surg 2010;29(4):204–9.
141. Thirlwell C, Nathan P. Melanoma–part 2: management. BMJ 2008;337:a2488.
142. Patel JK, Didolkar MS, Pickren JW, et al. Metastatic pattern of malignant melanoma. A study of 216 autopsy cases. Am J Surg 1978;135(6):807–10.
143. Patnana M, Bronstein Y, Szklaruk J, et al. Multimethod imaging, staging, and spectrum of manifestations of metastatic melanoma. Clin Radiol 2011;66(3): 224–36.
144. Friedman RJ, Rigel DS, Kopf AW. Early detection of malignant melanoma: the role of physician examination and self-examination of the skin. CA Cancer J Clin 1985;35(3):130–51.
145. Abbasi NR, Shaw HM, Rigel DS, et al. Early diagnosis of cutaneous melanoma: revisiting the ABCD criteria. JAMA 2004;292(22):2771–6.
146. Rigel DS, Russak J, Friedman R. The evolution of melanoma diagnosis: 25 years beyond the ABCDs. CA Cancer J Clin 2010;60(5):301–16.
147. Garbe C, Leiter U. Melanoma epidemiology and trends. Clin Dermatol 2009; 27(1):3–9.
148. Porras BH, Cockerell CJ. Cutaneous malignant melanoma: classification and clinical diagnosis. Semin Cutan Med Surg 1997;16(2):88–96.
149. Balch CM, Gershenwald JE, Soong SJ, et al. Final version of 2009 AJCC melanoma staging and classification. J Clin Oncol 2009;27(36):6199–206.
150. Au A, Ariyan S. Melanoma of the head and neck. J Craniofac Surg 2011;22(2): 421–9.
151. Zager JS, Hochwald SN, Marzban SS, et al. Shave biopsy is a safe and accurate method for the initial evaluation of melanoma. J Am Coll Surg 2011;212(4): 454–60.

152. Tuong W, Cheng L, Armstrong AW. Melanoma: epidemiology, diagnosis, treat-ment, and outcomes. Dermatol Clin 2012;30:113–24.
153. Duncan LM. The classification of cutaneous melanoma. Hematol Oncol Clin North Am 2009;23(3):501–13, ix.
154. Clark WH Jr, Mihm MC Jr. Lentigo maligna and lentigo-maligna melanoma. Am J Pathol 1969;55(1):39–67.
155. Markovic SN, Erickson LA, Rao RD, et al. Malignant melanoma in the 21st cen-tury, part 1: epidemiology, risk factors, screening, prevention, and diagnosis. Mayo Clin Proc 2007;82(3):364–80.
156. Coleman WP 3rd, Loria PR, Reed RJ, et al. Acral lentiginous melanoma. Arch Dermatol 1980;116(7):773–6.
157. Narayanan DL, Saladi RN, Fox JL. Ultraviolet radiation and skin cancer. Int J Dermatol 2010;49(9):978–86.
158. Bataille V, de Vries E. Melanoma–part 1: epidemiology, risk factors, and preven-tion. BMJ 2008;337:a2249.
159. Lin JS, Eder M, Weinmann S. Behavioral counseling to prevent skin cancer: a systematic review for the U.S. Preventive Services Task Force. Ann Intern Med 2011;154(3):190–201.
160. Cascinelli N. Margin of resection in the management of primary melanoma. Semin Surg Oncol 1998;14(4):272–5.
161. Perkins W. Who should have Mohs micrographic surgery? Curr Opin Otolar-yngol Head Neck Surg 2010;18(4):283–9.
162. Wheatley K, Ives N, Hancock B, et al. Does adjuvant interferon-alpha for high-risk melanoma provide a worthwhile benefit? A meta-analysis of the randomised trials. Cancer Treat Rev 2003;29(4):241–52.
163. Mocellin S, Pasquali S, Rossi CR, et al. Interferon alpha adjuvant therapy in pa-tients with high-risk melanoma: a systematic review and meta-analysis. J Natl Cancer Inst 2010;102(7):493–501.
164. Agarwala S. Improving survival in patients with high-risk and metastatic mel-anoma: immunotherapy leads the way. Am J Clin Dermatol 2003;4(5): 333–46.
165. Hodi FS, O'Day SJ, McDermott DF, et al. Improved survival with ipilimumab in patients with metastatic melanoma. N Engl J Med 2010;363(8):711–23.
166. Johnson H, Robles M, Kamino H, et al. Trichoepithelioma. Dermatol Online J 2008;14:5.
167. Salhi A, Bornholdt D, Oeffner F, et al. Multiple familial trichoepithelioma caused by mutations in the cylindromatosis tumor suppressor gene. Cancer Res 2004; 64:5113.
168. Zhang XJ, Liang YH, He PP, et al. Identification of the cylindromatosis tumor-suppressor gene responsible for multiple familial trichoepithelioma. J Invest Der-matol 2004;122:658–64.
169. Blake PW, Toro JR. Update of cylindromatosis gene (CYLD) mutations in Brooke–Spiegler syndrome: novel insights into the role of deubiquitination in cell signaling. Hum Mutat 2009;30:1025–36.
170. Hu G, Onder M, Gill M, et al. A novel missense mutation in CYLD in a family with Brooke–Spiegler syndrome. J Invest Dermatol 2003;121:732–4.
171. Arits AH, Parren LJ, van Marion AM, et al. Basal cell carcinoma and trichoepi-thelioma: a possible matter of confusion. Int J Dermatol 2008;47(Suppl 1): 13–7.
172. Koay JL, Ledbetter LS, Page RN, et al. Asymptomatic annular plaque of the chin: desmoplastic trichoepithelioma. Arch Dermatol 2002;138:1091–6.

173. Huang TM, Chao SC, Lee JY. A novel splicing mutation of the CYLD gene in a Taiwanese family with multiple familial trichoepithelioma. Clin Exp Dermatol 2008;34:77–80.

174. Sajben FP, Ross EV. The use of the 1.0 mm handpiece in high energy, pulsed CO_2 laser destruction of facial adnexal tumors. Dermatol Surg 1999;25:41–4.

175. Shaffelburg M, Miller R. Treatment of multiple trichoepithelioma with electrosurgery. Dermatol Surg 1998;24:1154–6.

176. Eisen DB, Michael DJ. Sebaceous lesions and their associated syndromes: part I. J Am Acad Dermatol 2009;61:549–60.

177. de Berker DA, Taylor AE, Quinn AG, et al. Sebaceous hyperplasia in organ transplant recipients: shared aspects of hyperplastic and dysplastic processes? J Am Acad Dermatol 1996;35:696–9.

178. Salim A, Reece SM, Smith AG, et al. Sebaceous hyperplasia and skin cancer in patients undergoing renal transplant. J Am Acad Dermatol 2006;55:878–81.

179. Boschnakow A, May T, Assaf C, et al. Ciclosporin A-induced sebaceous gland hyperplasia. Br J Dermatol 2003;149:198–200.

180. Short KA, Williams A, Creamer D, et al. Sebaceous gland hyperplasia, human immunodeficiency virus and highly active anti-retroviral therapy. Clin Exp Dermatol 2008;33:354–5.

181. Ito M, Motoyoshi K, Suzuki M, et al. Sebaceous gland hyperplasia on rabbit pinna induced by tetradecane. J Invest Dermatol 1985;85:249–54.

182. Rice JM, Anderson LM. Sebaceous adenomas with associated epidermal hyperplasia and papilloma formation as a major type of tumor induced in mouse skin by high doses of carcinogens. Cancer Lett 1986;33:295–306.

183. Fuciarelli K, Cohen PR. Sebaceous hyperplasia: a clue to the diagnosis of dermatofibroma. J Am Acad Dermatol 2001;44:94–5.

184. Requena L, Roo E, Sanchez Yus E. Plate-like sebaceous hyperplasia overlying dermatofibroma. J Cutan Pathol 1992;19:253–5.

185. Davis TT, Calilao G, Fretzin D. Sebaceous hyperplasia overlying a dermatofibroma. Am J Dermatopathol 2006;28:155–7.

186. Dalziel K, Marks R. Hair follicle-like change over histiocytomas. Am J Dermatopathol 1986;8:462–6.

187. Schoenfeld RJ. Epidermal proliferations overlying histiocytomas. Arch Dermatol 1964;90:266–70.

188. Pochi PE, Strauss JS, Downing DT. Age-related changes in sebaceous gland activity. J Invest Dermatol 1979;73:108–11.

189. Kumar P, Marks R. Sebaceous gland hyperplasia and senile comedones: a prevalence study in elderly hospitalized patients. Br J Dermatol 1987;117: 231–6.

190. Sehgal VN, Bajaj P, Jain S. Sebaceous hyperplasia in youngsters. J Dermatol 1999;26:619–20.

191. Schwartz RA, Torre DP. The Muir-Torre syndrome: a 25-year retrospect. J Am Acad Dermatol 1995;33:90–104.

192. Sciallis GF, Winkelmann RK. Multiple sebaceous adenomas and gastrointestinal carcinoma. Arch Dermatol 1974;110:913–6.

193. Finan MC, Connolly SM. Sebaceous gland tumors and systemic disease: a clinicopathologic analysis. Medicine 1984;63:232–42.

194. Prioleau PG, Santa Cruz DJ. Sebaceous gland neoplasia. J Cutan Pathol 1984; 11:396–414.

195. Zaballos P, Ara M, Puig S, et al. Dermoscopy of sebaceous hyperplasia. Arch Dermatol 2005;141:808.

196. Oztas P, Polat M, Oztas M, et al. Bonbon toffee sign: a new dermatoscopic feature for sebaceous hyperplasia. J Eur Acad Dermatol Venereol 2008;22:1200–2.
197. Berk DR, Bayliss SJ. Milia: a review and classification. J Am Acad Dermatol 2008;59:1050–63.
198. Risma KA, Lucky AW. Pseudoacne of the nasal crease: a new entity? Pediatr Dermatol 2004;21:427–31.
199. George DE, Wasko CA, Hsu S. Surgical pearl: evacuation of milia with a paper clip. J Am Acad Dermatol 2006;54:326.
200. Stefanidou MP, Panayotides JG, Tosca AD. Milia en plaque: a case report and review of the literature. Dermatol Surg 2002;28:291–5.
201. Ishiura N, Komine M, Kadono T, et al. A case of milia en plaque successfully treated with oral etretinate. Br J Dermatol 2007;157:1287–9.
202. Al-Mutairi N, Joshi A. Bilateral extensive periorbital milia en plaque treated with electrodesiccation. J Cutan Med Surg 2006;10:193–6.
203. White GM. Recent findings in the epidemiologic evidence, classification, and subtypes of acne vulgaris. J Am Acad Dermatol 1998;39(2 Pt 3):S34–7.
204. Thiboutot D, Gollnick H, Bettoli V, et al. New insights into the management of acne: an update from the Global Alliance to Improve Outcomes in Acne group. J Am Acad Dermatol 2009;60(Suppl 5):S1–50.
205. Burton JL, Cunliffe WJ, Stafford L, et al. The prevalence of acne vulgaris in adolescence. Br J Dermatol 1971;85:119–26.
206. Leyden JJ. New understandings of the pathogenesis of acne. J Am Acad Dermatol 1995;32:S15–25.
207. James WD, Berger TG, Elston DM. Acne. In: James WD, Berger TG, Elston DM, editors. Andrews' diseases of the skin: clinical dermatology. 11th edition. Philadelphia: Saunders; 2011.
208. Titus S, Hodge J. Diagnosis and treatment of acne. Am Fam Physician 2012;86: 734–40.
209. Layton AM. Disorders of sebaceous glands. In: Burns T, Breathnach S, Cox N, et al, editors. Rook's textbook of dermatology. Oxford (United Kingdom): Wiley-Blackwell; 2010.
210. Archer CB, Cohen SN, Baron SE. Guidance on the diagnosis and clinical management of acne. Clin Exp Dermatol 2012;37(Suppl 1):1–6.
211. Thielitz A, Abdel-Naser MB, Fluhr JW, et al. Topical retinoids in acne—an evidence-based overview. J Dtsch Dermatol Ges 2008;6:1023–31.
212. Thiboutot D, Zaenglein A, Weiss J, et al. An aqueous gel fixed combination of clindamycin phosphate 1.2% and benzoyl peroxide 2.5% for the once-daily treatment of moderate to severe acne vulgaris: assessment of efficacy and safety in 2813 patients. J Am Acad Dermatol 2008;59:792–800.
213. Strauss JS, Krowchuk DP, Leyden JJ, et al. American Academy of Dermatology/American Academy of Dermatology Association. Guidelines of care for acne vulgaris management. J Am Acad Dermatol 2007;56:651–63.
214. Böni R, Nehrhoff B. Treatment of gram-negative folliculitis in patients with acne. Am J Clin Dermatol 2003;4:273–6.
215. Neubert U, Jansen T, Plewig G. Bacteriologic and immunologic aspects of gram-negative folliculitis: a study of 46 patients. Int J Dermatol 1999; 38:270–4.
216. Leyden JJ, Marples RR, Mills OH Jr, et al. Gram-negative folliculitis – a complication of antibiotic therapy in acne vulgaris. Br J Dermatol 1973;88:533–8.
217. Kelly AP. Pseudofolliculitis barbae and acne keloidalis nuchae. Dermatol Clin 2003;21:645–53.

218. Brown LA. Pathogenesis and treatment of pseudofolliculitis barbae. Cutis 1983; 32:373–5.
219. Perry P, Cook-Bolden FE, Rahman Z, et al. Defining pseudofolliculitis barbae in 2001: a review of the literature and current trends. J Am Acad Dermatol 2002;46: 3113–9.
220. Brauner GJ, Flandermeyer KL. Pseudofolliculitis barbae. Medical consequences of interracial friction in the US Army. Cutis 1979;23:61–6.
221. Coquilla BH, Lewis CW. Management of pseudofolliculitis barbae. Mil Med 1995;160:263–9.
222. Crutchfield CE. The causes and treatment of pseudofolliculitis barbae. Cutis 1998;61:351–4.
223. Halder RM, Richards GM. Therapeutic approaches for pseudofolliculitis barbae. Cosmet Dermatol 2003;16:42–5.
224. Ribera M, Fernández-Chico N, Casals M. Pseudofolliculitis barbae. Actas Dermosifiliogr 2010;101:749–57.
225. Yang LP, Keam SJ. Retapamulin: a review of its use in the management of impetigo and other uncomplicated superficial skin infections. Drugs 2008;68:855–73.
226. Steer A, Danchin M, Carapetis J. Group A streptococcal infections in children. J Paediatr Child Health 2007;43:203–13.
227. Popovich KJ, Hota B. Treatment and prevention of community-associated methicillin-resistant Staphylococcus aureus skin and soft tissue infections. Dermatol Ther 2008;21:167–79.
228. Durupt F, Mayor L, Bes M, et al. Prevalence of Staphylococcus aureus toxins and nasal carriage in furuncles and impetigo. Br J Dermatol 2007;157:1161–7.
229. Cole C, Gazewood J. Diagnosis and treatment of impetigo. Am Fam Physician 2007;15:75.
230. Koning S, Verhagen A, van Suijlekom-Smit L, et al. Interventions for impetigo. Cochrane Database Syst Rev 2004;(2):CD003261.
231. George A, Rubin G. A systematic review and meta-analysis of treatments for impetigo. Br J Gen Pract 2003;53:480–7.
232. Morelli JG. Impetigo. In: Kliegman RM, Stanton BF, Geme JW, et al, editors. Nelson textbook of pediatrics. 19th edition. Philadelphia: Saunders; 2011. p. 2229–300.
233. Darmstadt GL. Impetigo: an overview. Pediatr Dermatol 1994;11:293–303.
234. Bangert S, Levy M, Hebert AA. Bacterial resistance and impetigo treatment trends: a review. Pediatr Dermatol 2012;29:243–8.
235. Koning S, van der Sande R, Verhagen AP, et al. Interventions for impetigo. Cochrane Database Syst Rev 2012;(1):CD003261.
236. Wilkin J, Dahl M, Detmar M, et al. Standard classification of rosacea: report of the National Rosacea Society Expert Committee on the classification and staging of rosacea. J Am Acad Dermatol 2002;46:584–7.
237. Crawford GH, Pelle MT, James WD. Rosacea: I. Etiology, pathogenesis, and subtype classification. J Am Acad Dermatol 2004;51:327–41.
238. Wilkin JK. Rosacea: pathophysiology and treatment. Arch Dermatol 1994;130: 359–62.
239. Heymann WR. Rosacea subtype directed therapy. J Am Acad Dermatol 2004; 51:90–2.
240. Pelle MT, Crawford GH, James WD. Rosacea: II. Therapy. J Am Acad Dermatol 2004;51:499–512.
241. Dahl MV, Katz HI, Krueger GG, et al. Topical metronidazole maintains remissions of rosacea. Arch Dermatol 1998;134:679–83.

242. Wilkinson DS, Kirton V, Wilkinson JD. Perioral dermatitis: a 12-year review. Br J Dermatol 1979;101(3):245–57.
243. Hogan DJ, Epstein JD, Lane PR. Peroral dermatitis: an uncommon condition? CMAJ 1986;134(9):1025–8.
244. Sneddon I. Perioral dermatitis. Br J Dermatol 1972;87(5):430–4.
245. Peralta L, Morais P. Perioral dermatitis—the role of nasal steroids. Cutan Ocul Toxicol 2012;31(2):160–3.
246. Hall CS, Reichenberg J. Evidence based review of perioral dermatitis therapy. G Ital Dermatol Venereol 2010;145(4):433–44.
247. Rietchel RL, Fowler JF. Fisher's contact dermatitis. 5th edition. Philadelphia: Lipincott Williams & Wilkins; 2001.
248. Champion RH, Burton JL, Burns DA. Rook/Wilkinson/Ebling textbook of dermatology. 6th edition. Oxford: Blackwell Science Inc; 1998.
249. Rogers RS, Bekic M. Diseases of the lips. Semin Cutan Med Surg 1997;16: 328–36.
250. Castanedo-Tardan MP, Zug KA. Patterns of cosmetic contact allergy. Dermatol Clin 2009;27:265–80.
251. Zoli V, Silvani S, Vincenzi C, et al. Allergic contact cheilitis. Contact Dermatitis 2006;54:296–7.
252. Francalanci S, Sertoli A, Giorgini S, et al. Multicenter study of allergic contact cheilitis from toothpastes. Contact Dermatitis 2000;43:216–22.
253. Lim SW, Goh CL. Epidemiology of eczematous cheilitis at a tertiary dermatological referral center in Singapore. Contact Dermatitis 2000;43:322–6.
254. Freeman S, Stephens R. Cheilitis: analysis of 75 cases referred to a contact dermatitis clinic. Am J Contact Dermatitis 1999;10:198–200.
255. Zug KA, Kornik R, Belsito DV, et al. Patch-Testing North American lip dermatitis patients: data from the North American Contact Dermatitis Group, 2001 to 2004. Dermatitis 2008;19(4):202–8.
256. Naldi L, Rebora A. Seborrheic dermatitis. N Engl J Med 2009;360:387–96.
257. Xu J, Saunders CW, Hu P, et al. Dandruff-associated Malassezia genomes reveal convergent and divergent virulence traits shared with plant and human fungal pathogens. Proc Natl Acad Sci U S A 2007;104:18730–5.
258. Tajima M, Sugita T, Nishikawa A, et al. Molecular analysis of Malassezia microflora in seborrheic dermatitis patients: comparison with other diseases and healthy subjects. J Invest Dermatol 2008;128:345–51.
259. DeAngelis YM, Gemmer CM, Kaczvinsky JR, et al. Three etiologic facets of dandruff and seborrheic dermatitis: malassezia fungi, sebaceous lipids, and individual sensitivity. J Investig Dermatol Symp Proc 2005;10:295–7.
260. Foley P, Zuo Y, Plunkett A, et al. The frequency of common skin conditions in preschool-aged children in Australia: seborrheic dermatitis and pityriasis capitis (cradle cap). Arch Dermatol 2003;139:318–22.
261. Coopman SA, Johnson RA, Platt R, et al. Cutaneous disease and drug reactions in HIV infection. N Engl J Med 1993;328:1670–4.
262. Mahé A, Simon F, Coulibaly S, et al. Predictive value of seborrheic dermatitis and other common dermatoses for HIV infection in Bamako, Mali. J Am Acad Dermatol 1996;34:1084–6.
263. Hay RJ. Malassezia, dandruff and seborrhoeic dermatitis: an overview. Br J Dermatol 2011;165(Suppl 2):2–8.

Pediatric Soft Tissue Oral Lesions

Andres Pinto, DMD, MPH, FDS RCSEd[a],*,
Christel M. Haberland, DDS, MS[b], Suher Baker, BDS, DMD, MS[c]

KEYWORDS

- Children • Oral lesions • Soft tissue • Color changes • Nodules

KEY POINTS

- Oral mucosal lesions in children may present as ulcers, color changes, and alterations in size and configuration of oral anatomy.
- Leukoedema is a benign white lesion found bilaterally or unilaterally on the buccal or labial mucosa.
- Pseudomembranous candidiasis, a common condition in children, is an opportunistic fungal infection caused by *Candida albicans*, more likely to occur in children who had a recent use of antibiotics, corticosteroids, or extended exposure to pacifier.
- Melanotic nevus is an alteration of mucosal color. Nevi may be congenital or develop over the life span and mostly represent deviations of normal anatomy.
- Nodular vascular anomalies are currently classified into either benign tumors or vascular malformations based on the clinical presentation and evolution of the lesion and its histopathologic features.

PEDIATRIC SOFT TISSUE ORAL LESIONS

Oral mucosal lesions in children may present as ulcers, color changes, alterations in size, and configuration of oral anatomy. This article presents a broad overview of oral conditions that affect children, focusing on abnormalities of color and nodular changes. Ulcerative disorders are covered extensively in other readily accessible literature.

MUCOSAL CHANGES (COLOR)
White Lesions

Frictional keratosis (Morsicatio buccarum)
The constant rubbing of the mucosa may cause white patches that can disappear if the causative agent habit is discontinued. Habits causing this finding include traumatic

The authors do not report any significant financial disclosures.
[a] Department of Oral and Maxillofacial Medicine and Diagnostic Sciences, University Hospitals Case Medical Center and Case Western Reserve School of Dental Medicine, 2124 Cornell Road, Rm 1190, Cleveland, OH 44106, USA; [b] Yale Hamden Dental Center, Yale School of Medicine, Yale-New Haven Hospital, 2560 Dixwell Avenue, Hamden, CT 06514, USA; [c] Pediatric Dentistry Residency Program, Department of Dentistry, Yale School of Medicine, Yale-New Haven Hospital, 1 Long Whart Drive, Suite 403, New Haven, CT 06511, USA
* Corresponding author.
E-mail address: andres.pinto@uhhospitals.org

Dent Clin N Am 58 (2014) 437–453
http://dx.doi.org/10.1016/j.cden.2013.12.003
0011-8532/14/$ – see front matter © 2014 Elsevier Inc. All rights reserved.

tooth brushing (toothbrush keratosis) and forcefully rubbing the tongue against the teeth (tongue thrust keratosis). The prevalence of frictional keratosis has been reported between 0.26% and 1.89% in children.[1,2]

Clinical presentation The condition is observed as a corrugated, gray or white lesion that may be smooth or rough and occasionally irregular with small loose tags of epithelium on the surface. The site of appearance is mostly the buccal mucosa.

Treatment Removal of intraoral irritants and discontinuation of causative habits usually resolves this lesion.

Leukoedema
Leukoedema is a benign white lesion found bilaterally or unilaterally on the buccal or labial mucosa. The etiology is unknown but associations with tobacco smoking, local irritation, and malocclusion have been made. The prevalence differs in adults depending on the population examined and ranges between 0.96% and 58.00%,[3,4] with the highest prevalence noted in African Americans.

Clinical presentation Leukoedema is characterized by a diffuse white opacification that resolves when the mucosa is stretched.

Treatment No treatment is needed, as this condition is benign.

Linea alba
This condition is a benign finding located on the buccal mucosa across the commissures and extending posteriorly toward the molars. The prevalence is 1.5% in children[5] and up to 5.3% in adolescents.[6]

Clinical presentation Linea alba presents as a distinct white linear area on the buccal mucosa opposing the plane of occlusion (**Fig. 1**). Occasionally, it has also been recognized on the lateral border of the tongue.

Treatment No treatment is needed, as this condition is benign.

Hairy tongue
Hairy tongue is a benign condition that arises from abnormal elongation of the filiform papillae of the tongue (1–12 mm) or the proliferation of bacteria that release pigments

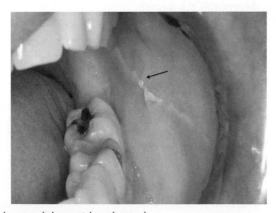

Fig. 1. Linea alba in an adolescent boy (*arrow*).

on them. This condition may also be caused by intrinsic factors, such as antibiotics (erythromycin), antipsychotics (olanzapine), iron supplements, or radiation therapy. Extrinsic causative factors are primarily related to diet (coffee, tea), poor oral hygiene, mouth washes, or smoking, a concern in adolescent patients.[7,8] The prevalence of hairy tongue in children is unknown.[1]

Clinical presentation Papillary elongation gives the appearance of thick, hairylike surface on the dorsal tongue. The condition may present with superficial coating that blunts the hairy appearance (**Fig. 2**).

Treatment Good oral hygiene, diet restriction, smoking cessation, or tobacco counseling and brushing with 1% to 2% hydrogen peroxide solution or diluted sodium hypochloride has been suggested.[9]

Pseudomembranous candidiasis
This common condition in children is an opportunistic fungal infection caused by *Candida albicans*, more likely to occur in children who had a recent use of antibiotics, corticosteroids, or extended exposure to pacifier.[10–13] It is a hallmark oral finding in children with systemic conditions, such as endocrine disorders, leukemia, chemotherapy, radiation therapy, transplantation, prematurity, and malnutrition.[14–17] The prevalence is 0.99% to 8.57% in children[2,11] and 37.00% of infants.

Clinical presentation This condition is presented as superficial white plaques on the mucous membranes that can be wiped off.[18–20] These white plaques can be seen on the buccal and labial mucosa, hard and soft palate, tongue, and oropharynx.

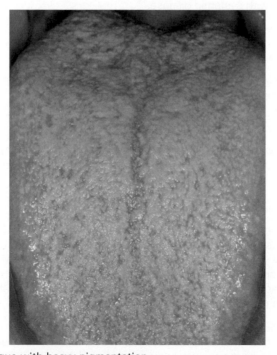

Fig. 2. Dorsal tongue with heavy pigmentation.

Treatment Treatment usually includes gentian violet or topical nystatin for infants, and nystatin (topical) or topical clotrimazole for older children. Systemic fluconazole, ketoconazole, or itraconazole may be used for children who are at risk of developing systemic infection or are intolerant to topical therapy.[21,22]

White sponge nevus

White sponge nevus is a benign asymptomatic condition due to an autosomal dominant inheritance. Lesions clinically present as bilateral white plaques that are thickened, spongy, and folded. The buccal mucosa is the most frequent site but the condition also may be seen on the labial mucosa, floor of the mouth, and gingiva. They are usually present at birth or in early childhood and may occasionally develop in adolescence. The prevalence is 1.54%.[11]

Clinical presentation White, raised, folded unilateral or bilateral tissue on tongue or buccal mucosa. The tissue cannot be removed. The differential diagnosis may include leukoplakia, chemical burns, trauma, tobacco, and *Candida* infections.

Treatment No treatment is necessary unless masticatory function is compromised.

RED AND/OR WHITE LESIONS
Petechiae, Purpura, Ecchymosis

These red lesions are commonly caused by trauma affecting the underlying vasculature. They are frequently a sign of bleeding disorders, such as thrombocytopenia or hemophilia, and may occasionally be associated with leukemia and anemia. The prevalence of vascular lesions is 1.89% to 8.39% in children[1,2] and may be up to 42.8% in children with systemic disease.[11]

Clinical presentation

The lesions are predominantly seen on the lips, tongue, hard palate, and gingiva and are classified as follows:

- Petechiae: pinpoint hemorrhages
- Purpura: 2-mm to 2-cm hemorrhages
- Ecchymosis: >2 cm hemorrhages

Treatment

Treatment includes the initial investigation of the source of the trauma to rule out child abuse. All other lesions associated with medical conditions or medications must be referred for further medical workup.

Erythematous Candidiasis

The etiology of the symptomatic form is often linked to vitamin B12 and folate deficiency, as well as recent antibiotic or steroid therapy. The asymptomatic form is characterized by chronic erythema of tissues covered by prostheses, such as dentures and retainers. Lesions are commonly seen on the palate and occasionally on the mandibular tissue. The prevalence in children is unknown. It is presumed to be lower than the prevalence of pseudomembranous candidiasis.

Clinical presentation

Red macular lesions that are usually asymptomatic or occasionally symptomatic with a burning sensation on the tongue or mouth and a bright red appearance.

Treatment

See pseudomembranous candidiasis.

Angular Chelitis

This disorder is a chronic inflammation of the skin and labial mucosa at the corners of the mouth. The etiology may be due to nutritional deficiencies (riboflavin, folate), anemia (iron deficiency) allergy, infections, physical irritation, low socioeconomic status,[23] and bruxism.[5,6,24,25] The prevalence is 3% in children[5] and 9% in adolescents.[6]

Clinical presentation

Angular chelitis is characterized by the presence of painful cracking, fissuring, and erythema on bilateral commissures. Hemorrhage may be a concomitant finding.

Treatment

See pseudomembranous candidiasis.

Erythema Migrans (Benign Migratory Glossitis)

Also known as geographic tongue, erythema migrans is a benign condition affecting the dorsum of the tongue. The etiology is unknown, but studies have suggested an association with atopy, psoriasis, and fissured tongue and included a genetic linkage between the 2 conditions.[26–29] Geographic tongue is also more prevalent in allergic patients.[30,31] Prevalence ranges between 0.37% and 14.3%[2,5] in pediatric patients depending on the populations examined and may be up to 40.6% in children with systemic disease.[11]

Clinical presentation

Clinically, benign migratory glossitis appears as a well-configured maplike appearance due to the well-defined depapillated erythematous regions that are surrounded by white borders (**Fig. 3**).

Treatment

No treatment is necessary, other than reassurance. In adults, zinc, topical anesthetics, steroid gels, and antihistamine mouth rinses have been suggested for symptomatic cases.[32]

Median Rhomboid Glossitis

This particular fungal infection has predisposing factors, such as *Candida* infections, and immunosuppressive diseases, such as diabetes. Other risk factors reported in the literature, but have inconsistent results include age, smoking, and removable prostheses.[33,34] Prevalence in pediatric patients has been reported between 0% and 1.23%.[1,35–37]

Clinical presentation

The condition presents as a well-circumscribed central papillary atrophy of the tongue, typically located in the midline on the dorsum of the tongue anterior to the circumvallate papillae (**Fig. 4**). The surface of the lesion is smooth and glossy and is asymptomatic in most patients; however, pain, irritation, and pruritus have been reported. Tongue lesions may occasionally present with palatal inflammations or kissing lesions that are considered a marker for HIV infection.[35]

Treatment

Because this is an asymptomatic lesion, treatment is not indicated. However, the lesion often responds to antifungal treatment with nystatin, fluconazole, or clotrimazole as a suspension or oral troches.

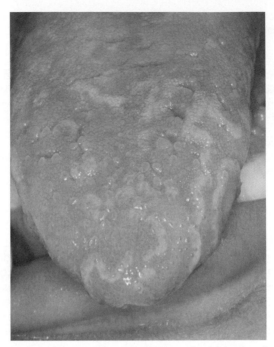

Fig. 3. Geographic tongue in a 12-year-old girl. Note the white borders surrounding the lesions.

BROWN-BLACK LESIONS
Physiologic Pigmentation

This pigmentation is the most common form of diffuse and bilateral pigmentation that arises from the increased production of melanin in dark-skinned populations (Middle Eastern, African American, and occasionally Asians).[38,39] In general, conditions that increase the prevalence of this pigmentation are race/ethnicity, increased age, smoking, pregnancy, endocrine syndromes, and hormonal changes. Atypical cases have been reported in newborns.[40] Peutz-Jeghers syndrome is an autosomal dominant trait

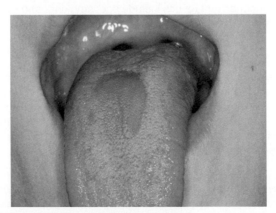

Fig. 4. Central papillary atrophy in an 8-year-old child.

that is associated with multiple intraoral and perioral pigmentations, most of which do not require treatment and involute after the first decade of life.[7,39,41–45] However, the early establishment of a diagnosis is critical for a gastroenterology workup for intestinal polyps and hamartomas that have a 2% to 3% tendency for malignant transformation.[46] Addison disease or adrenal insufficiency is an autoimmune disease resulting in insufficient secretion of glucocorticoids and mineralocorticoids. Initial symptoms include diffuse bronzing of the skin and mucous membranes. In the oral cavity, the pigmentation is commonly located on the gingiva, tongue, buccal mucosa, and hard palate. Occasionally, isolated macules maybe present. Oral surfaces frequently exposed to trauma may develop the pigmentation more frequently. The prevalence of oral pigmentation in children is 13.5%[38] with an onset in the first/second decades.[11]

Clinical presentation
The pigmentation is commonly found on the attached gingiva. Occasionally, the buccal mucosa, palate, and lips, as well as the dorsal surface of the tongue are affected.

Treatment
Treatment is not required. Intraoral pigments associated with Peutz-Jeghers syndrome require monitoring and evaluation by a gastroenterologist for the development of mucosal gastric malignancies.

Amalgam Tattoo/Graphite

This disorder occurs as sequelae of surgical oral interventions or removal of amalgam restorations. The prevalence in children is 1.3%.[47]

Clinical presentation
Amalgam tattoo is a localized flat blue-gray solitary or multiple lesions of variable sizes and shapes (0.1–2.0 cm). It is commonly found on the attached and alveolar mucosa next to teeth restored with amalgam, and may be occasionally seen dispersed in the buccal mucosa or the floor of the mouth. Graphite pigmentation is a common finding in the anterior palatal area in children due to trauma. It appears clinically as an ill- defined flat gray/black pigmentation.[47,48]

Treatment
No biopsy is indicated in most cases unless a confirmation of amalgam is needed when the patient's medical history suggests susceptibility to dermatologic malignancy.[7,42]

Melanotic Nevus

Melanotic nevus is an alteration of mucosal color. Nevi may be congenital or develop over the life span and mostly represent deviations of normal anatomy. It is important to mention the histologic classification of nevi, as it may impact lesion prognosis:[49–56]

1. Junctional: proliferation of the nevus cells at the tips of the rete pegs that are close to the surface and are confined in the epithelium.
2. Compound: proliferation of nevus cell into the epithelium and connective tissue.
3. Intradermal/intramucosal: nevus cells are located in the lamina propria and do not contact the basement membrane. These lesions are dome shaped, typically light brown in color and are commonly seen on the gingiva, and labial and buccal mucosa.[57,58]
4. Blue nevi: proliferation of spindle cells within the deep connective tissue and remotely from the surface epithelium. This lesion is commonly seen on the hard

palate. They are further classified into atypical blue nevus, locally aggressive blue nevus, and congenital giant melanotic nevus with nodular growth.[59]

5. Other melanotic nevi include the combined nevus and the Spitz nevus, which may be located on the palate or tongue.[60–62]

6. The congenital melanotic nevi with large nodules.[63]

The prevalence of oral nevi in children is unknown, and published figures include older patients.[57]

Clinical presentation

Melanotic nevi present as localized brown, blue, gray, black, or colorless macule or papule and rarely polypoid[57,58] that range from 0.1 to 3.0 cm (**Fig. 5**).[57,58] The nevi are commonly located on the hard palate, buccal mucosa, and gingiva at 41.0%, 12.0%, and 11.5% respectively.[47,57,58]

Treatment

Treatment includes excisional biopsy to rule out mucosal melanoma, especially if the lesion is located in the palate. Transformation of pigmented nevi to melanoma is not well documented in the literature.[64–66]

Soft Tissue Nodules

Most reports establish that 90% to 98% of soft tissue biopsies in children are diagnosed as benign.[67–74] These benign lesions can be divided into 2 categories according to their etiology: inflammatory/reactive lesions and benign neoplasms. Malignancies are uncommon in children; however, because when they occur they cannot be clinically distinguished from benign lesions, these must be biopsied to establish a definitive diagnosis.

Inflammatory/reactive lesions

Mucocele (mucous extravasation phenomenon) A mucocele is a lesion that results from the extravasation of mucous into the connective tissue of the oral mucosa secondary to the rupture of a minor salivary gland duct. The prevalence of mucoceles in children has been reported between 0.04% and 1.00%.[75]

Clinical presentation Mucoceles appear most frequently as slightly bluish nodules measuring smaller than 1.5 cm, most of which have a history of increasing and decreasing in size.[76] On palpation, they can be fluctuant or firm. If the extravasated

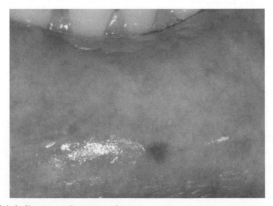

Fig. 5. Macular labial discrete pigmentation.

mucous is located in the deeper connective tissue, they may appear as pink nodules. The most common location is the lower labial mucosa, which is a site that is frequently traumatized by biting.[77] Other common locations include the floor of the mouth, ventral tongue, and buccal mucosa (**Fig. 6**).

Treatment Occasionally mucoceles have been reported to rupture spontaneously. For those that persist, treatment consists of surgical excision with removal of the associated minor salivary glands to prevent recurrence.[78] Other treatment modalities include cryosurgery, electrosurgery, CO_2 laser removal, or laser vaporization.[79] Mucoceles located on the floor of the mouth (ranulas) are treated by marsupialization or removal of the lesion and the associated salivary gland.[80]

Irritation fibroma Irritation fibromas represent a fibrous connective tissue hyperplasia that occurs secondary to chronic trauma to the oral mucosa.[81] Although they are the most common benign soft tissue lesion seen in adults, they can also be found in children. The prevalence of fibromas in children is unknown.

Clinical presentation Fibromas appear clinically as nodules with a smooth surface or sometimes an ulcerated surface. Their color is that of the surrounding mucosa and they feel firm on palpation. The most frequent locations are mucosal sites that are easily traumatized, such as the buccal mucosa, the labial mucosa, and the lateral tongue (**Fig. 7**).[82]

Treatment Conservative excision is the treatment of choice if the lesion interferes with normal oral functions and to obtain a definitive diagnosis. If the source of chronic trauma is not eliminated, the lesion may recur.

Peripheral ossifying fibroma Peripheral ossifying fibromas are benign neoplasms thought to arise from cells in the periodontal ligament or periosteum; therefore, they are seen almost exclusively on the gingiva. They are reported to be the most common gingival lesion seen in children, comprising 9.6% of all gingival lesions, occurring in the second decade of life.[83]

Clinical presentation This lesion presents as a sessile nodule on the gingiva, especially the anterior maxillary gingiva. Depending on the amount of calcification, it can be soft to palpation to firm or hard. Their color is usually that of the surrounding mucosa, but occasionally can appear red or with surface ulceration. It is more prevalent in younger patients and has a predilection for female patients (3:2).[84]

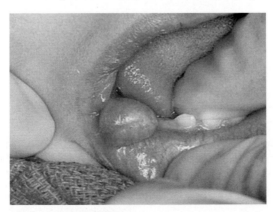

Fig. 6. Labial mucocele in a 1-year-old boy.

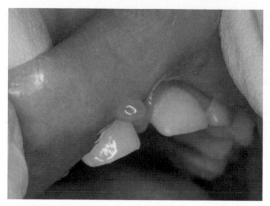

Fig. 7. Irritation fibroma on upper lip of a 6-year-old boy.

Treatment Surgical excision of the lesion, including the periodontal ligament, is thought to reduce the possibility of recurrence, but can lead to gingival defects. The recurrence rate for this lesion is 16% to 20%. Use of laser excision has also been effective.[85]

Pyogenic granuloma Pyogenic granuloma is a benign soft tissue lesion that is thought to result from chronic irritation, trauma, and hormonal factors.[86] Despite its name, it is a vascular proliferation and not a true granuloma.[87] Recently, the International Society for the Study of Vascular Anomalies has classified pyogenic granulomas as vascular tumors, but this classification is still not widely used.[88] The prevalence of pyogenic granulomas has been reported as high as 52% of reactive lesions, which are most of the oral lesions in children.[87]

Clinical presentation Oral pyogenic granulomas present as sessile or pedunculated nodules, ranging in size from a few millimeters to 2 cm, with a bright red color and a smooth or ulcerated surface (**Fig. 8**). In some cases, they can rapidly increase in size, mimicking a malignancy and causing increased concern to the patient or clinician. The most common site is the gingiva, especially the maxillary anterior labial gingiva. Other common sites are the lips, tongue, buccal mucosa, and palate.[89]

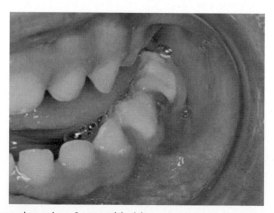

Fig. 8. Pyogenic granuloma in a 9-year-old girl.

Treatment Surgical excision of the lesion is recommended, but other modalities, such as cryosurgery, electrosurgery, and laser excision have been used. In gingival lesions, the excision should extend down to the periosteum. Intralesional steroid therapy has been used for recurrent lesions. A recurrence rate of up to 16% has been reported.[86]

Peripheral giant cell granuloma Peripheral giant cell granuloma is a benign lesion of unknown origin characterized by the presence of giant cells. It presents in patients of all ages, including children, and has a female predilection. Because it is thought to arise from the cells in the periodontal ligament or periosteum, it is seen exclusively in the gingiva secondary to local irritation or trauma.[90,91]

Clinical presentation This lesion appears clinically as a soft tissue nodule with a pedunculated or sessile base and either a smooth or ulcerated surface. It is located usually in the interproximal dental papillae on the buccal or lingual aspect and measures approximately 2 cm. In some cases, it can surround a tooth and produce displacement of the adjacent teeth and even some saucerization of the underlying bone.[92–94]

Treatment Complete surgical excision and curettage of underlying bone is the preferred treatment. A recurrence rate of 10% has been reported.[95] Early diagnosis and treatment is important to minimize risk of bone or tooth loss.[96]

Benign neoplasms
Squamous papilloma There are more than 100 human papilloma virus (HPV) types and they are known to cause lesions in human mucosal sites. In the oral cavity, the most frequent lesion induced by HPV types 6 and 11 is the squamous papilloma.[97] In addition, squamous papillomas represent 8% of all soft tissue masses in children.[71]

Clinical presentation Squamous papilloma presents as a small pedunculated or sometimes sessile papule with papillary "fronds" and may be the same color of mucosa or appear white.[98] They usually appear as a single lesion measuring approximately 0.5 cm. Squamous papillomas can occur anywhere in the oral mucosa but are commonly seen on the soft palate and tongue. Oral condylomas, on the other hand, clinically appear larger in size (average of 3 cm), have a sessile base, and occur more commonly in labial mucosa, lingual frenum, or soft palate.[99]

Treatment The treatment of choice is either conventional scalpel surgical excision or laser ablation, and recurrence has been rarely reported.[100,101] The recent introduction of a vaccine against HPV types 6, 11, 16, and 18 could potentially impact the prevalence of squamous papillomas in children, preventing the occurrence of these lesions.[102]

Hemangioma/vascular malformations Nodular vascular anomalies are currently classified into either benign tumors or vascular malformations based on the clinical presentation and evolution of the lesion and its histopathologic features.[103] The prevalence of hemangiomas is 1% of newborns in the United States and the head and neck area accounts for 60% of these lesions.[104,105] Hemangiomas can be a clinical feature of multiple syndromes.[104] Alternatively, vascular malformations are considered congenital structural anomalies of blood vessels that are non-neoplastic.[106] They do not proliferate or undergo involution; however, they may expand secondarily to stimuli, such as trauma, endocrine changes, or infection.[103]

Clinical presentation Hemangiomas appear as either as a red or purple/red macule or nodule with a smooth or lobulated surface. The more superficial lesions appear red in color, whereas the deeper lesions appear purple. Approximately 90% of hemangiomas will resolve by age 9.[103] Common locations in the head and neck area are the parotid and the orbit.[107] Vascular malformations are present at birth and do not involute but persist and are classified according to the vessel type (capillary, venous, lymphatic, or arteriovenous). Port wine stains are a common capillary malformation that occurs in 0.3% to 1.0% of newborns. Other malformations can present initially as flat macules that blanch under pressure and slowly become more nodular or cobblestoned in appearance.[103]

Treatment It is important to differentiate between a hemangioma and a vascular malformation because their treatment modalities differ.[108] Because hemangiomas can spontaneously involute during infancy, treatment is deferred until the lesion has involuted. For any remaining lesion, corticosteroid injections have been used to decrease the size and surgical modalities include the use of lasers and scalpel excision.[109,110]

In summary, color changes and soft tissue lesions are relevant findings in the pediatric population. Oral health practitioners should be aware of the clinical characteristics of these findings and the need for further workup or referral in select cases.

REFERENCES

1. Shulman JD. Prevalence of oral mucosal lesions in children and youths in the USA. Int J Paediatr Dent 2005;15(2):89–97.
2. Bessa CF, Santos PJ, Aguiar MC, et al. Prevalence of oral mucosal alterations in children from 0 to 12 years old. J Oral Pathol Med 2004;33(1):17–22.
3. Pindborg JJ, Kalapessi HK, Kale SA, et al. Frequency of oral leukoplakias and related conditions among 10,000 Bombayites. Preliminary report. J All India Dent Assoc 1965;37(7):228–9.
4. Martin JL. Epidemiology of leukoedema in the Negro. J Oral Med 1973;28(2): 41–4.
5. Vieira-Andrade RG, Martins-Junior PA, Correa-Faria P, et al. Oral mucosal conditions in preschool children of low socioeconomic status: prevalence and determinant factors. Eur J Pediatr 2013;172(5):675–81.
6. Parlak AH, Koybasi S, Yavuz T, et al. Prevalence of oral lesions in 13- to 16-year-old students in Duzce, Turkey. Oral Dis 2006;12(6):553–8.
7. Eisen D. Disorders of pigmentation in the oral cavity. Clin Dermatol 2000;18(5): 579–87.
8. Ioffreda MD, Gordon CA, Adams DR, et al. Black tongue. Arch Dermatol 2001; 137(7):968–9.
9. Newman CC, Wagner RF. Images in clinical medicine. Black hairy tongue. N Engl J Med 1997;337(13):897.
10. Garcia-Pola MJ, Garcia-Martin JM, Gonzalez-Garcia M. Prevalence of oral lesions in the 6-year-old pediatric population of Oviedo (Spain). Med Oral 2002; 7(3):184–91.
11. Majorana A, Bardellini E, Flocchini P, et al. Oral mucosal lesions in children from 0 to 12 years old: ten years' experience. Oral Surg Oral Med Oral Pathol Oral Radiol Endod 2010;110(1):e13–8.
12. Manning DJ, Coughlin RP, Poskitt EM. Candida in mouth or on dummy? Arch Dis Child 1985;60(4):381–2.
13. Fotos PG, Hellstein JW. Candida and candidosis. Epidemiology, diagnosis and therapeutic management. Dent Clin North Am 1992;36(4):857–78.

14. Gonzalez Gravina H, Gonzalez de Moran E, Zambrano O, et al. Oral candidiasis in children and adolescents with cancer. Identification of *Candida* spp. Med Oral Patol Oral Cir Bucal 2007;12(6):E419–23.

15. Fotos PG, Vincent SD, Hellstein JW. Oral candidosis. Clinical, historical, and therapeutic features of 100 cases. Oral Surg Oral Med Oral Pathol 1992;74(1):41–9.

16. Shetty SS, Harrison LH, Hajjeh RA, et al. Determining risk factors for candidemia among newborn infants from population-based surveillance: Baltimore, Maryland, 1998-2000. Pediatr Infect Dis J 2005;24(7):601–4.

17. Epstein JB, Gorsky M, Caldwell J. Fluconazole mouthrinses for oral candidiasis in postirradiation, transplant, and other patients. Oral Surg Oral Med Oral Pathol Oral Radiol Endod 2002;93(6):671–5.

18. Dilley DC, Siegel MA, Budnick S. Diagnosing and treating common oral pathologies. Pediatr Clin North Am 1991;38(5):1227–64.

19. Silverman RA. Diseases of the mucous membranes in children. Clin Dermatol 1987;5(2):137–56.

20. Goins RA, Ascher D, Waecker N, et al. Comparison of fluconazole and nystatin oral suspensions for treatment of oral candidiasis in infants. Pediatr Infect Dis J 2002;21(12):1165–7.

21. Garcia-Pola Vallejo MJ, Martinez Diaz-Canel AI, Garcia Martin JM, et al. Risk factors for oral soft tissue lesions in an adult Spanish population. Community Dent Oral Epidemiol 2002;30(4):277–85.

22. Patton LL, Bonito AJ, Shugars DA. A systematic review of the effectiveness of antifungal drugs for the prevention and treatment of oropharyngeal candidiasis in HIV-positive patients. Oral Surg Oral Med Oral Pathol Oral Radiol Endod 2001;92(2):170–9.

23. Crivelli MR, Aguas S, Adler I, et al. Influence of socioeconomic status on oral mucosa lesion prevalence in schoolchildren. Community Dent Oral Epidemiol 1988;16(1):58–60.

24. Arendorf TM, van der Ross R. Oral soft tissue lesions in a black pre-school South African population. Community Dent Oral Epidemiol 1996;24(4):296–7.

25. Vieira-Andrade RG, Zuquim Guimaraes Fde F, Vieira Cda S, et al. Oral mucosa alterations in a socioeconomically deprived region: prevalence and associated factors. Braz Oral Res 2011;25(5):393–400.

26. Darwazeh AM, Pillai K. Prevalence of tongue lesions in 1013 Jordanian dental outpatients. Community Dent Oral Epidemiol 1993;21(5):323–4.

27. Redman RS. Prevalence of geographic tongue, fissured tongue, median rhomboid glossitis, and hairy tongue among 3,611 Minnesota schoolchildren. Oral Surg Oral Med Oral Pathol 1970;30(3):390–5.

28. Chosack A, Zadik D, Eidelman E. The prevalence of scrotal tongue and geographic tongue in 70,359 Israeli school children. Community Dent Oral Epidemiol 1974;2(5):253–7.

29. Ghose LJ, Baghdady VS. Prevalence of geographic and plicated tongue in 6090 Iraqi schoolchildren. Community Dent Oral Epidemiol 1982;10(4):214–6.

30. Marks R, Czarny D. Geographic tongue: sensitivity to the environment. Oral Surg Oral Med Oral Pathol 1984;58(2):156–9.

31. Sigal MJ, Mock D. Symptomatic benign migratory glossitis: report of two cases and literature review. Pediatr Dent 1992;14(6):392–6.

32. Gonsalves WC, Chi AC, Neville BW. Common oral lesions: Part I. Superficial mucosal lesions. Am Fam Physician 2007;75(4):501–7.

33. Tapper-Jones LM, Aldred MJ, Walker DM, et al. Candidal infections and populations of *Candida albicans* in mouths of diabetics. J Clin Pathol 1981;34(7):706–11.

34. Willis AM, Coulter WA, Fulton CR, et al. Oral candidal carriage and infection in insulin-treated diabetic patients. Diabet Med 1999;16(8):675–9.
35. Rogers RS 3rd, Bruce AJ. The tongue in clinical diagnosis. J Eur Acad Dermatol Venereol 2004;18(3):254–9.
36. Joseph BK, Savage NW. Tongue pathology. Clin Dermatol 2000;18(5):613–8.
37. Goregen M, Miloglu O, Buyukkurt MC, et al. Median rhomboid glossitis: a clinical and microbiological study. Eur J Dent 2011;5(4):367–72.
38. Amir E, Gorsky M, Buchner A, et al. Physiologic pigmentation of the oral mucosa in Israeli children. Oral Surg Oral Med Oral Pathol 1991;71(3):396–8.
39. Gaeta GM, Satriano RA, Baroni A. Oral pigmented lesions. Clin Dermatol 2002; 20(3):286–8.
40. Anavi Y, Mintz S. Unusual physiologic melanin pigmentation of the tongue. Pediatr Derrnatol 1992;9(2):123–5.
41. McGrath DR, Spigelman AD. Preventive measures in Peutz-Jeghers syndrome. Fam Cancer 2001;1(2):121–5.
42. Lenane P, Powell FC. Oral pigmentation. J Eur Acad Dermatol Venereol 2000; 14(6):448–65.
43. Kauzman A, Pavone M, Blanas N, et al. Pigmented lesions of the oral cavity: review, differential diagnosis, and case presentations. J Can Dent Assoc 2004; 70(10):682–3.
44. Cicek Y, Ertas U. The normal and pathological pigmentation of oral mucous membrane: a review. J Contemp Dent Pract 2003;4(3):76–86.
45. Meleti M, Vescovi P, Mooi WJ, et al. Pigmented lesions of the oral mucosa and perioral tissues: a flow-chart for the diagnosis and some recommendations for the management. Oral Surg Oral Med Oral Pathol Oral Radiol Endod 2008; 105(5):606–16.
46. Boardman LA, Thibodeau SN, Schaid DJ, et al. Increased risk for cancer in patients with the Peutz-Jeghers syndrome. Ann Intern Med 1998;128(11):896–9.
47. Buchner A, Hansen LS. Amalgam pigmentation (amalgam tattoo) of the oral mucosa. A clinicopathologic study of 268 cases. Oral Surg Oral Med Oral Pathol 1980;49(2):139–47.
48. Owens BM, Johnson WW, Schuman NJ. Oral amalgam pigmentations (tattoos): a retrospective study. Quintessence Int 1992;23(12):805–10.
49. Page LR, Corio RL, Crawford BE, et al. The oral melanotic macule. Oral Surg Oral Med Oral Pathol 1977;44(2):219–26.
50. Weathers DR, Corio RL, Crawford BE, et al. The labial melanotic macule. Oral Surg Oral Med Oral Pathol 1976;42(2):196–205.
51. Ho KK, Dervan P, O'Loughlin S, et al. Labial melanotic macule: a clinical, histopathologic, and ultrastructural study. J Am Acad Dermatol 1993;28(1):33–9.
52. Gupta G, Williams RE, Mackie RM. The labial melanotic macule: a review of 79 cases. Br J Dermatol 1997;136(5):772–5.
53. Buchner A, Hansen LS. Melanotic macule of the oral mucosa. A clinicopathologic study of 105 cases. Oral Surg Oral Med Oral Pathol 1979;48(3): 244–9.
54. Buchner A, Merrell PW, Carpenter WM. Relative frequency of solitary melanocytic lesions of the oral mucosa. J Oral Pathol Med 2004;33(9):550–7.
55. Kaugars GE, Heise AP, Riley WT, et al. Oral melanotic macules. A review of 353 cases. Oral Surg Oral Med Oral Pathol 1993;76(1):59–61.
56. Laskaris G, Kittas C, Triantafyllou A. Unpigmented intramucosal nevus of palate. An unusual clinical presentation. Int J Oral Maxillofac Surg 1994;23(1): 39–40.

57. Buchner A, Hansen LS. Pigmented nevi of the oral mucosa: a clinicopathologic study of 36 new cases and review of 155 cases from the literature. Part II: analysis of 191 cases. Oral Surg Oral Med Oral Pathol 1987;63(6): 676–82.
58. Buchner A, Hansen LS. Pigmented nevi of the oral mucosa: a clinicopathologic study of 36 new cases and review of 155 cases from the literature. Part I: a clinicopathologic study of 36 new cases. Oral Surg Oral Med Oral Pathol 1987; 63(5):566–72.
59. Gonzalez-Campora R, Galera-Davidson H, Vazquez-Ramirez FJ, et al. Blue nevus: classical types and new related entities. A differential diagnostic review. Pathol Res Pract 1994;190(6):627–35.
60. Pinto A, Raghavendra S, Lee R, et al. Epithelioid blue nevus of the oral mucosa: a rare histologic variant. Oral Surg Oral Med Oral Pathol Oral Radiol Endod 2003;96(4):429–36.
61. Nikai H, Miyauchi M, Ogawa I, et al. Spitz nevus of the palate. Report of a case. Oral Surg Oral Med Oral Pathol 1990;69(5):603–8.
62. Dorji T, Cavazza A, Nappi O, et al. Spitz nevus of the tongue with pseudoepitheliomatous hyperplasia: report of three cases of a pseudomalignant condition. Am J Surg Pathol 2002;26(6):774–7.
63. Rose C, Kaddu S, El-Sherif TF, et al. A distinctive type of widespread congenital melanocytic nevus with large nodules. J Am Acad Dermatol 2003;49(4):732–5.
64. Meleti M, Mooi WJ, Casparie MK, et al. Melanocytic nevi of the oral mucosa—no evidence of increased risk for oral malignant melanoma: an analysis of 119 cases. Oral Oncol 2007;43(10):976–81.
65. Hicks MJ, Flaitz CM. Oral mucosal melanoma: epidemiology and pathobiology. Oral Oncol 2000;36(2):152–69.
66. Eisen D, Voorhees JJ. Oral melanoma and other pigmented lesions of the oral cavity. J Am Acad Dermatol 1991;24(4):527–37.
67. Zuniga MD, Mendez CR, Kauterich RR, et al. Paediatric oral pathology in a Chilean population: a 15-year review. Int J Paediatr Dent 2013;23(5):346–51.
68. Shah SK, Le MC, Carpenter WM. Retrospective review of pediatric oral lesions from a dental school biopsy service. Pediatr Dent 2009;31(1):14–9.
69. Maaita JK. Oral tumors in children: a review. J Clin Pediatr Dent 2000;24(2): 133–5.
70. Keszler A, Guglielmotti MB, Dominguez FV. Oral pathology in children. Frequency, distribution and clinical significance. Acta Odontol Latinoam 1990; 5(1):39–48.
71. Das S, Das AK. A review of pediatric oral biopsies from a surgical pathology service in a dental school. Pediatr Dent 1993;15(3):208–11.
72. Al-Khateeb T, Al-Hadi Hamasha A, Almasri NM. Oral and maxillofacial tumours in north Jordanian children and adolescents: a retrospective analysis over 10 years. Int J Oral Maxillofac Surg 2003;32(1):78–83.
73. Sklavounou-Andrikopoulou A, Piperi E, Papanikolaou V, et al. Oral soft tissue lesions in Greek children and adolescents: a retrospective analysis over a 32-year period. J Clin Pediatr Dent 2005;29(2):175–8.
74. Skinner RL, Davenport WD Jr, Weir JC, et al. A survey of biopsied oral lesions in pediatric dental patients. Pediatr Dent 1986;8(3):163–7.
75. Baurmash HD. Mucoceles and ranulas. J Oral Maxillofac Surg 2003;61(3): 369–78 United States.
76. Nico MM, Park JH, Lourenco SV. Mucocele in pediatric patients: analysis of 36 children. Pediatr Dermatol 2008;25(3):308–11.

77. Chi AC, Lambert PR 3rd, Richardson MS, et al. Oral mucoceles: a clinicopathologic review of 1,824 cases, including unusual variants. J Oral Maxillofac Surg 2011;69(4):1086–93.
78. Minguez-Martinez I, Bonet-Coloma C, Ata-Ali-Mahmud J, et al. Clinical characteristics, treatment, and evolution of 89 mucoceles in children. J Oral Maxillofac Surg 2010;68(10):2468–71.
79. Wu CW, Kao YH, Chen CM, et al. Mucoceles of the oral cavity in pediatric patients. Kaohsiung J Med Sci 2011;27(7):276–9.
80. Sigismund PE, Bozzato A, Schumann M, et al. Management of ranula: 9 years' clinical experience in pediatric and adult patients. J Oral Maxillofac Surg 2013; 71(3):538–44.
81. Dayan D, Bodner L, Hammel I, et al. Histochemical characterization of collagen fibers in fibrous overgrowth (irritation fibroma) of the oral mucosa: effect of age and duration of lesion. Arch Gerontol Geriatr 1994;18(1):53–7.
82. Barker DS, Lucas RB. Localised fibrous overgrowths of the oral mucosa. Br J Oral Surg 1967;5(2):86–92.
83. Buchner A, Shnaiderman A, Vared M. Pediatric localized reactive gingival lesions: a retrospective study from Israel. Pediatr Dent 2010;32(7):486–92.
84. Buchner A, Hansen LS. The histomorphologic spectrum of peripheral ossifying fibroma. Oral Surg Oral Med Oral Pathol 1987;63(4):452–61.
85. Kendrick F, Waggoner WF. Managing a peripheral ossifying fibroma. ASDC J Dent Child 1996;63(2):135–8.
86. Jafarzadeh H, Sanatkhani M, Mohtasham N. Oral pyogenic granuloma: a review. J Oral Sci 2006;48(4):167–75.
87. Gordon-Nunez MA, de Vasconcelos Carvalho M, Benevenuto TG, et al. Oral pyogenic granuloma: a retrospective analysis of 293 cases in a Brazilian population. J Oral Maxillofac Surg 2010;68(9):2185–8.
88. Puttgen KB, Pearl M, Tekes A, et al. Update on pediatric extracranial vascular anomalies of the head and neck. Childs Nerv Syst 2010;26(10):1417–33.
89. Saravana GH. Oral pyogenic granuloma: a review of 137 cases. Br J Oral Maxillofac Surg 2009;47(4):318–9.
90. Giansanti JS, Waldron CA. Peripheral giant cell granuloma: review of 720 cases. J Oral Surg 1969;27(10):787–91.
91. Ozalp N, Sener E, Songur T. Peripheral giant cell granuloma and peripheral ossifying fibroma in children: two case reports. Med Princ Pract 2010;19(2):159–62.
92. Mighell AJ, Robinson PA, Hume WJ. Peripheral giant cell granuloma: a clinical study of 77 cases from 62 patients, and literature review. Oral Dis 1995; 1(1):12–9.
93. Chaparro-Avendano AV, Berini-Aytes L, Gay-Escoda C. Peripheral giant cell granuloma. A report of five cases and review of the literature. Med Oral Patol Oral Cir Bucal 2005;10(1):53–7, 48–52.
94. Buchner A, Shnaiderman-Shapiro A, Vered M. Relative frequency of localized reactive hyperplastic lesions of the gingiva: a retrospective study of 1675 cases from Israel. J Oral Pathol Med 2010;39(8):631–8.
95. Motamedi MH, Talesh KT, Jafari SM, et al. Peripheral and central giant cell granulomas of the jaws: a retrospective study and surgical management. Gen Dent 2010;58(6):e246–51.
96. Flaitz CM. Peripheral giant cell granuloma: a potentially aggressive lesion in children. Pediatr Dent 2000;22(3):232–3.
97. Pinheiro Rdos S, de Franca TR, Ferreira Dde C, et al. Human papillomavirus in the oral cavity of children. J Oral Pathol Med 2011;40(2):121–6.

98. Carneiro TE, Marinho SA, Verli FD, et al. Oral squamous papilloma: clinical, histologic and immunohistochemical analyses. J Oral Sci 2009;51(3):367–72.
99. Kui LL, Xiu HZ, Ning LY. Condyloma acuminatum and human papilloma virus infection in the oral mucosa of children. Pediatr Dent 2003;25(2):149–53.
100. Abbey LM, Page DG, Sawyer DR. The clinical and histopathologic features of a series of 464 oral squamous cell papillomas. Oral Surg Oral Med Oral Pathol 1980;49(5):419–28.
101. Boj JR, Hernandez M, Espasa E, et al. Laser treatment of an oral papilloma in the pediatric dental office: a case report. Quintessence Int 2007;38(4):307–12.
102. Smith EM, Swarnavel S, Ritchie JM, et al. Prevalence of human papillomavirus in the oral cavity/oropharynx in a large population of children and adolescents. Pediatr Infect Dis J 2007;26(9):836–40.
103. Ethunandan M, Mellor TK. Haemangiomas and vascular malformations of the maxillofacial region—a review. Br J Oral Maxillofac Surg 2006;44(4):263–72.
104. Adams DM, Lucky AW. Cervicofacial vascular anomalies. I. Hemangiomas and other benign vascular tumors. Semin Pediatr Surg 2006;15(2):124–32.
105. Couto RA, Maclellan RA, Zurakowski D, et al. Infantile hemangioma: clinical assessment of the involuting phase and implications for management. Plast Reconstr Surg 2012;130(3):619–24.
106. Correa PH, Nunes LC, Johann AC, et al. Prevalence of oral hemangioma, vascular malformation and varix in a Brazilian population. Braz Oral Res 2007;21(1):40–5.
107. Buckmiller LM, Munson PD, Dyamenahalli U, et al. Propranolol for infantile hemangiomas: early experience at a tertiary vascular anomalies center. Laryngoscope 2010;120(4):676–81.
108. Nair SC, Spencer NJ, Nayak KP, et al. Surgical management of vascular lesions of the head and neck: a review of 115 cases. Int J Oral Maxillofac Surg 2011;40(6):577–83.
109. Theologie-Lygidakis N, Schoinohoriti OK, Tzerbos F, et al. Surgical management of head and neck vascular anomalies in children: a retrospective analysis of 42 patients. Oral Surg Oral Med Oral Pathol Oral Radiol 2014;117(1):e22–31.
110. Buckmiller LM, Richter GT, Suen JY. Diagnosis and management of hemangiomas and vascular malformations of the head and neck. Oral Dis 2010;16(5):405–18.

Index

Note: Page numbers of article titles are in **boldface** type.

A

Acne vulgaris, 416–417
Acyclovir, in herpes virus infection, 268
Amalgam tatto/graphite, 443
Antibiotics, topical, in recurrent aphthous stomatitis, 290
Antiinflammatory agents, in oral mucositis, 347
Antimicrobial agents, in oral mucositis, 347–348
Aphthous stomatitis, recurrent, **281–297**
    causes of, 281
    classification of, 282
    clinical manifestation and pathogenesis of, 289
    epidemiology of, 282, 283
    etiologic factors in, allergic, 287
        hereditary and genetic, 286–287
        immunologic, 287–288
        local, 283–284
        microbial, 284–285
        nutritional, 288
        psychological stress as, 288
        underlying disease as, 285–286, 287
    herpetiform, 282
    management of, 282, 289–292
    minor, 282
    types of, 282, 283

B

Basal cell carcinoma, 407–408
Bisphosphonate, in osteonecrosis of jaw, 370, 372, 378, 379

C

Cancer, of head and neck, incidence of, 315, 316
    oral, **315–340**
        5-year survival rate in, 315–316
        classification of, 318
        clinical assessment of, 322
        delay in diagnosis of, 326–327
        genomics and proteomics and, 328–329
        human papilloma virus and, 322
        immune system and, 320

Dent Clin N Am 58 (2014) 455–461
http://dx.doi.org/10.1016/S0011-8532(14)00011-1
0011-8532/14/$ – see front matter © 2014 Elsevier Inc. All rights reserved.

dental.theclinics.com

Moving?

Make sure your subscription moves with you!

To notify us of your new address, find your **Clinics Account Number** (located on your mailing label above your name), and contact customer service at:

Email: journalscustomerservice-usa@elsevier.com

800-654-2452 (subscribers in the U.S. & Canada)
314-447-8871 (subscribers outside of the U.S. & Canada)

Fax number: 314-447-8029

Elsevier Health Sciences Division
Subscription Customer Service
3251 Riverport Lane
Maryland Heights, MO 63043

*To ensure uninterrupted delivery of your subscription, please notify us at least 4 weeks in advance of move.